Also by Simon Elmer

The Colour of the Sacred: Georges Bataille and the Image of Sacrifice

The Sorcerer's Apprentice, 2008-2014

The Costs of Estate Regeneration

Inequality Capital

Fight and Flight: Poems 2012-2021

The Road to Fascism: For a Critique of the Global Biosecurity State

The New Normal: Selected Articles on the UK Biosecurity State, Vol. 2

and with Geraldine Dening

Architects for Social Housing, 2015-2022

The Truth about Grenfell Tower

Central Hill: A Case Study in Estate Regeneration

For A Socialist Architecture: Under Capitalism

Saving St. Raphael's Estate: The Alternative to Demolition

Simon Elmer

Virtue and Terror

Selected Articles on the UK Biosecurity State

Volume 1

Published in Great Britain in 2023 by

Architects for Social Housing
Fairford House
Kennington Lane
London SE11 4HW
e-mail: info@architectsforsocialhousing.co.uk
website: www.architectsforsocialhousing.co.uk

ISBN 978-1-4709-4171-0 (clothbound)
ISBN 978-1-4709-0203-2 (paperbound)

Cover design by Architects for Social Housing

For the unafraid

Contents

Fear, fear: you speak of fear.
What is this fear? Is it the fear we dare not fear,
That fear of fear itself, or fear of other's fear,
Such fear as ends
In passionate untruth, self-justifying falsehood without end?
Demonic fear
Of individual guilt, of being caught, of doing wrong,
And fear of failure or of being found a fool,
And fear of anything that might contrast with me
And thus reveal my insufficiency,
My lack, my weakness, my inferiority,
In showing up my difference from itself;
Fear of uncertainty and loss, fear of all change,
Fear of all strangeness and all strangers; and above all else the fear
Of Love, of being loved, of being asked for love,
Of being loved yet knowing one has no love to return;
Fear of forgiveness —
Fear of that love which is so great it can forgive
And the exhausting fear of Death and Mystery,
The Mystery of Death, of Life and Death,
The huge appalling Mystery of everything;
Arid fear of Nothing,
Yes, after all the fear of Nothing really,
Fear of Nothing, Nothing

Fear of Nothing, Nothing, absolutely Nothing.

— David Gascoyne, *Night Thoughts*, 1956

Introduction

'If the mainspring of popular government in peacetime is virtue, the mainspring of popular government during a revolution is both virtue and terror; virtue, without which terror is fatal; terror, without which virtue is powerless. Terror is nothing but swift, severe, inflexible justice; it is therefore an emanation of virtue. It is less a principle in itself than a consequence of the general principle of democracy, applied to our nation's most pressing needs.'

— Maximilien Robespierre, *On the Principles of Political Morality*, 1794

The past three years have exposed the structural flaw in Western democracy with more disastrous consequences for its populations than at any time in recent history. It's generally known that democracy, from the Ancient Greek *dēmokratia*, means 'rule by the people'; but it is perhaps less widely known that the fifth-century city-state of Athens on which the West modelled its democracy was a slave-owning society in which only adult males and hereditary citizens comprising maybe 10-15 per cent of the population had the right to vote. The universal suffrage we have in the UK today was only attained through centuries of political struggle, and is predicated, at least in principle, on an equally universal education. One of the arguments against extending rights of suffrage that were originally restricted to landowners, then to property owners, then to heads of households, then to men over twenty-one, then to propertied women over thirty, and only eventually made a universal right, was that according equal votes to individuals with vastly unequal levels of education, influence and understanding of policy was politically suicidal. The counter argument, which eventually won out, is that those who, because of their wealth or education or age or gender, had the right to vote, were unlikely to do so against their interests, making their political franchise a guarantee of political hegemony. The eventual concession to universal suffrage, however, gave those who grudgingly conceded it ample time to turn this threat to their advantage, and make the vastly expanded electorate the object of demographically targeted political strategies. It was from this necessity, and from the opportunity it afforded, that the modern mass media were born.

A century later, universal suffrage has produced not the Platonic ideal of a universally educated, socially conscientious and politically informed *demos* but, to the contrary, a people governed by virtue and terror. It is not only in the interests of a Government and its beneficiaries to keep the electorate both ignorant and stupid; it is necessary in order to maintain its grip on power — and not only a sitting Government but every political party that hopes to form one. This hardly needs to be argued, as the evidence of the erasure of our politics, which every year descends to new lows of populism, is denied only by those who strut on its stages, script its tragedies and direct their endings from behind the scenes.

For the same reason, universal education, which has always served to indoctrinate citizens into the dominant ideology, has been transformed into more or less explicit propaganda for the changing values and pressing needs of Western capitalism far beyond how we vote. Globalism, multiculturalism, political correctness, identity politics, environmental fundamentalism, the orthodoxies of woke and now the dogma and cultic practices of biosecurity are all products of the neoliberalisation of our education, media and culture industries. The result of this ideological co-ordination of every sector of our society is that the most educated demographic in human history, the middle classes of the West, is now the most easily manipulated populace in history. A century and more of universal suffrage and education has created not 'rule by the people' but a *demos* in thrall to the ever-expanding technologies of biopower.

The systemic exploitation of this flaw in our democracy means that our lives are now effectively ruled by the most gullible, the most afraid, the most obedient and the most compliant members of our society, on the grounds that they constitute a democratic consensus. It is not by chance that every crisis manufactured to justify removing our freedoms is turned into a 'health' crisis. Just as our human rights, discarded on the justification of the health and safety of the 'people', have become the means by which our lives have been taken into the protective custody of the state, so too our democracy has become the means by which the institutions and processes of democratic oversight and accountability have been dismantled and replaced by the rule of a global technocracy implementing a totalitarian system of governance. How this was done, by whom, for whose benefit and to what ends is the subject of the articles collected in these two volumes.

1. The Great Reset

Let me start — by way of an introduction — with some questions about where we are now, offer some cursory answers about how we got here, and then sketch a brief picture of where we are heading. This, if you like, is my 'State of the Nation' address, and it paints a very different picture of the UK in 2023 to that presented by our unelected Prime Minister.[1]

First, how did they do it? How was it was possible for the Bank of England to create a quantitative easing programme that by November 2020 had reached £895 billion in government and corporate bonds, and yet two years later the UK Chancellor, Jeremy Hunt, can dismiss the ensuing and inevitable inflation, that in the Consumer Price Index has reached a 45-year high of nearly 12 per cent, as the result of the coronavirus 'pandemic' and 'Russia's invasion of Ukraine'?[2]

How was it possible that, during two years of restrictions on our previously universal, indivisible and inalienable human rights and freedoms, the UK Government was allowed to transform the UK from a parliamentary democracy into a constitutional dictatorship in which 537 coronavirus-justified Statutory Instruments containing thousands of regulations were made into UK law by Government Ministers before being laid before Parliament for scrutiny or approval, and without proof of their justification or proportionality or assessment of their impact?[3]

How was it possible that, under cover of a politically declared 'emergency period' it was in its power to extend indefinitely, the Government, by the end of March 2022, could spend £376 billion of present and future British taxpayers' money on so-called COVID-19 'measures' — including £147 billion on support for businesses, £89 billion for health and social care, £75 billion for other public services and emergency responses, £60 billion in support for individuals, £3 billion for 'other' support, and £2 billion for operational costs — on the justification of

---

1. See Rishi Sunak, 'PM speech on building a better future' (4 January 2023).

2. See Bank of England, 'Quantitative Easing' (last updated 15 December, 2022); and HM Treasury, 'Open letters between HM Treasury and Bank of England, December 2022 (15 December, 2022).

3. See Hansard Society, 'Coronavirus Statutory Instruments Dashboard, 2020-2022' (9 April, 2020-17 June 2022).

combatting the spread of a virus with the infection fatality rate of seasonal influenza?[4]

How was it possible for the Government, on the justification of waging 'war' on a virus that represents a significant threat exclusively to the elderly and already ill, to impose scientifically meaningless and largely illegal medical 'measures' of surveillance, registration, inspection, prohibition, exclusion, quarantine, incarceration and punishment not employed in Europe since the Seventeenth Century on the whole of the British public, causing poverty, unemployment, bankruptcy, psychological damage, and the ongoing deaths of tens of thousands of UK citizens denied medical diagnosis, care and treatment by two years of 'social distancing', 'lockdown', mandatory 'masking' and 'vaccination'?[5]

How was it possible that multiple injections with a mix of experimental adenovirus vector and mRNA gene therapies that introduce DNA sequences into our cells — the clinical trials for which are still incomplete, whose developers and producers have admitted they do nothing to stop transmission of the coronavirus, that have demonstrably failed either to protect the injected from infection or to lessen the symptoms of disease, and which have already killed thousands of Britons, caused millions of serious injuries, and are having long-term negative consequences for the health and lives of unknown millions of people across the globe — could be made a condition of restoring our constitutional rights and freedoms under UK and international law, and despite all the data on their lack of effectiveness and dangers are still being injected into the UK public, having recently been extended to children as young as 6 months old on the justification of protecting them from a disease to which they are statistically immune?[6]

How is it possible that the British people, like the populations of every Western nation, are being forcibly subjected to a process of deliberate impoverishment and erasure of our rights and freedoms through policies for which

---

4. See National Audit Office, 'COVID-19 cost tracker' (last updated 23 June, 2022); and John P. A. Ioannidis, 'The infection fatality rate of COVID-19 inferred from seroprevalence data', *MedRxiv* (13 May, 2020).

5. See John P. A. Ioannidis, 'Infection fatality rate of COVID-19 in community-dwelling populations with emphasis on the elderly: An overview' (13 July, 2021); and Michel Foucault, *Discipline and Punish: The Birth of the Prison*; translated from the French by Alan Sheridan (Penguin Books, 1977), pp. 195-200.

6. See Medicines and Healthcare products Regulatory Agency, 'Pfizer/BioNTech COVID-19 vaccine authorised for use in infants and children aged 6 months to 4 years' (6 December, 2022);

our Government does not have a mandate from the electorate, which have not been voted for by our democratically elected representatives in Parliament, or even been debated in the national media, on the spurious justification of 'saving the planet' from a constantly deferred environmental catastrophe about whose nature or cause or threat or imminence or even existence there is no scientific consensus, but for the lobbying, marketing and promotion of which there has been vast corporate and government investment?[7]

How is it possible that, following the lead of the London Mayor's road closure scheme and an Ultra-Low Emission Zone that this year will encompass the entire capital, the municipal authorities of Oxford City and Canterbury City have announced they are going to enforce restrictions on the movement of motorists in and out of their civic jurisdiction, in violation of our freedom of movement under Protocol No. 4, Article 2 of the European Convention on Human Rights, but in compliance with the concept of the '15-minute city' formulated by the World Economic Forum, a privately-funded think-tank without democratic mandate or legal jurisdiction?[8]

How is it possible that, on the justification of 'tackling' numerous manufactured health, environmental, energy, food, security and geopolitical 'crises', the elected national governments of Western states are openly and even insistently forming what the French President, Emmanuel Macron, recently called a 'Single Global Order' fronted by unelected transnational organisations like the United Nations, the European Council, the World Health Organization, the World Economic Forum and the International Panel on Climate Change, but whose policies are being dictated by global financial institutions like the US Federal Reserve, the Bank for International Settlements, the World Bank, the International Monetary Fund, the European Central Bank, and US-based asset management firms like BlackRock, Vanguard Group and State Street Global Advisors?[9]

---

7. See Chris Morrison, '"There is no Climate Emergency": Hundreds More Sign the World Climate Declaration, Including 20 Professors', *The Daily Sceptic* (31 October, 2022).

8. See Rhoda Wilson, 'Council claims it is a "Victim of Abuse" following new Policy to enforce Climate Lockdowns without consent of the Public', *The Exposé* (9 December, 2022); and Janez Potocnik and Julia Okatz, 'How Europe can reshape its cities to boost vibrancy, resilience and climate action', *World Economic Forum* (16 December, 2022).

9. See 'Macron calls for "a single global order" to combat China', news.com.au on *YouTube* (19 November, 2022).

How is it possible that the biologically nonsensical, socially unaccepted, medically mutilating, child abusing, violently misogynist and implicitly homophobic orthodoxies of so-called 'trans-rights', formulated by a previously marginal subculture associated with body dysmorphia, gender dysphoria and self-harming, are being written into more and more UK policy and legislation, indoctrinated into children without parental approval, normalised by our institutions of education, propagated by our institutions of art, culture and entertainment, imposed on employees through intellectually vacuous but now mandatory programmes such as 'unconscious bias' and 'equality, diversity and inclusion' training, and enforced on the non-compliant through new police powers?[10]

How is it possible that, on the justification of combatting the invasion of the Ukraine by Russia in a proxy war waged by a government installed in 2014 by a US-engineered coup, which until recently was denounced across the West as Neo-Nazi, and whose puppet President has banned opposition political parties, worker unions and independent media platforms and issued hit lists on journalists and academics who have criticised its actions, the UK Government has not only committed £4.6 billion in military, financial and humanitarian aid to the Ukraine but has collaborated in US acts of sabotage against Russia's Nord Stream pipeline to Europe, increasing our financial dependence on US energy sources and entrenching its political hegemony over the West?[11]

How is it possible that private companies already making billions of pounds in profit from the privatisation of our utilities by successive neoliberal governments

---

10. It was recently revealed that £7 billion of public money is being spent by the UK Government on woke programmes of indoctrination, including £557 million a year on 'Equality, Diversity and Inclusivity' training for workers. These include such Arts Council programmes as 'unlearning whiteness'. See Tony Diver, 'Jeremy Hunt faces Tory rebellion over £7bn government spending on "woke" projects', *The Telegraph* (10 December, 2022). The Gender Recognition Reform (Scotland) Bill, which was made into law on 22 December, 2022, empowers a child as young as 16 and a man of any age to attain a Gender Recognition Certificate without a diagnosis of gender dysphoria.

11. See Abdul Rahman, 'Opposition political parties banned in Ukraine and "unified information policy" imposed', *Peoples Dispatch* (21 March, 2022); Vanessa Beeley, 'Assassinated for telling the truth about Ukraine', *The Wall Will Fall* (17 April, 2022); Seymour Hersh, 'How America took out the Nord Stream pipeline', *Peoples Dispatch* (10 February, 2023); Prime Minister's Office, 'UK will match record Ukraine support in 2023' (20 September, 2022) and 'US and UK announce new energy partnership' (7 December, 2022).

have been allowed to raise the price of energy in the UK to the extent that, this year, an estimated 65 per cent of UK households, over 45.5 million people, will be driven into fuel poverty — which means spending 10 per cent of their net income on fuel after housing costs?[12]

How is it possible that environmental fundamentalist organisations like Extinction Rebellion, Insulate Britain and Just Stop Oil that are funded by, among other corporate backers financing the Climate Emergency Fund, the heir to the J. Paul Getty oil fortune, are given free rein by the UK Government, municipal authorities, police forces and security services to block the country's roads and bridges, cause criminal damage to the UK offices of some of the world's most powerful and high-security companies, and enter and vandalise the nation's political, cultural and artistic institutions?[13]

How is it possible that, nearly three years into the 'pandemic', when a Member of Parliament finally found the courage to point out that more people have reported adverse reactions to mRNA 'vaccines' for COVID-19 than had from all the other vaccines combined over the previous forty years and called on the Prime Minister to halt the UK 'vaccination' programme, his comments were condemned by his fellow MPs first as 'dangerous' and then as 'anti-Semitic', and he himself was dismissed as a 'conspiracy theorist', suspended from Parliament and eventually expelled from his Party?[14]

How is it possible that the worst and most corrupt Parliament in modern British history, and the three Governments it has failed to scrutinise or hold to account during the biggest changes to our society and politics since at least the Second World War, have permitted the outsourcing of the authority and duties of the UK state to multinational corporations, including the right of information

---

12. See Jasper Jolly and Jessica Elgot, 'Profits at world's seven biggest oil forms soar to almost £150bn this year', *The Guardian* (27 October, 2022); and Child Poverty Action Group, 'Fuel poverty estimates for April 2023 following the Autumn statement' (23 November, 2022).

13. See Aileen Getty, 'I fund climate activism — and I applaud the Van Gogh protest', *The Guardian* (22 October, 2022); and Climate Emergency Fund, 'Protest movements are the fastest, most cost-effective way of creating transformative change'.

14. See Andrew Bridgen, 'List of supporting references used in vaccine harms debate speech' (16 December, 2022); Martina Bet, 'Tory MP urged to apologise and correct record on "dangerous" Covid vaccine claim', *The Independent* (7 December, 2022); and Paul Seddon and Rachel Schraer, 'Andrew Bridgen suspended as Tory MP over Covid vaccine comments', *BBC News* (11 January, 2023).

technology companies, under the Online Safety Bill, to censor anything Western governments and the international technocracies they form want silenced, creating the basis for a new form of totalitarian surveillance and control over our freedom of thought and expression?[15]

How is it possible that, in less than three years, our political, state and civil institutions have not only not opposed, but have willingly collaborated, in the revolution in the governance of Western democracies from the nation state, in which the actions of the executive are overseen by the legislature and judiciary, into global governance by international technocracies of corporate board members, bankers and unelected government bureaucrats appointed outside of any democratic process of election, scrutiny or accountability?

How is it possible that, under cover of unprecedented levels of public expenditure in response to a public health 'crisis' they were responsible for manufacturing, the financial institutions and governments of Western capitalism have overseen the greatest transfer of wealth from the poor to the rich in modern history, with the wealth of the world's 2,668 billionaires rising from $8.6 trillion to $13.8 trillion over the two years of lockdown restrictions in which 250 million people were driven into extreme poverty?[16]

How is it possible that our latest Prime Minister, Rishi Sunak, who was not elected by the British people or even by his own political party but was appointed to the role following the disapproval of his predecessor by unknown figures in the financial sectors of the UK, Europe or the world, no sooner took office than he unilaterally announced the 'roll-out' of Central Bank Digital Currency (CBDC) employing blockchain technology to log every transaction we ever make, and which is programmable with restrictions and limits on expenditure contingent on our biosecurity status, carbon footprint and social compliance?[17]

---

15. See Matthew Feeney, 'A Censor's Charter? The case against the Online Safety Bill', *Centre for Policy Studies* (September 2022).

16. See Anna Cooban, 'Billionaires added $5 trillion to their fortunes during the pandemic', *CNN Business* (16 January, 2022); and Oxfam International, '"Terrifying prospect" of over a quarter of a billion more people crashing into extreme levels of poverty and suffering this year' (12 April, 2022).

17. See 'New UK Prime Minister Rishi Sunak Pushes Heavily to Introduce CBDC', *Unlock Media* (25 October, 2022).

How is it possible that, in response to a campaign of fear orchestrated by the UK media, the police and the Home Secretary, Her Majesty's Loyal Opposition can declare that, in order to control illegal immigration and as a condition of access to the rights of citizenship in the UK — including our freedom of movement and, under future 'crises', our freedom of association and assembly, and perhaps, if the COVID faithful have their way, our right to education, work, medical treatment and liberty — the never realised threat of 'vaccine' passports should be expanded into a programme of Digital Identity containing our biometric data, including our compliance with the constantly updated requirements to be injected as many times and with whatever the state tells us?[18]

How is it possible that, after the clinical trial on the population of the world lasting three years has irrefutably demonstrated that face masks do absolutely nothing to stop the spread of a virus one-ten-thousandth of a millimetre wide, and in the face of the overwhelming evidence of their physical and psychological harms — in particular to the mental health and development of infants and children — the COVID-faithful, including numerous medical professionals, continue not only to wear them but to call for their enforced imposition on the populations of the world, in some cases on a permanent basis?[19]

How is it possible that, three years since the 'pandemic' was officially declared by the World Health Organization on 11 March 2020, we have implemented or are on the cusp of implementing the programmes and technologies of a Global Biosecurity State, including not only Digital ID and CBDC, but also Universal Basic Income for the millions of workers, primarily from white-collar jobs, who will be made redundant by the new technologies, markets and programmes of the Fourth Industrial Revolution and the Great Reset of Western capitalism it has enabled; a system of Social Credit modelled on that currently employed in the People's Republic of China, in which individuals and companies

18. See Jamie Grierson, 'Labour revives ID cards idea to reduce irregular immigration', *The Guardian* (8 November, 2022); David Shaw, 'Vaccination status and intensive care unit triage: Is it fair to give unvaccinated Covid-19 patients equal priority?', *Bioethics* (7 August, 2022); Chartered Institute of Personnel and Development, 'COVID-19 vaccination: guide for employers' (7 March, 2022); and Sean Adi-Tabatabal, 'Sean Penn: "It's Time To Send Unvaccinated Citizens to Jail"', *News Punch* (20 December, 2022).

19. See Emily Craig, 'Return of the Masks: Health chiefs urge people to wear face coverings and say anyone feeling ill should "stay at home" in echo of pandemic era — as medics claim the NHS is under more pressure than at the height of Covid', *Daily Mail* (3 January, 2023).

are given a rating based on their compliance not only with the laws but also with the behavioural norms of the state, all of which will be established through access to our online browsing, search and purchase history; the Pandemic Prevention, Preparedness and Response Treaty that will allow national governments to justify imposing lockdowns, masking, 'vaccine' mandates and other programmes of biosecurity as the technical decisions of an international health technocracy; Smart Cities, in which our freedom of movement, assembly, association, access, business, consumption, ownership, privacy, expression and thought will be monitored, analysed and controlled by artificial intelligence algorithms linking the Internet of Things by which we are surrounded to the Internet of Bodies by which we are connected to it; and facial recognition technology that identifies citizens not compliant with regulations of biosecurity made not by our governments but by international technocracies overseeing global finance, expenditure, consumption, health, agriculture, animal husbandry, education and war?

Behind their health-and-safety, planet-saving, Putin-defeating branding, all these programmes are instruments of the new global technocracy and the international corporations, central banks and transnational institutions that compose it. We know who these are, because on 11 March, 2020, the same day the World Health Organization declared the 'pandemic', the World Economic Forum launched the COVID-19 Action Platform, a coalition of over 1,100 of the world's most powerful businesses.[20] This is the prototype for what it calls 'stakeholder capitalism', the new political economy of Western capitalism, through which our democratically elected governments are being replaced as the

---

20. See World Economic Forum, '1500 organizations working together in the COVID Action Platform' (6 May, 2020). For a list of the businesses partnered with the WEF, of which there are currently 1,112, see World Economic Forum, 'Our Partners' (2023). Notable members include, in banking and capital markets: Agricultural Bank of China, Allianz, Bank of America, Bank of China, Bank Santander, Barclays, China Construction Bank, China Merchants Group, Citi, Credit Suisse, Deutsche Bank, Goldman Sachs, Hong Kong Exchanges and Clearing, HSBC, Industrial Commercial Bank of China, JPMorgan Chase, Lloyds Banking Group, London Stock Exchange Group, Mastercard, Morgan Stanley, Nasdaq, PayPal, Qatar National Bank, Qatar Investment Authority, Qatar Financial Centre Regulatory Authority, Saudi National Bank, State Bank of India, UBS and Visa; in asset management: BlackRock, Bridgewater Associates, Fidelity International, and State Street Global Advisors; in healthcare: American Heart Foundation, AstraZeneca, Bayer, the Bill & Melinda Gates Foundation, Johnson & Johnson, Moderna, Merck, Novartis, Pfizer, Roche, Serum Institute of India, Sanofi, Thermo Fisher Scientific and the Wellcome Trust; in information technology: Accenture, Amazon, Apple, Dell, Google, IBM, Intel, Meta, Microsoft, Yoti and Zoom.

final arbiters of the policies of the nation state and the rights and freedoms of its citizens, and in their place international corporations and financial institutions, through their macro-management of the global economy, will constitute a new form of global governance.[21] Based on this technocratic model, the programmes of the Great Reset of Western capitalism are being implemented as mere upgrades in the technological infrastructure of the nation state; but in practice they are bringing about a qualitative and perhaps irreversible shift in the power of the state over the population and the unaccountability of the rulers to the ruled. And yet, all this is being implemented as I write, largely without the knowledge and certainly without the vote of the British people.[22]

So, how did it come to this? In response, I will try to offer some preliminary answers that are not given in the articles collected in these two volumes, which focus on the manufacture of the coronavirus 'crisis', but which are founded on their analysis and findings.

2. The Politics of Fundamentalism

As the restrictions and obligations of biosecurity have mostly but not entirely been lifted since March 2022 — while still being suspended over our necks like the axe of the *fasces* — their replacement by their equally fundamentalist environmental equivalents has shown the arbitrariness of the crises on which the Global Biosecurity State is being imposed — and their shared end. Last year's COP27, the United Nations Climate Change Conference 2022, is a demonstration and model of how the forms of global governance that have assumed so much power over our lives on the justification of responding to numerous manufactured 'crises'

---

21. World Economic Forum, 'Measuring Stakeholder Capitalism: Towards Common Metrics and Consistent Reporting of Sustainable Value Creation' (2023).

22. See Cabinet Office, 'Consultation on draft legislation to support identify verification' (4 January, 2022); Bank of England, 'UK central bank digital currency' (last updated 1 September, 2022); Francis Hobson and Aaron Kulakiewicz, 'Research Briefing: Potential merits of a universal basic income', *House of Commons Library* (13 June, 2022); Patrick Butchard and Bukky Balogun, 'Research Briefing: What is the proposed WHO Pandemic Preparedness Treaty?', *House of Commons Library* (18 May, 2022); Lydia Harriss and Philippa Kearney, 'Research Briefing: Smart Cities', *UK Parliament* (22 September, 2021); UK Government Chief Scientific Advisor, 'The Internet of Things: Making the most of the Second Digital Revolution' (December 2014); and Home Office, 'Guidance: Automated Facial Recognition: ethical and legal use' (25 October, 2021).

will operate outside of any democratic representation or accountability. Held from 6-18 November 2022 in Egypt, COP27 was the twenty-seventh such conference held annually since the first UN climate agreement in 1992. This led to the Kyoto Protocol of 1997 and the Paris Agreement of 2015 that committed participating nations to unquestionable orthodoxies. These included what it called the 'scientific consensus' 1) that global warming is occurring, and 2) that man-made carbon dioxide (CO_2) emissions are driving it.[23] The effect of this political agreement is that anyone, including climatologists, meteorologists or geologists, who asserts or presents evidence to the contrary is categorised and branded as a 'climate-change denier' — exactly as those who question the equally authoritarian and unquestionable orthodoxies of the coronavirus 'crisis' are branded as 'COVID deniers'.[24]

Parties to this fundamentalist orthodoxy, and the economic obligations and policies to which it commits them, include — by order of the size of their economy — the USA, China, Japan, Germany, India, the UK, France, Brazil, Italy, Canada and 182 other countries, which is to say, almost the whole world. To address what it melodramatically calls the 'existential threat' of climate change, the UK Government has committed to spending £11.6 billion of British taxpayers' money on international climate finance, with funding for what it calls 'climate adaptation' tripling from £500m in 2019 to £1.5 billion in 2025. £150 million of that funding will go to 'protecting' rainforests, including in the Amazon and the Congo Basin, the sites of some of the world's largest reserves of the copper and cobalt required for electric batteries; £65 million to the Nature, People and Climate Investment Fund in Egypt, with a focus on hydrogen and wind power; and a further £2 billion to the

---

23. See United Nations, 'Kyoto Protocol to the United Nations Framework Convention on Climate Change' (1998).

24. See Global Climate Intelligence Group, 'World Climate Declaration: There is no climate emergency' (1 October, 2022), signatories to which now number 1,410 scientists and energy industry professionals from Argentina (1), Australia (154), Austria (5), Bangladesh (1), Barbados (1), Belgium (31), Bolivia (1), Brazil (16), Bulgaria (1), Canada (111), Chile (1), China and Hong Kong (2), Costa Rica (1), Croatia (2), Cyprus (1), the Czech Republic (9), Denmark (11), Estonia (1), Ecuador (1), Finland (4), France (97), Germany (66), Greece (11), Guatemala (1), Hungary (6), India (3), Indonesia (1), Ireland (20), Israel (5), Italy (176), Japan (4), Malaysia (1), Mexico (4), the Netherlands (132), New Zealand (23), Norway (27), Paraguay (1), the Philippines (1), Poland (4), Portugal (5), Russia (7), Saudi Arabia (1), Serbia (1), Singapore (1), Slovenia (2), South Africa (9), South Korea (2), Spain (9), Sweden (42), Switzerland (11), Turkey (1), the UK (111), the USA (277), and Vietnam (1).

UK-Kenya Strategic Partnership for 'clean and green' investment in geothermal, solar energy and hydroelectric power projects.[25]

All this public financing will go to private companies selected by the international technocracies formed to do so in accord with the UN's Sustainable Development Goals (SDG), a Miss-World list of humanitarian objectives ranging from abolishing world hunger and poverty to peace, justice and gender equality that was adopted by the United Nations in 2015 under the rubric of Agenda 2030.[26] In reality and practice, however, Sustainable Development Goals allocate the flow of global capital, investment and preferential treatment to governments and corporations according to their compliance with the Environmental, Social and corporate Governance (ESG) criteria.[27] Despite their UN branding, these are formulated and imposed by immensely wealthy international corporate asset managers, the most powerful of which, BlackRock, the Vanguard Group and State Street Global Advisor, between them hold 20 per cent of shares and with it something like government authority over the 500 largest companies on the New York Stock Exchange.[28] Far from saving the planet from exploitation by predatory corporations, Sustainable Development Goals are designed to increase the monopoly of wealthy Western economies and international companies able to meet their criteria over poorer countries, and in doing so create the financial framework for purchasing their UN-assigned quota of emissions in carbon credits.[29] On the same justification, developing countries will be loaded with debt by financial organisations like the World Bank and the International Monetary Fund in order to fulfil these goals, and those unable to meet repayments through increased taxation and spending cuts to their already impoverished populations will be compelled to hand over their land and natural resources to their creditors.[30]

---

25. Prime Minister's Office, 'UK announces major new package of climate support at COP27' (7 November 2022).

26. See United Nations, 'Transforming our world: the 2030 Agenda for Sustainable Development' (Resolution adopted by the General Assembly on 25 September, 2015).

27. See UK Cabinet Office, 'Implementing Sustainable Development Goals' (15 July, 2022).

28. See Gibson Dunn Lawyers, 'BlackRock, Vanguard, State Street Update Corporate Governance and ESG Policies and Priorities for 2022' (25 January, 2022).

29. See Jason Hickel, 'The World's Sustainable Development Goals Aren't Sustainable', *Foreign Policy* (30 September, 2020).

30. See Iain Davis and Whitney Webb, 'Sustainable Debt Slavery', *Unlimited Hangout* (13 September, 2022).

Indeed, both SDG and ESG criteria are predicated on monetising the natural world, which has recently been estimated by the New York Stock Exchange at $4 quadrillion ($4,000,000,000,000,000).[31] Monetised nature is the basis of a new form of corporation called a Natural Asset Company, the purpose of which is to maximise what it calls 'ecological performance' and the production of 'ecosystem services', over the management of which these corporations will, of course, have legal rights and authority.[32] Behind their 'green' credentials, therefore, these programmes, like those implemented on the justification of the coronavirus 'crisis', are instruments of stakeholder capitalism.

By the end of 2022, the total value of contracts awarded to companies by the UK Government in response to the coronavirus 'crisis' was £47.3 billion. This included £22.8 billion on the utterly useless 'Test and Trace' programme; £14.7 billion on largely unusable or undelivered personal protection equipment; £3.8 billion on medicines and the almost entirely unused 'Nightingale' hospitals; £5 billion on 'other' supplies and services; and £1 billion on the totally useless and increasingly dangerous 'vaccines'.[33] This vast expenditure of public money on the justification of combatting a manufactured threat to public health is a microcosm of how the UN's Sustainable Development Goals, on the justification of combatting global warming, will allocate the national wealth of the countries party to its obligations to the international companies able to meet the criteria they themselves have imposed. In this respect, the trillions of dollars to which the workers of the West have been placed in debt by their governments on the justification of combatting a 'pandemic' declared by the World Health Organization — an agency of the UN funded by Western governments and private companies and subject to lobbying from both — is an example and model of how the equally manufactured environmental 'crisis' is designed to impoverish their

---

31. Ellen Brown, 'Conservation or Land Grab? The Financialization of Nature', *The Web of Debt Blog* (5 November, 2021).

32. See Intrinsic Exchange Group, 'Be Invested' (2022).

33. See Henry Thompson, 'Latest Updates on UK Government COVID-19 Contracts and Spending', *Tussell* (29 March, 2022); Andrew Woodcock, 'Scathing report blasts "unimaginable" £37bn cost of coronavirus test and trace system', *Independent* (10 March, 2021); Ben Quinn, 'What has happened to England's seven Nightingale hospitals?', *The Guardian* (8 October, 2020); and Gareth Iacobucci, 'Covid-19: Government writes off £10bn on unusable, overpriced, or undelivered PPE', *BMJ* (3 February, 2022).

populations and enrich the architects of both this crisis and the power grab it is enabling.[34]

All this vast expenditure, which is loading still more debt onto the future of our children, is being implemented at a time when the UK public is facing £60 billion in tax rises and spending cuts; when the price cap on annual energy costs for a typical household has been set at £2,500, 96 per cent higher than the previous year, and will increase to £3,000 from April this year; has experienced a 16.4 per cent rise in food prices over the past year, the highest rate since at least 1977; and when 22 per cent of the population, 14.5 million people, are already living in poverty.[35]

Creating public compliance for this transfer of billions of pounds from the national taxpayer to international corporations without mandate from the electorate or oversight of how it is spent, by whom or on what, has been achieved by a vast international campaign of propaganda. One of the forms this has taken is the protests by corporate-funded environmental fundamentalist groups like Extinction Rebellion, Insulate Britain and Just Stop Oil, which our Government, municipal authorities and police forces have granted the freedom to shut down UK roads for hours, and whose promotion by the antics of a handful of 'activists' receive millions of pounds of media coverage denied to the millions of UK citizens who marched in protest against illegal lockdown and 'vaccine' mandates.

I am not claiming that these activists are hired actors or not sincere in their infantile beliefs. The best salesman is someone who believes in their product, and there is no need to hire crocodile tears when a generation of lachrymose kids and apocalyptic 'greens' will shed theirs for free. Indeed, Just Stop Oil's imperious declaration on its website that 'If you are not in resistance you are appeasing evil' is typical of the religious rhetoric of these environmental fundamentalists, and as authoritarian as Black Lives Matter's motto that 'silence is violence', or Extinction

---

34. See Katheryn N. Russ, Phillip Baker, Manho Kang and David McCoy, 'Corporate Lobbying on U.S. Positions Toward the World Health Organization: Evidence of Intensification and Cross-Industry Coordination', *Global Health Governance*, Vol XVII, No. 1 (Spring 2022).

35. See HM Treasury, 'Autumn Statement 2022' (17 November, 2022); Trading Economics, 'United Kingdom Food Inflation' (December 2022); Paul Bolton and Iona Stewart, 'Domestic Energy Prices', *House of Commons Library* (25 November, 2022); and Joseph Rowntree Foundation, 'Overall UK Poverty Rates' (2022).

Rebellion's demand for 'zero carbon'.[36] Only a demographic as politically naive as the Western middle classes could believe that the globalists, international bankers and corporate CEOs implementing Agenda 2030 will 'save the planet'; but their absolutist rhetoric makes it clear that they are willing to impoverish the rest of the world to realise their fundamentalist religious beliefs.

Of course, we've seen this before, and I don't mean the suicide bombers and iconoclasts of Islamic fundamentalist groups. There's a parallel between the fanciful 'solutions' proposed to avert the imminent prospect of environmental disaster and the belief in the effectiveness of wearing medical masks designed to be used within a sterilised operating theatre, or standing two metres apart when outside, or placing acetate screens between tables in indoor venues, or washing our hands in antibacterial gel at the entrance and exit to every building, and in all the other stage props in the theatre of biosecurity invented to 'combat' the virus.

Last April, the Intergovernmental Panel on Climate Change declared that annual greenhouse gas emissions must be reduced by 43 per cent by 2030 and reach 'net zero' emissions by 2050.[37] This will supposedly be achieved not only by enforced restrictions on our energy and food consumption but also through our embrace of highly inefficient technologies like wind turbines, solar panels and electric batteries, in the illusory belief that, over the next three decades, these supposedly renewable sources of energy, which currently provide just 2 per cent of global energy, can replace coal, petroleum and natural gas, which provide 82 per cent. The problem is, unlike the silicon technologies that have transformed computer power exponentially over the past decades, the energy required to move people, drive machines, produce heat or grow food is determined by properties of nature whose boundaries are set by the laws of gravity, inertia, friction, mass, and thermodynamics. Even the vast resources of propaganda disposed of by the World Economic Forum cannot overcome the reality that it takes the energy equivalent of one-hundred barrels of oil to fabricate the batteries to store the energy equivalent of a single barrel of oil.[38]

---

36. See Just Stop Oil, 'Campaign Background' (2023).

37. See Paul Collins, 'IPCC climate report 2022 summary: The key findings', *Climate Consulting by Selectra*, 2022.

38. See Mark P. Mills, 'The "New Energy Economy": An Exercise in Magical Thinking', *Manhattan Institute* (26 march, 2019); and British Petroleum, 'Statistical Review of World Energy' (71st edition, 2022).

In reality, the energy produced by these new technologies is a new commodity, the promotion of which suppresses the fact that producing millions of electric vehicles to replace the existing ones taxed and fined out of use, or erecting hundreds of thousands of wind turbines with a 20-year life-span, or demolishing millions of homes to make way for so-called 'passive housing', or mining the lithium, cobalt and copper for the vast increase in the number of batteries required to harness these energy sources, is far more destructive to our environment and the people who live in it but far more lucrative to the companies and governments with access to the technology and natural resources of other countries.[39] The refusal to see the environmental, social, economic and even political costs of the total cycle of extraction, construction, transportation, demolition and disposal within which these new technologies operate 'sustainably' is part of the willing blindness with which the chimera of 'net zero' has been conjured into being.[40] The truth is, these are new markets requiring new relations of production, new rights of ownership, new regulations of distribution and new controls of consumption enforced by an authoritarian reduction not only of our standard of living but also of our rights and freedoms, and with them the sovereignty of governments over their national wealth, assets and resources.

It's unclear what the environmental fundamentalists hope to achieve with their demands, which if realised will condemn hundreds of millions in the global south to starvation and billions more to increased poverty; but their naivety about the ends to which their beliefs are being put is the legacy of this generation. Born into austerity and identity politics, raised by iPhones and social media, in debt £30,000 for a degree nobody wants, graduated to masks, lockdown and gene therapy: they're so alienated from themselves and the world they experience through social media they don't know what sex they are, yet they think they can 'save the planet'. They're the new compliant. The recent images of hysterical, weeping children, chained to bridges or glued to a painting, accusing an imaginary father-figure of stealing their future through the screens of smart phones, the footage from which is then sent around the world by international media

---

39. See Iain Davis, 'SDG7: The Impossible Energy Transformation', *Unlimited Hangout* (6 January, 2023).

40. On estimating carbon cost not only on operational performance but on the total economy of a system, see Simon Elmer and Geraldine Dening, 'Lecture 2. The Environmental Sphere' in *For a Socialist Architecture: Under Capitalism* (Architects for Social Housing, 2021), pp. 73-103.

companies promoting Agenda 2030, is the new model of citizenship in the Global Biosecurity State.

Like all arguments that use the threat of a 'crisis' to justify coercive action by the forces of the state, the effect of environmental fundamentalism is to circumvent critical thinking, silence questions and pathologise disagreement as 'denial'.[41] And like the equally manufactured health, energy, food and geopolitical 'crises' with which we are threatened today, it's purpose is to dismantle our institutions of democracy, erase our human rights, remove our freedoms, automate our jobs and bankrupt our businesses, leaving us impoverished and defenceless against the predations of capital and the authority of the state.

But these organisations also serve another function, of which the religious acolytes only too ready to offer themselves for arrest appear to be equally ignorant. Just as Black Lives Matter and Extinction Rebellion were cited as justification for the Police, Crime, Sentencing and Courts Act 2022, so the vandalism by Just Stop Oil and Insulate Britain, whose activists have apparently unimpeded access to the city with the highest level of security in Europe, are cited by the Government as justification for the Public Order Bill that, when passed, will remove even more of our freedoms.[42] This is why environmentalist activists can shut down Oxford Street, Westminster Bridge or Trafalgar Square, spray paint across the Houses of Parliament, shatter the windows of JP Morgan's City offices, empty milk bottles across the floor of Harrods, or glue themselves to priceless works of art in the National Gallery, and the police refuse to arrest them; when a few months before UK citizens were carried off by the same police for holding a sheet of paper saying 'Not my King', and a few months before that violently assaulted for not wearing a mask or leaving their homes without permission.[43]

The Metropolitan Police Service is one of the largest, best equipped and well-funded police forces in the world, with 43,000 personnel and an annual budget of £3.8 billion. If it didn't want Just Stop Oil activists blocking roads in London, they

---

41. On the ideological reach of environmental fundamentalism over the British public, see House of Lords Environment and Climate Change Committee, 'In our hands: behaviour change for climate and environmental goals', 1st Report of Session 2022-2023 (12 October, 2022).

42. See UK Public General Acts, 'Police, Crime, Sentencing and Courts Act 2022' (28 April, 2022); and Home Office, 'Public Order Bill: factsheet' (28 October, 2022).

43. See 'Arrest of UK anti-royal protesters raises free speech concerns', *Al Jazeera* (13 September, 2022).

wouldn't be able to do so. The UK also has the highest density of CCTV cameras in Europe, with 1 for every 18 people in London. If the security of Goldman Sachs, the National Gallery and Westminster Palace was so easy to circumvent, it wouldn't be these innocents who made their way inside, but organisations with a far greater reason to resent the UK state. They can because their protests are corporate-funded advertisements for Agenda 2030. They're there by invitation.

In stark contrast to which, the millions of UK citizens who, in the Spring and Summer of 2021, protested without trespass or vandalism against the illegal lockdowns, 'vaccine' mandates and 'vaccine' passports on which the 'Zero-COVID/Zero-carbon' demands are founded, received a very different welcome from the Metropolitan Police Service, were universally censored by the media, ignored by those they had elected to represent them in Parliament, and threatened by the Government with increased powers of arrest, fines and criminal sanctions.[44]

Despite their radical rhetoric, therefore, and whether they know it or not, Just Stop Oil are the paid promoters of the UN's Agenda 2030 and its goal to financialise the natural world. This is why their website, their professionally-printed banners and their media-covered protests combine the slick look of consumer advertising with the language of revolution. Like Insulate Britain, Animal Rebellion, Extinction Rebellion, Black Lives Matter, The People's Assembly, Momentum and all the other 'grass roots' movements astro-turfing for their political and corporate backers, Just Stop Oil has appropriated street protest for the political agenda of globalists. Between 2015 and 2019, I watched the UK Labour Party turn council residents protesting against the demolition of their housing estates into voters for the Party whose councils were demolishing them, and then blame Labour's neoliberal housing policies on Tory austerity.[45] This is a similar lie but with far greater resources and on a global scale. Indeed, this nexus of environmental fundamentalism, biosecurity restrictions, woke ideology, corporate takeover of national governments and managed economic decline is what the governments of Western nations, only a few months into the 'pandemic', informed us was to be 'The New Normal'. What they didn't tell us is to what end.

---

44. See Simon Elmer, 'March for Freedom: London, 29 May, 2021', *Architects for Social Housing* (30 May, 2021).

45. See Simon Elmer, 'Stand Up To Labour: The Denials of Momentum', *Architects for Social Housing* (10 October, 2016).

3. The Western Oligarchy

One of the obstacles to understanding the managed and apparently deliberate destruction of the small and medium-sized businesses that in the UK have decreased in number by half a million since 2020 and the removal of our national sovereignty on the justification of saving us from, by turns, a health crisis, an environmental crisis, an energy crisis or a cost-of-living crisis, is the question of how anyone can benefit from doing so.[46] It's always difficult to look into the future and predict what is going to happen, but we can look back on and try to learn from the recent past. If we want to know where this impoverishment and disenfranchisement of the British people is leading and who will benefit, we could do worse than look at what happened to Russia in the 1990s.

When Mikhail Gorbachev became General Secretary of the Communist Party of the Soviet Union in March 1985, he immediately began his programme of *perestroika* ('restructuring') the economic and political policy of the USSR. Five years later, in September 1990, under the policy reform called *glasnost* ('openness'), the Soviet Parliament granted Gorbachev, now the newly elected President of the USSR, emergency powers of privatisation. This included the authority to transform state-owned enterprises into joint-stock companies with shares offered on stock exchanges. After Gorbachev's resignation and the formal dissolution of the USSR in December 1991, the first Russian President, Boris Yeltsin, initiated a programme of privatisation that sought to compress twenty years of Western neoliberalism into a few years in a country whose population had no experience of how finance capitalism works. Two years later, more than 85 per cent of Russian small businesses and more than 82,000 Russian state-owned companies, about one-third of the total in existence, had been privatised.[47]

One of the first initiatives was Voucher Privatisation, which between 1992 and 1994 distributed 144 million vouchers that could be converted into stock shares in more than 100,000 state-owned companies among 98 per cent of the Russian population, in principle giving each citizen a share of the national wealth. However, the Russian worker, impoverished and increasingly unemployed by the rapid dismantling of the Soviet economy, had little understanding of shareholder

---

46. See Department for Business, Energy and Industrial Strategy, 'Business population estimates for the UK and regions 2022: statistical release' (6 October, 2022).

47. See Facts and Details, 'Russian Privatization and Oligarchs' (last updated May 2016).

capitalism, and these vouchers were almost entirely bought up for a few rubles by Russian bureaucrats, who had a clearer idea of the state of the Russian economy, state-owned company directors, who had a better grasp of the value of Russian resources, and the mafia, who after years of trading Western commodities on the Soviet black market had a better idea of the future value of these shares. By the end of June 1994, ownership of 70 per cent of Russia's large and medium-sized companies and about 90 per cent of its small businesses had been transferred into private hands.

In 1995, with the Government facing a fiscal deficit and in return for funding his re-election campaign, Yeltsin initiated the Loans for Shares scheme, through which state industrial assets in petroleum, gas, coal, iron and steel were auctioned for loans by commercial banks. Since these loans were never returned, largely because they were used to pay off the interest on existing Government debt, and because the auctions were rigged by political insiders, the state assets were effectively sold for a fraction of their value. Yukos Oil, for example, worth around $5 billion, was sold for $310 million; Sibneft, the third-largest producer of oil in Russia and worth $3 billion, was sold for $100 million; and Norilsk Nickel, which produced a quarter of the world's nickel, sold for $170 million, half as much as a competing bid.[48]

This scheme created a new class of oligarchs (from the Ancient Greek *oligarkhía*, 'the rule of the few'), industrialists and bankers who now controlled not just the Russian economy but also its Government. Conscious, however, that future governments might reverse Yeltsin's carpet-sale of the nation's wealth, the oligarchs, instead of investing in these industries, immediately set about stripping their assets to increase their equity. The vast wealth they accumulated from doing so was invested abroad, largely in Swiss banks, but also into UK property through the largest money-laundering service in the world, the City of London.[49]

This flight of capital out of the country left the Government unable to collect taxes, leading to it defaulting on debt repayments and ultimately to the Russian

---

48. See Alessandro Stanley, 'Russian Banking Scandal Poses Threat to Future of Privatization', *New York Times* (28 January, 1996); and Marshal I. Goldman, 'Putin and the Oligarchs', *Council on Foreign Relations* (November-December, 2004).

49. It is estimated that around £100 billion of dirty money enters the UK every year, the largest amount from Russia and the Ukraine. See Transparency International, 'At Your Service: Investigating how UK businesses and institutions help corrupt individuals and regimes launder their money and reputations' (October 2019).

financial crisis of 1998. When foreign investors began to pull out of the market, selling Russian currency and assets, the Central Bank of Russia, which had only been founded in July 1990, had to spend its foreign reserves to defend Russia's currency, expending approximately $27 billion of its US dollar reserves. This led to the most cataclysmic peacetime economic collapse of an industrial country in history. By 1999, the gross domestic product of Russia had fallen by more than 40 per cent, and hyperinflation that hit 2,500 per cent had wiped out what personal savings the Russian people had accumulated. A decline in meat consumption was mirrored by a huge increase in crime, corruption and mortality, the latter of which reached the highest in history of an industrial country not at war. Unemployment in a country where it had previously been unknown reached 13 per cent. Inflation peaked at 85.7 per cent. Government debt reached 135 per cent of GDP, and Russia, consequently, became the largest borrower from the International Monetary Fund, with loans totalling $20 billion in the 1990s. Little of this served its ostensible purpose, however. A quarter of this sum, some $5 billion, was stolen upon its arrival in Russia on the eve of the financial crisis, and disappeared into an anonymous account registered in the offshore tax jurisdiction of Jersey.

If all this sounds familiar, Yeltsin's reforms were based on the Washington Consensus, ten principles of economic neoliberalisation first implemented in Augusto Pinochet's Chile and by the Argentinian Junta in the 1970s, and imposed by the International Monetary Fund, the World Bank and the US Treasury as a condition of receiving loans. These include redirecting public spending from funding state services to investment in pro-growth services like education and healthcare; eliminating restrictions on import trade and foreign investment; abolishing regulations on safety, health and polluting the environment that impede the market; and above all privatising state industries. As a result of these reforms, on October 1998, the Government of Russia, despite being the largest exporter of natural gas and oil reserves in the world, had to appeal for international humanitarian aid. It was a long way but only a short time since the Soviet Union had been one of two world superpowers, and a lesson in how quickly the wealth and national assets of a country can be stripped when its population is exposed naked to the predations of finance capitalism.[50]

---

50. See Janine R. Wedel, 'The Harvard Boys Do Russia', *The Nation* (14 May, 1998).

Although it has 'recovered' to the extent that today — particularly following the rise in energy prices consequent upon the sanctions — Russia is in the top ten largest economies in the world by nominal GDP, per capita it drops to 53rd.[51] A decade ago, the gap between rich and poor in Russia was the largest of any country in the world, with 35 per cent of the wealth of a country of 144 million people owned by just 110 billionaires, with much of that wealth stored in offshore financial jurisdictions.[52] In 2021, the 500 richest Russians, each with a net worth of more than £100 million and making up just 0.001 per cent of the total population, still controlled 40 per cent of the country's entire household wealth — more than the poorest 99.8 per cent, 114.6 million people, combined.[53] This is what finance capitalism does to a nation and a people without the political and institutional means to protect themselves.

Today, across the neoliberal democracies of the West, national governments in thrall to the new forms of global governance formed on the justification of addressing multiple manufactured 'crises' are implementing equivalent programmes of managed economic collapse devised by the same international institutions of global macro-economic management. Instead of *Perestroika, Glasnost*, Voucher Privatisation and Loans for Shares, these programmes of economic and political 'reform' are called Agenda 2030, Sustainable Development Goals, Universal Basic Income and Central Bank Digital Currency. And although these are being implemented not on the collapse of a centralised command economy like that of the Soviet Union but in neoliberal economies facing the second Global Financial Crisis in twelve years, the aim of these programmes is the same: impoverishment of national populations, bankruptcy of independent businesses, expropriation of national land and resources, instalment of puppet governments to present a facade of democracy to technocratic rule, and an economic and political power-grab by a financial ruling class.

The removal of our rights, driving down of our standard of living, reduction in our food and energy consumption, spiralling inflation and the economic sanctions

---

51. See 'Russia enters the top ten economies in the world for GDP at current prices', *Nova News* (31 December, 2022); and World Population Review, 'GDP per Capita by Country 2023'.

52. Ron Synovitz, 'Russia Has Highest Level Of Wealth Inequality', *Radio Free Europe Radio Liberty* (10 October, 2013).

53. 'Russia's 500 Super Rich Wealthier Than Poorest 99.8% – Report', *The Moscow Times* (10 June, 2021).

and programmes enforcing these, are all designed to transfer our national and personal assets into the hands of this global elite. Just as happened in Russia in the 1990s, the Bank of England has increased its quantitative easing programme to bail out the UK economy, recently spending £19.3 billion buying up Government bonds to prop up the failing pound, with the commitment to spend £65 billion if necessary.[54] With the number of company insolvencies in 2022 the highest in 13 years, small businesses driven into bankruptcy by two years of government-enforced lockdown and rocketing energy prices have had their market share bought up by corporate monopolies.[55] Inflation was predicted by the Bank of England to reach 13 per cent in early 2023, with some estimates predicting a high of 18 per cent.[56] And the duties and authority of the UK state continue to be outsourced by our Government to international companies, who are being empowered by new legislation to set the limits of our previously inalienable rights and freedoms. Finally, our new globalist Prime Minister has been elected not by UK voters or even by his own parliamentary party, but by the international financiers and technocrats who, just as they do in Russia, now dictate not only our economic policies but also our politics.

Let me clarify what I mean and don't mean by this comparison. I am not saying that post-Soviet Russia is a mirror of the UK in 2023. The differences between the historical circumstances and the economies of the two countries are too great. What I'm arguing is that the managed destruction of the Russian economy after the dissolution of the Soviet Union is an image of where we are heading and why we are being driven to such an end. The Russian and Ukrainian oligarchs weren't only motivated by the wealth they could take out of their countries and into offshore tax jurisdictions managed by financial advisers in the City of London; they were, and are, interested in the political power that wealth gave them. And just as they chose Vladimir Putin to be the successor to the shambling Boris Yeltsin, so too our oligarchs have chosen Rishi Sunak as the successor to the shambling Boris Johnson.

---

54. See 'Bank of England ceases bond-buying after spending £19.3bn', *Sky News* (14 October, 2022).

55. See Office for National Statistics, 'Commentary — Monthly Insolvency Statistics October 2022' (15 November, 2022).

56. See Alex Lawson and Rowena Mason, 'UK inflation will hit 18% in early 2023, says leading bank Citi', *The Guardian* (22 August, 2022).

The UK hasn't been a democratic state since at least March 2020, when the country was placed in a *de facto* State of Emergency and thousands of regulations stripping us of our rights and freedoms were made by ministerial decree without oversight or approval by our elected representatives in Parliament. But in the wake of those restrictions having largely been lifted in March 2022 — while still being imposed by private and public companies, including airlines and the National Health Service, as a condition of access, service or employment — Sunak's unilateral decision to impose the programmes of biosecurity and Agenda 2030 outside of any democratic process is the brazen admission that we are now ruled by international technocracies of global governance run by corporate CEOs, international bankers and government appointed technocrats. And although today we call them 'philanthropists', 'entrepreneurs' and 'global investors', the actions of these unelected globalists are every bit as criminal as those of the Russian and Ukrainian oligarchy in the 1990s, except that they're acting on a far greater stage and with far more damaging consequences for their by turns outraged or applauding but always deceived audience.

The economic and cultural sanctions placed on Russia and the immense financial and military investment in the Ukraine by this global government since March 2022 are instrumental to the financial war these Western globalists are waging against Russia's oligarchs; but contrary to the rhetoric of our politicians and actors, they are doing so not to defend the human rights of Ukrainians and a puppet government installed by the US for precisely this reason, but rather to emulate, replace and surpass that oligarchy in wealth, political influence and above all control over the immense natural resources of Russia and, more immediately, of the Ukraine.

The recent announcement by President Volodymyr Zelensky, following the €100 billion in military, financial and humanitarian aid the West handed over to his Government in 2022, that BlackRock will 'coordinate' its investment in the Ukraine and its natural resources — not only in grain, oil and gas but also in minerals and the lithium that is the primary component in electric batteries — should demonstrate to all but the most fervent blue-and-yellow-flag-waving zealots what interest the West has in this manufactured geopolitical, military and energy crisis.[57]

---

57. See Professor Christophe Trebesch, Katelyn Bushnell, Lukas Franz, Andre Frank, Bharath Kumar and Ivan Kharitonov, 'Ukraine Support Tracker', Kiel Institute for the World Economy (7

If we want an image of where we are being led by this globalist coup — which is being implemented on the spurious justifications of protecting our health from a deadly new virus, defending Europe from 'Mad Vlad' Putin, and saving the planet from man-made global warming — the economic inequality, financial corruption and political disenfranchisement of the Russian people and, closer in time, the puppet Government of the Ukraine and its dance-contestant President, is a good place to look. This is an image of our future.

4. Truth and Lies

These articles are a record of how, with the collaboration of a terrorised and virtuous public, a threat to public health that never existed was turned into a 'crisis', and on the justification of combatting it the experimental 'vaccination' programme was implemented, laying the foundations for the UK biosecurity state of today. Published in two volumes titled, respectively, *Virtue and Terror* and *The New Normal*, they have been selected from the two-dozen or so that first appeared on the website of Architects for Social Housing in the eighteen months between April 2020 and October 2021. These received a far more positive response than I had reason to expect at the time, having been visited on our website by over 300,000 readers from 190 countries. Indeed, I have previously made collections of all these articles, which were distributed as pdf files to those who wanted to read them in a different format to the scroll of an online text. So why publish them now, 18 months and more later? The answer, partly, is in order to capitalise on the unexpected success of my book, *The Road to Fascism: For a Critique of the Global Biosecurity State*, which I published last September, and which gives me the chance to bring these articles to a wider audience now that more ears and eyes are opening to the information and arguments they contain. But there is another, more pressing, reason.

As the evidence of the immense and increasing damage of both lockdown and the UK 'vaccination' programme has become too overwhelming for all but the COVID faithful to ignore, those who called loudest for their enforcement —

December, 2022); Ben Norton, 'Ukraine's Zelensky sends love letter to US corporations, promising "big business" for Wall Street', *Scheerpost* (27 January, 2023); and Geeta Mohan, 'Are Ukraine's vast natural resources a real reason behind Russia's invasion?' *Business Today* (25 February, 2022).

politicians, journalists and doctors — have claimed not only that they did not know what the consequences would be but that nobody else knew either, and have made plaintive appeals for an 'amnesty' between the financially ruined, psychologically traumatised, 'vaccine' injured and bereaved and those responsible for their suffering and loss.[58] I'm happy to say that these appeals have been almost universally rejected and denounced for what they are: denials of culpability by cowards and criminals.[59] The data and analysis contained in these articles are a reminder and historical record that those who took the time to look knew almost from the start that the coronavirus 'crisis' had been manufactured, that closing down the economy for two years would impoverish millions and enrich a few, that printing hundreds of billions of pounds in quantitative easing to save it from collapse would lead to rampant inflation, that withdrawing medical diagnosis, care and treatment for 68.8 million people for two years would cause the deaths of tens of thousands of UK citizens, and that injecting 170 million doses of experimental gene therapies into a terrorised public would kill thousands, injure millions, and go on to have still unknown consequences for the health and lives of the British people.

It is a convention of the House of Commons that Members of Parliament can (and do) lie through their teeth to their honourable friends but cannot accuse another MP of doing the same, and the UK media and publishing industry obediently follows this gentleman's agreement; but if we are to expose and oppose the Great Lie we have been living since March 2020, we'll have to overthrow more entrenched conventions than this. We can start by calling a lie a 'lie' when we hear or read one. To claim ignorance of the consequences of these medieval health 'measures' is a lie, and the articles collected in these volumes, like many others written by other independent researchers, are the proof of that lie. I am neither a medical doctor nor an actuary, yet anyone who had the courage

---

58. See, for example, Jeremy Warner, 'Only now are the crippling costs of lockdown becoming fully apparent', *The Telegraph* (20 August, 2022); Ed Conway, 'Cost of Living: Bank of England shares responsibility for crisis, former governor says', *Sky News* (20 May, 2022); Chris Smyth, 'Chris Whitty warns of high death rates due to Covid delays', *The Times* (1 December, 2022); World Council for Health, 'Press Conference: Dr. Aseem Malhotra's New Peer-Reviewed Paper Calls for Immediate and "Complete Suspension" of Covid-19 Vaccine' (27 September, 2022); Emily Oster, 'Let's Declare a Pandemic Amnesty', *The Atlantic* (31 October, 2022).

59. See Rhoda Wilson, 'Covid Vaccine News: How much longer can Covidians keep up appearances?', *The Exposé* (4 January, 2023).

to analyse the impact of lockdown on both the economy and medical services of the UK and other countries, or what should have been the ample safety signals about the dangers and risks of these injections, and of the complete absence of medical, scientific or rational basis to either, knew that this was a lie. If the guilty are now protesting their ignorance, they are doing so to absolve themselves of responsibility for what they collaborated in doing or enabling, to deny culpability for the damage and deaths, and to avoid retribution from a public coming to the realisation that we have been the object of a campaign of impoverishment and genocide being waged against us by the UK state and its global partners, and in which large portions of the population continue to be complicit.[60]

The truth is not merely a statement of fact — that, for example, this chair is made of wood, or that all men are mortal. The truth is always stated in the face of the attempt and threat of powerful forces to silence it and those who dare to speak it. Totalitarianism is not only the agreement but the dogmatic insistence of the vast majority of the population of a society and all those in positions of power that what is clearly, evidently and demonstrably false is true. When a mother insists that the child she persuaded or allowed to be injected wasn't killed by the experimental gene therapy that was injected into it a few hours earlier she is, understandably, trying to deny her complicity in the naivety and stupidity that led her to agree to allow someone to expose her child to such a risk. But she is also silencing what is impossible for her, at that moment, to entertain as a possibility: that the National Health Service she has been raised to regard as a secular Church, the pharmaceutical industry and her Government not only don't care about whether her child and everybody else she knows lives or dies, but may even be intentionally trying to kill them. Between this realisation and denial of the reality

---

60. The United Nations defines genocide as a) 'killing members of the [persecuted] group'; b) causing serious bodily or mental harm to members of the group; c) deliberately inflicting conditions of life calculated to bring about its physical destruction in whole or in part; d) imposing measures intended to prevent births within the group, e) forcibly transferring children of the group to another group. See the United Nations, 'Convention on the Prevention and Punishment of the Crime of Genocide', Article II (9 December, 1948). As demonstrated by the order of the Auckland High Court to take into custody the sick child of New Zealand parents who wanted the doctors performing the child's heart surgery to use blood transfusions from people who had not been injected with mRNA gene therapies, and for which the parents had found uninjected donors, the UN's fifth definition of an act of genocide is what is coming next for those who do not comply. See 'New Zealand takes custody of ill baby from anti-vaccine parents', *Manila Standard* (7 December, 2022).

of everything she knows, has seen, learned and experienced in her life, it is the latter that she and the vast majority of people in this country as in others have chosen to believe; or if not to believe themselves then to insist others believe, even on pain of being silenced, fined, imprisoned and worse for not believing. It is on this mutual agreement to insist on the truth of a lie that nobody believes that a totalitarian society is made. This describes, precisely, the society we are living in now.

Everything — every last thing without exception — that we've been told about the 'pandemic' over the last three years has been a lie. Nothing we have been told is true. Whether we did or do choose to believe it is not a question of opinion, or what we grandly call 'our' politics, or even of our trust in authority. Those in authority in our society, as in every other across the world and throughout history, didn't get there by telling the truth: they got there by lying — among other and worse things. If we chose to believe them — and as a 'people' the British did so in overwhelming numbers — it was because we were scared, and our fear made us stupid, it made us compliant, it made us weak, it made us turn to the liars in authority and ask them to tell us what to do — worse, to demand that they tell us what to do, and not only us but everybody else too. No-one who wanted to could not have failed to realise, very early on, that we were being lied to. There were and are no grey areas between what was and wasn't true. The truth was and still is there for anyone who wants to find it. The lies were and are easier to listen to, for they are everywhere, in every mouth, across every screen, loud and stupid and unbelievable except by an act of will — not to truth but to believe easy lies. But the difficult truth is that only cowards believed them, that only cowards can possibly choose to continue to believe them after three years of unrelenting and universal lying. It is on this collective cowardice, and on the acceptance and repetition of lies to the point that they are now accepted and enforced by the authorities as truth, even when secretly scarcely anyone still believes them, that the New Normal has been constructed. And the unpleasant truth is that this tells us something about where we are, in the UK, as a society and perhaps, in the West, as a civilisation, as well as about the terrible place we are heading.

The accusation of 'conspiracy theorist' by which anyone opposing or even questioning Government policy continues, still, to be dismissed by our representatives in Parliament, slandered in mainstream and social media, and now criminalised by our Government, judiciary and police forces, is the dark seed of our postmodernity come to fruition. Where modernity understood the truth to be concealed beneath the surface reality of things and sought to excavate it from beneath the lies of the powerful, postmodernity views reality itself as constituted by those surfaces, beneath which there is only the abyss of competing opinions, whose will to power produces a truth that is therefore always contingent, always a product of power, regardless of any purchase that truth may have on the world.

Not only truth, therefore, but reality itself now is up for grabs. A man in a dress is now a woman if those with the legislative power to punish us for denying it say he is. Gene therapies that do nothing to stop transmission of the virus but instead destroy the human immune system can be injected into the population of the globe as a 'vaccine' if governments accord themselves the power to lock us in our homes until enough of us comply. A global pandemic which leaves little or no trace on the overall mortality of the populations infected is the excuse for removing our human rights and freedoms under a permanent State of Emergency and dismantling our democracies for a constitutional dictatorship if there are enough police to enforce it and the media machinery to make people believe it. The imminence of an environmental catastrophe for which there is little and contested evidence is the justification for the revolution into the new totalitarianism of global governance if the financial institutions, international corporations and national governments that form it want it to happen. And they do. Totalitarianism is a dictatorship in which everyone is complicit, in which everyone collaborates, because everyone believes the reality for whose consensus they lost the struggle. The outcome of our struggle is still not decided — not yet, not quite — but on its triumph or defeat will depend the fate of the West, and perhaps even of humankind.

When I look back on the last three years and the memories that most capture its insanity and obscenities, I recall the elderly residents of Porlock, a village on the North Coast of Somerset I visited on the first summer of lockdown, shuffling through the sweltering streets with their terrified faces covered not only with masks but with plastic visors. Or of the dozens of virtuous members of the public who, in pubs, shops, supermarkets or on country walks, have screamed at me for not keeping my distance or wearing a mask. And, most horrifying of all, the recorded videos, too numerous to recall, of men and women, young and old, shaking uncontrollably, too weak to walk or even stand, lying in hospital beds, their skin covered in rashes, some with their limbs amputated, their eyes blank and staring, coming to terms with what they've done.

But the memory that haunts me most is only tangentially connected to the effects of lockdown restrictions or the experimental gene therapies. Recently, I saw a small child, no more than a year old, sitting in a pram in the entrance to a supermarket. Admittedly, there was little for him to look at beside the wall-to-wall adverts with which we are surrounded in the city today, but even these were withdrawn from his attention. For the child's mother had placed in front of his face a screen, in size an infant's equivalent to the laptop on which I write these words, but across which a parade of brightly-coloured, digitally-generated images that bore no relation to the world flashed before his transfixed gaze. I don't know if this is typical of the practices of child-raising in the UK today, and whether this machine is the latest digital upgrade to what we in the UK call 'dummies' and in the US they call 'pacifiers'; but it was clearly doing the latter and producing the former. Not once, as I stood there watching this new model of the human being being made, did this infant look up at the world around him, or appear to make any distinction between that world and the virtual one into whose navigation and eventual mergence he was being subliminally trained. These are minds that can learn languages and skills in months that would take adults years of study and training; and it's to the digital, virtual and augmented world over which the enemies of humanity have complete control that our children are being raised, not the material, real and natural world from which they want to ban us, in order to possess and control its resources.

It is not by chance that the target and primary object of the trans-human programmes, technologies, ideology and agenda of the Global Biosecurity State is our children, whom they are doing their best to take away from the protection of their parents and families and into the control of the state. Only a generation raised by their iPhones into a childhood of austerity and national decline, educated by social media into the orthodoxies of identity politics and woke ideology, and which graduated to masks, lockdown and medical mandates, could possibly view the image of the future being created for them by the World Economic Forum as something desirable. Only a generation terrorised by an endless succession of civilisation-ending crises could swap their freedoms, their rights, their agency and their humanity for the promise of an all-encompassing 'safety'. The dystopian horror of that future is our greatest weapon in the fight to stop it becoming a reality. It is up to us, who are guilty of handing our children's education over to globalists, propagandists, ideologues, fanatics and preachers of the apocalypse, to convince them of the falseness of their fears, and that the only end of the world they are facing is that being built on their belief in those fears and obedience to those who have fabricated them. To this end, we need to paint a different image of the future they might one day inhabit if together we defeat the threats we face today. Not since the First Industrial Revolution have there been more profound and far-reaching changes to our world. Not since the Second World War has there been a greater threat to the freedoms of the people of the world. The battle is engaged. For the sake of the future in which all children will live out their lives either in some degree of freedom or in a totalitarian system the like of which has never been seen before, we need to win it.

Finally, there is a positive, hopeful, even happy reason to publish these articles in book form. Unlike an electronic text, a book is an object that enters and moves about in the real world. The author never knows where it will go, who will pick it up and read it, and what effect it may have. No one can monitor what you read in it or punish you for doing so. No one can tell you it's misinformation or censor the words or thoughts of which they don't approve. No one can suspend your bank account for what you learn in its pages. The printed word can't be deleted online, altered to fit woke ideology or fact-checked by corporate liars. Not the least joy of publishing these books independently is that no editor has meddled with them. Every word is as I wrote it, and both volumes are available uncensored by a publisher or the information technology companies handed the authority to adjudicate over our freedom of thought and expression. It's an inevitability, however, that sometime in the near future the Intergovernmental Panel on Climate Change or some other fundamentalist organisation will declare that, since books are made from carbon dioxide-absorbing trees, they are 'killing the planet', and reading them, therefore, is a crime. The spectacle of the virtuous burning books will return — this I prophesy! But while the last days of freedom remain to us, books are freedom.

— January 2023

Virtue and Terror

1. Giorgio Agamben and the Biopolitics of COVID-19

Today I want to talk about the contemporary Italian philosopher, Giorgio Agamben. Why? You ask. For two reasons. The first is because, since the coronavirus 'crisis' began, Agamben, who lives in Italy, has been writing commentaries and reflections that have been published by *Quodlibet*, and — amid the almost universal parroting of government propaganda by our so-called intellectuals — they are rare in openly questioning the official narrative on the coronavirus.[1] He's a philosopher, and not an easy one, so understanding what he writes may be difficult at first; but keep at it, as I have done, because they are some of the best responses I've read since this crisis-event was initiated, and accords with my own views about what is being done and how.

The second reason is to look at how Agamben's writings about the coronavirus panic have been met, which has been with howls of indignation, violent denunciations and contemptuous attempts to pathologise and dismiss the 78-year-old philosopher as an out-of-touch old man who should be censored for endangering the lives of others. In other words, the response has been the same that has greeted anyone, including myself, who has dared to question and challenge the government and media narrative about the coronavirus.

1. Biopolitics

We'll get back to that later, but before I get to Agamben's latest text — simply called 'A Question', and in that alone it has raised the ire of the unquestioning — I want to say a little about why we should be reading and listening to him at this time.

Giorgio Agamben is one of the foremost exponents of the theory of 'biopolitics'. This is a term most closely associated today with the work of the French philosopher and historian of ideas, Michel Foucault, who died in 1984. In

---

1. See Giorgio Agamben, *Quodlibet: Una voce, rubrica di Giorgio Agamben* (February 2020-October 2022); selections from which have been translated by Valeria Dani in *Where Are We Now? The Epidemic as Politics*; second updates edition (Eris, 2021).

a succession of studies, including *Madness and Civilisation: A History of Insanity in the Age of Reason* (1961), *The Birth of the Clinic: An Archaeology of Medical Perception* (1963), *The Order of Things: An Archaeology of the Human Sciences* (1966), *Discipline and Punish: The Birth of the Prison* (1975) and *The History of Sexuality* (1976-84), Foucault showed how various discourses — of knowledge, of madness, of education, of discipline, of punishment, of policing, of medicine, of sexuality, of subjectivity and of death — situate the body in relation to power; or, more accurately, how what Foucault called 'biopower' is manifested by and through this situating of the body within discourse. This marked a radical addition to the Marxist identification of power with the economic, political and legal structures of capitalism, and a refinement of how the sphere of ideology works. Crucial in this constitution of human subjectivity within the relations of power is the state's control over the biology of its population. Foucault called this a new technology of power that was an 'indispensable element in the development of capitalism'.[2]

This, so to speak, is where the work of Giorgio Agamben picks up. In a series of ten books published over more than twenty years under the collective title of *Homo Sacer*, which began with *Homo Sacer: Sovereign Power and Bare Life* (1995), and includes *Remnants of Auschwitz: The Witness and the Archive* (1998), *State of Exception* (2003) and *Stasis: Civil War as a Political Paradigm* (2015), Agamben has shown how, by reducing our human rights as citizens to the protection of what he calls our 'bare life', the institutions and technologies disposed of by the state have been able to subject us to a biopolitics that has become the paradigm for modern government. The key form of this biopolitics, and the one through which Agamben is viewing the coronavirus 'crisis', is the State of Exception in which the state suspends, removes or otherwise ignores our human rights and civil liberties, and with them the division between executive, legislative and juridical powers on which liberal democracy has been based, however imperfectly. In a State of Exception, the government assumes executive power without legislative oversight or approval, our civil liberties are suspended

---

2. The seminal exposition of 'biopower' is in Michel Foucault, 'Right of Death and Power over Life', part five of *The Will to Knowledge*, volume 1 of *The History of Sexuality*, translated by Robert Hurley (Penguin Books, 1998), 133-159.

indefinitely and our human rights are removed — all on the justification of protecting our biological existence or 'bare life'.

Whether we are being protected from a terrorist attack, a political extremist or a mysterious virus, and therefore on the justification of our safety, our security or our health, the State of Exception has been used, and continues to be used, to build a form of totalitarianism that, under new and renewed crisis-events, has become the norm. The so-called 'War on Terror' that followed the destruction of the World Trade Centre in September 2001 ushered in what the US calls the 'Security State' in which we have all lived for the past two decades. In France, the State of Emergency declared in November 2015 in response to terrorist attacks in Paris didn't expire, after no less than five extensions, until November 2017, two years later, when it was replaced by a raft of repressive measures embedded into ordinary law.[3] And as we are seeing now in the response of the UK Government to the so-called threat of COVID-19, this surveillance state, which is transnational and therefore transcends the sovereignty of the nation state and parliamentary legislation, is built on the total surveillance and control of the population. This is being implemented through the use of tracking, location and monitoring devices in our phones and other communication technologies, and imposed with new police powers to enforce so-called health and safety regulations that have had neither parliamentary scrutiny nor legislative approval.

While the UK Parliament is suspended indefinitely and we sit at home like frightened rabbits, both this surveillance and the regulations for its police enforcement are being developed by the UK Government in collaboration with tech companies like BT, EE and O2, using data collected through automatic number-plate recognition cameras by the Department for Transport, and through developing apps with Google and Apple to trace anyone infected with SARS-CoV-2 and share that information with other tracking devices.[4] All this has been done with the blessing of the Information Commissioner's Office, the UK's supposed privacy watchdog, on the grounds that sharing our private data will protect us

---

3. See Marco Perolini, 'France's Permanent State of Emergency', *Amnesty International* (26 September, 2017).

4. See NetPol undercover research group, 'Policing the corona state: a diary of security and surveillance during Britain's state of emergency'; Simon Chandler, 'U.K. Government Is Using Coronavirus As Excuse To Ramp Up Surveillance', *Forbes* (2 April, 2020); Leo Kelion, 'Coronavirus: UK confirms plan for its own contact tracing app', *BBC* (12 April, 2020).

against 'serious threats to public health'.[5] Once again, therefore, our citizenship and the rights deriving from it have been reduced to the biological existence of our bare life. This is the biopolitics of what has quickly been dubbed and accepted as our 'New Normal'.

All this, however, is in contravention of Article 8 of the European Convention on Human Rights on the 'Right to respect for private and family life, home and correspondence'. In the Guide to the enforcement of this right by the European Court of Human Rights dated August 2019, it states:

¶214. The court has found that the collection and storage of a person's health-related data for a very long period, together with the disclosure and use of such data for purposes unrelated to the original reasons for their collection, constituted a disproportionate interference with the right to respect for private life.

¶218. The mere existence of legislation which allows a system for the secret monitoring of communications entails a threat of surveillance for all those to whom the legislation may be applied. While domestic legislatures and national authorities enjoy a certain margin of appreciation in which to assess that system of surveillance is required, the Contracting States do not enjoy unlimited discretion to subject persons within their jurisdiction to secret surveillance.

¶219. Collection, through a GPS device attached to a person's car, and storage of data concerning that person's whereabouts and movements in the public sphere was also found to constitute an interference with private life.[6]

Certain human rights lawyers have expressed their concern that the Emergency Powers handed to the police by both the Coronavirus Act 2020 and The Health Protection (Coronavirus, Restrictions) (England) Regulations 2020 interfere not only with our right to private and family life under Article 8, but also with our right to liberty, as protected by Article 5 of the Convention; and that restrictions on gatherings potentially pose a threat to our rights to freedom of

---

5. See Mark Sweney, 'Watchdog approves use of UK phone data to help fight coronavirus', *The Guardian* (27 March, 2020).

6. See European Court of Human Rights, 'Guide on Article 8 of the European Convention on Human Rights' (August 2019, last updated 2022).

expression (Article 10) and our rights of assembly and association (Article 11).[7] This is why the various European governments theoretically subject to these conventions have declared a State of Emergency — either officially, as in Italy and Spain, or *de facto*, as in France, Germany and the UK — suspending our human rights for as long as the executive decides a State of Emergency caused by the coronavirus pertains.

As evidence of this, the Memorandum to the Joint Committee on The Coronavirus Bill, dated 20 March, addressed its infringement of our rights under the following articles and protocols of the Human Rights Act 1998, which incorporated the European Convention articles and protocols into British Law:

- Article 2. Right to life
- Article 3. Freedom from torture, inhuman and degrading treatment
- Article 5. Right to liberty and security
- Article 6. Right to a fair trial
- Article 8. Right to respect for private and family life
- Article 9. Freedom of thought, conscience and religion
- Article 10. Freedom of expression
- Article 11. Freedom of assembly and association
- Article 14. Prohibition of discrimination
- Protocol 1. Right to peaceful enjoyment of his possessions
- Protocol 2. Right to education
- Protocol 3. Right to free elections[8]

The general consideration of the unnamed lawyers writing this Memorandum was that the proposed police powers are, in their opinion, necessary in order to protect public health, and that any interference they have with our human rights is therefore 'justified, proportionate and lawful'. They duly concluded that the Coronavirus Bill was 'compatible' with the Human Rights Act 1998.

---

7. See UK Public General Acts, 'Coronavirus Act 2020' (25 March, 2020); UK Statutory Instruments, 'The Health Protection (Coronavirus, Restrictions) (England) Regulations 2020' (26 March, 2020); and Sidley Austin LLP, 'COVID-19 Control Measures — UK Police Powers' (31 March, 2020).

8. See UK Parliament, 'Memorandum to the Joint Committee on the Coronavirus Bill' (20 March, 2020).

What these Government lawyers didn't explain is why, under Section 89 of the Coronavirus Act when it is made into law, these police powers will be in existence for at least 2 years, with the option, under Section 90, to extend them another 6 months, and, under Section 92, to make 'consequential modifications' to them. One chambers briefing observed that:

> Although technically approval is still required within 28 days, as Parliament is now in recess this will not happen prior to the first review which is due by 16 April 2020. This effectively means there will be no parliamentary scrutiny of Regulations which on their face impose extraordinary and draconian restrictions on freedom of movement backed by increased powers of arrest and prosecution. If this is a sign of things to come it does not bode well.[9]

In *State of Exception*, which everybody trying to understand this moment should be reading, Giorgio Agamben has pointed out that, under the Chancellorship and then Leadership of Adolf Hitler, the Constitution of the Weimar Republic was never abolished but merely suspended by the Decree of the Reich President for the Protection of People and State issued in February 1933 — which under Article 48 of the Constitution suspended a raft of human rights, including the right of public assembly and of free association, the privacy of postal, telegraphic and telephonic communications, the freedom of expression and the freedom of the press, as well as *habeas corpus* — and the subsequent Law to Remedy the Distress of People and State — which legally handed Hitler dictatorial powers.[10] From a juridico-political point of view, therefore, the twelve years of the National Socialist Government were administered under a State of Exception.

The same State of Exception has been applied by three successive US governments to the Guantanamo Bay prison camp, where so-called 'enemy combatants' are detained indefinitely outside of international law, the Geneva convention and even US criminal law without charge or trial, suspended in a state of bare life which means that even those who try to kill themselves through hunger

---

9. Louise Hooper, 'Briefing on the Health Protection (Coronavirus, Restrictions) (England) Regulations 2020', Garden Court Chambers (27 March, 2020).

10. See Giorgio Agamben, *State of Exception*, Homo Sacer II, 1; translated by Kevin Attell (University of Chicago Press, 2005), Chapter 1, 'The State of Exception as a Paradigm of Government', pp. 1-31.

strikes are force-fed. In this we can see repeated the practices of the Margaret Thatcher governments against IRA prisoners denied political status and also force fed when on hunger protests, as well as the anticipation of the extrajudicial imprisonment and torture of the journalist, Julian Assange, by the current UK Government. But we can also see the medical practice of keeping dying patients suspended in a state of vegetative life in which they have been deprived even of the right to die; and, most recently, the enforced, painful and ultimately futile ventilation of elderly and sick patients, who would otherwise be administered palliative care, simply because they have tested positive for SARS-CoV-2.

This is the context in which, on 13 April, Giorgio Agamben published his text titled 'A Question' — the question being: 'How could it happen that an entire country, without realising what was happening, collapsed both politically and ethically in the face of an illness?'[11] To answer this, Agamben presents several examples of this collapse, which include not only allowing loved ones to die alone, but allowing the bodies of the dead to be burned without a funeral; allowing our freedom of movement and therefore our relationships of friendship and love with each other to be limited to an extent greater even than when Italy was under curfew during the Second World War; and — which he identifies as the root of this compliance — allowing the unity of lived experience to be divided into, on the one hand, a social, political and spiritual life that has been denied to us, and, on the other, a purely biological entity. Rejecting the justification that these are purely temporary measures and divisions and that life will return to how it was before, Agamben reminds the reader that, to the contrary, even one month into lockdown, the authorities that declared the State of Emergency and imposed the restrictions were already declaring these restrictions will be the 'new organising principle of society'. In their failure to prevent this collapse, Agamben indicts both the Church and the Law and their failure to defend either society or the constitution; for the priests, he says, like the lawyers, are silent. Finally, he addresses the argument that the sacrifice of our freedoms has been made in the name of moral principles. Recalling that Adolf Eichmann made the same defence of his obedience to the orders implementing the so-called 'Final Solution of the Jewish Problem' in Europe, Agamben concludes:

---

11. See Giorgio Agamben, 'A Question', *Quodlibet* (13 April, 2020); collected in *Where Are We Now?*, pp. 34-37.

A rule which states that good must be renounced in order to save the good is just as false and contradictory as that which, in order to protect freedom, orders us to renounce freedom.

In the rest of this article I want to look at how this and other commentaries by Agamben on the coronavirus 'crisis' have been greeted, for it tells us a lot about how the biopolitics of COVID-19 is being deployed.

2. The Assumption of Evidence

Agamben is the author of over forty book-length works. He's one of the most interesting and — until he questioned the extraordinary restrictions imposed by governments in response to the coronavirus — one of the most respected of philosophers in the West. We might think, given that he has been read for the past quarter of a century precisely because his writings have addressed and analysed exactly the situation in which we find ourselves now, that we would listen to what he has to say. But we would, of course, be wrong. What has actually happened has been the exact opposite.

Agamben's first commentary, titled 'The Invention of an epidemic', was published by *Il Manifesto* on 26 February. I won't quote the whole thing here, but he concluded by writing:

This disproportionate response to something the CNR [National Research Council] considers to be not too different from the normal influenzas that recur every year is absurd. It is almost as if, with terrorism exhausted as a cause for exceptional measures, the invention of an epidemic offers the ideal pretext for increasing them beyond all known limits.

The other, no less disturbing, factor is the state of precarity and fear that in recent years has been systematically cultivated in people's minds, and which has resulted in a genuine need for situations of collective panic for which the epidemic provides, once again, the ideal pretext. . . . Thus, in a perverse and vicious cycle, the limitations of freedom imposed by governments are being accepted in the name of a desire for safety that has been created by the same governments that are now intervening to satisfy it.[12]

This brought forth paroxysms of online rage and contempt, only some of which I shall briefly list here, placing the key terms in their attacks in italics.

- On 5 March, the journal of psychoanalysis, *Antinomie*, published an article by Sergio Benvenuto, an Italian psychoanalyst, in which he described Agamben's commentaries as *'paranoiac* interpretations of history.'[13]
- On 13 March, the Hannah Arendt Center for Politics and Humanities published an article by Roger Berkowitz, a Professor of Political Studies and Human Rights, titled 'When Philosophers are Blinded by Theory', in which he accuses Agamben of 'blindness to reality that can come from a too-strong love for one's own theoretical *fantasies*.'[14]
- On 16 March, *MicroMega* published an article by Paolo Flores d'Arcais, an Italian philosopher and journalist, titled 'Philosophy and Virus: The *Ravings* of Giorgio Agamben'.[15]
- On 23 March, the *Chronicle of Higher Education* published an article by Anastasia Berg, a postdoctoral Junior Research Fellow in Philosophy, titled 'Giorgio Agamben's Coronavirus Cluelessness', in which she claimed 'the Italian philosopher's interventions are *symptomatic* of theory's collapse into *paranoia*.'[16]
- On 26 March, *Critical Legal Thinking* published an article titled 'Must Society be Defended from Agamben?' by Tim Christaens, a Ph.D. student in Philosophy writing his dissertation on Agamben, in which he writes of Agamben's texts: 'If the reader thinks that makes Agamben sound like

---

12. Giorgio Agamben, 'The Invention of an Epidemic', *Il Manifesto* (26 February, 2020); translated in *Where Are We Now?*, pp. 11-13.

13. Sergio Benvenuto, 'Benvenuto in clausura', *Antinomie* (5 March, 2020).

14. Roger Berkowitz, 'When Philosophers are blinded by theory', *The Hannah Ardent Center for Politics and Humanities* (18 March, 2020).

15. Paolo Flores d'Arcais, 'Filosofia e virus: le farneticazioni di Giorgio Agamben', *MicroMega* (16 March, 2020).

16. Anastasia Berg, 'Giorgio Agamben's Coronavirus Cluelessness', *The Chronicle of Higher Education* (23 March, 2020).

coronavirus *denialists* such as Bolsonaro or Trump, then I must confess they are right.'[17]

- On 29 March, *Verso* published an article titled 'States of Emergency, Metaphors of Virus, and COVID-19' by Joseph Owen, another Ph.D. student, who dismissed Agamben as an '*elderly* and misguided sage' whose 'theoretical dispositions have *clouded* his judgement'.[18]
- In its March/April edition, the *New Left Review* published an article by Marco d'Eramo, an Italian journalist, titled 'The Philosopher's Epidemic', in which he accused Agamben of 'coronavirus *denialism*', and argued that the likelihood of security services benefiting from the pandemic 'does not justify a leap to *paranoid conspiricism*'.[19]

Despite the extraordinary arrogance of these judgements, they are not the ravings of Twitter trolls. All the authors are highly educated people writing in authoritative forums. And yet, as can be seen, in all their attempts to dismiss Agamben the authors resort to the same convergence of medicine and politics they are denying is applicable to a biopolitical understanding of the current 'crisis', and whose medical separation of the patient's body from the patient's person Foucault analysed in *The Birth of the Clinic*. Through this discourse of biopower, Agamben is repeatedly diagnosed as 'paranoid', a theoretical 'fantasist', his judgement 'clouded' by age, his thoughts reduced to 'symptoms' of his 'paranoid theorising' and 'ravings', himself in 'denial' brought on by the lockdown, and a fermenter of 'conspiracy theories'. Indeed, the full panoply of medical and psychiatric discourse is employed to justify — if not yet the sectioning and incarceration of one of the most influential philosophers of the past quarter of a

---

17. Tim Christaens, 'Must Society be Defended from Agamben?', *Critical Legal Thinking* (26 March, 2020).

18. Joseph Owen, 'States of Emergency, Metaphors of Virus, and COVID-19', *Verso* (31 March, 2020).

19. Marco d'Eramo, 'The Philosopher's Epidemic', *New Left Review* (March/April 2020). To this collection of fools, cowards and collaborators employing the discourse of biopower, I would like to add the more recent contribution of the former translator of some of Agamben's books, Adam Kotsko, 'What Happened to Giorgio Agamben?', *Slate* (20 February, 2022), in which he describes Agamben's pandemic writings as 'paranoiac', 'embarrassing' and 'screeds', claims they sound 'disturbingly like a right-wing crank', and arrives at the biopolitical diagnosis that 'excessive distrust of any state authority has blinded him'.

century — then certainly his dismissal outside the realms of rational discourse. That this is being done irrationally — without the authors needing to argue why Agamben's arguments, in their opinion, are flawed — is characteristic of all such *ad hominem* attacks, which have come to characterise the forums of Twitter, Facebook, the BBC and the UK Parliament, if not yet the discursive practices of philosophical thought.

However, there is another aspect of these attempts to pathologise Agamben that I want to draw attention to in this article, and one which has a far wider application in spreading the orthodoxy on coronavirus than this attempt to silence an Italian philosopher of whom most people will not have heard.

Perhaps the most disappointing of these, because it is written by an old friend and comrade of Agamben, is by the French philosopher, Jean-Luc Nancy, for whose writings on community I have great respect. I cite his response here to show how, even in the most subtle of minds, there has taken hold what the French semiologist and critic, Roland Barthes, called the '*doxa*' of ideology. By this he meant that which, because it has been so widely accepted as given, has become invisible to interrogation. On 27 February, in response to Agamben's text, Nancy, taking exception with Agamben's description of coronavirus as 'not too different from the normal influenzas', wrote — again in the psychoanalytical journal *Antinomie:*

> 'Normal' flu always kills several people, while coronavirus, against which there is no vaccine, is evidently capable of causing far higher levels of mortality. The difference (according to sources of the same type as those Agamben uses) is about 1 to 30: it does not seem insignificant to me.[20]

This assumption of 'evidence' is what has become most pervasive in the debates — if one can call them that, more accurately in the pronouncements, official and unofficial, on mainstream and social media — by governments and journalists alike. This assumption is that some contemptuous few of us, such as Donald Trump and Boris Johnson, assumed that the coronavirus was just another flu, and even recommended herd immunity as the proper response, but that now we know better. Now, is the assumption, we have the evidence. Now we have

---

20. See Jean-Luc Nancy, 'Eccezione virale', *Antinomie* (27 February, 2020).

'The Science', as Microsoft founder and billionaire vaccine investor Bill Gates said this week when announcing his plans to immunise the world.[21] Now we have the justification to declare a State of Exception that the UK Government is considering maintaining for the two years they initially extended — to everyone's initial surprise — to the powers handed to the police by the Coronavirus Act 2020. We were wrong, but now we understand — and accept — why parliamentary scrutiny must be suspended, why legislative approval is not necessary for our politics, why Health Protection Regulations in contravention of our human rights must be enforced by police officers, community support officers, local authorities, and anyone else the Secretary of State authorises to do so.

To take just one example that must stand in for many of how consensus for these dictatorial powers has been assumed: in one of the most widely-read, copied, shared and commented-upon of these assumptions, *The Sunday Times* last week published an article titled 'Coronavirus: 38 Days when Britain sleepwalked into disaster.'[22] Significantly, the article is an attack on Boris Johnson, with the implication being that anyone who disagrees with its assumptions is therefore 'on the side' of the much reviled UK Prime Minister. But in making its claim that COVID-19 is 'one of the worst infections of the most deadly virus to have hit the world in more than a century', the authors cite a study published on 24 January in the medical journal *The Lancet*, which they claim suggested the potential lethality of coronavirus 'was comparable to the 1918 Spanish flu pandemic, which killed up to 50 million people.'[23] In fact, the *Lancet* study said nothing of the kind, and the authors of *The Sunday Times* article fail to cite the huge amount of subsequent evidence correcting these wild speculations, as if we know nothing more about the virus than we did three months ago. But it's too late. This emotive, fear-mongering, factually inaccurate, deliberately deceptive and hugely irresponsible article has now become the default official history of the coronavirus in the UK, spread through the viral network of social media into everyone's laptop.

---

21. See Bill Gates, 'Transcript: Bill Gates speaks to the FT about the global fight against coronavirus', *Financial Times* (9 April, 2020).

22. See Jonathan Calvert, George Arbuthnott and Jonathan Leake, 'Coronavirus: 38 days when Britain sleepwalked into disaster', *The Times* (18 April, 2020).

23. See Chen Wang, Peter W. Horby, Frederick G. Hayden and George F. Gao, 'A novel coronavirus outbreak of global health concern', *The Lancet* (15 February, 2020).

On the day I publish this article, 25 April 2020, with all the inaccuracies built into how most countries, and certainly those in Europe and the United States, are recording deaths 'with' COVID-19 — which includes anyone who died testing positive for SARS-CoV-2; or anyone to whose death the doctor filling out the certificate thought COVID-19 might have been a possible or contributing cause; or simply anyone who displayed similar symptoms to COVID-19 but wasn't tested — even with this systemic inaccuracy by which so-called 'COVID-19 deaths' are being hugely exaggerated in number, there have been 216,870 deaths officially attributed to the disease across the world since the first official deaths in China four months ago.[24] To put this figure into context, so far this year, 18.6 million people have died across the world: 2,598,000 of them from cancer; 1,581,000 from smoking; 532,000 from HIV/AIDS; 427,000 from traffic accidents; 339,000 from suicide; 310,000 from malaria; and 154,000 from seasonal flu — all in the last four months.

In the UK, the official number of deaths attributed to COVID-19 by the Department of Health and Social Care and its executive agency, Public Health England, according to the criteria listed above is 19,500. Yet, according to a much-quoted and retweeted article published this week in the *Financial Times*, which extrapolates future 'COVID-19 deaths' as a percentage of overall excess deaths recorded by the Office for National Statistics, it may be as many as 41,000, more than twice as much.[25] In this exaggeration it parallels the claim of 50,000 deaths for the seasonal influenza of 2016-17, also drawing on figures from the ONS, in an article published in November 2018 in the *Daily Mail*.[26] In actual fact, only 18,000 deaths were associated with seasonal influenza in England in 2016-17, which is a similar proportion of fact to media report (more than double).[27] As chance would have it, the same day as the *Financial Times* article, 22 April, Giorgio

---

24. See Worldometer, 'COVID-19 Coronavirus Pandemic'.

25. See Chris Giles, 'UK coronavirus deaths more than double official figure, according to FT study', *Financial Times* (22 April, 2020).

26. See Vanessa Chalmers, 'Winter death toll highest since 1975: Failure of flu jab to combat severe outbreak resulted in more than 50,000 extra people dying in England and Wales last year', *Daily Mail* (30 November, 2018).

27. See Public Health England, 'Surveillance of influenza and other respiratory viruses in the UK: Winter 2016 to 2017', *The National Archives* (May 2017).

Agamben published his most recent text on the coronavirus, an interview titled 'New Reflections', in which he calmly observed:

> Anyone with some knowledge of epistemology cannot fail to be surprised by the fact that the media for all these months have released figures without any scientific criterion, not only without relating them to the annual mortality for the same period, but without even specifying the cause of death. I am not a virologist or a doctor, but I limit myself to verbally citing reliable official sources. 21,000 deaths from COVID-19 seem and are certainly an impressive figure. But if you put them in relation with the annual statistical data, things, as is right, take on a different aspect. The president of the National Institute of Statistics, Dr. Gian Carlo Blangiardo, communicated the numbers of last year's mortality a few weeks ago: 647,000 deaths (therefore 1,772 deaths per day). If we analyse the causes in detail, we see that the latest available data for 2017 record 230,000 deaths from cardiovascular diseases, 180,000 deaths from cancer, at least 53,000 deaths from respiratory diseases. I quote the words of Dr. Blangiardo: 'In March 2019 the deaths from respiratory diseases were 15,189 and the year before had been 16,220. Incidentally, it is noted that they are more than the corresponding number of deaths for COVID-19 (12,352) reported in March 2020.'[28]

The official and universal assumption about the exceptional fatality rate of coronavirus has, in fact, no empirical or statistical basis, neither the deaths nor the figures recording them. On the contrary, what has been assumed is precisely what is disproved by the facts. What is 'evident', to use Nancy's word, is that the fatality rate of coronavirus is very much comparable to the seasonal influenza in Italy in 2016-17, when there were nearly 25,000 excess deaths attributable to influenza-related illnesses; in Germany in 2017-18, when there were over 25,000 excess deaths, in England in 2014-15, when there were over 28,300 excess deaths; or as recently as 2017-18, when there were 26,400 excess deaths.[29] I've

---

28. See Giorgio Agamben, 'New Reflections', *Quodlibet* (22 April, 2020); collected in *Where Are We Now?*, pp. 43.

29. See Aldo Rosano, Antonino Bella, Francesco Gesualdo, Anna Acampora, Patrizio Pezzottia, Stefano Marchetti, Walter Ricciardi, Caterina Rizzoa, 'Investigating the impact of influenza on excess mortality in all ages in Italy during recent seasons (2013/14–2016/17 seasons)', *International Journal of Infectious Diseases* (8 August, 2019); Robert Koch Institute, 'Bericht zur

quoted these figures before, and will continue to quote them as evidence for my reasoned deduction — against the blind orthodoxy of assumption — that SARS-CoV-2 and the symptoms that maybe 1 in 10 of those infected with it will develop, and which according to recent estimates kills maybe 0.1 per cent of those infected and most likely less, is very much comparable and equivalent to seasonal influenza, as the monitoring of excess deaths in Europe shows.[30]

Imagine a camp in which 770 people are lying on 770 separate bunks, stacked one on top of the other. This represents the 12.2 million people and 18 per cent of the population in the UK that are over 65. One of them, aged 82, and therefore more than 2 years over the average life expectancy for a man in the UK, has died. At the time of dying he tested positive for SARS-CoV-2, possibly contracted in the camp infirmary in which he has been a patient for the past 16 days, half of them while sedated on a ventilator that took over his breathing, causing rapid weight loss and atrophy of his muscles. This is a proportional representation of the 15,850 people over 60 who have died from COVID-19 in England and Wales. But it is also an image of the painful, unnecessary and cruel biopolitics of the crisis our response to those deaths has created, in which elderly and sick citizens have been deprived of the palliative care they should be receiving in their passage to death in order to justify the lockdown not only of the other 769 people in the camp, but also of the other 4,277 people under the age of 65 living in 6 other camps, all under the surveillance and control of our police and security forces, aided and abetted by a growing body of citizen enforcers and informers.

The widespread belief — and all but universal assertion in our mainstream and social media — that the threat presented by coronavirus justifies imposing a State of Exception on 2.9 billion people across the globe is a product, first, of World Health Organization and UK Government guidelines on identifying and attributing deaths to COVID-19 that that would otherwise be listed as a respiratory disease such as bronchopneumonia or pneumonia; and, second, of the reporting and exaggeration of those already exaggerated numbers outside of any context

---

Epidemiologie der Influenza in Deutschland Saison 2018/19' (2019); Public Health England, 'Surveillance of influenza and other respiratory viruses in the United Kingdom: Winter 2014 to 2015', *The National Archives* (May 2015) and 'Surveillance of influenza and other respiratory viruses in the UK: Winter 2017 to 2018', *The National Archives* (May 2018).

    30. See Jason Oke, Carl Heneghan, 'Global Covid-19 Case Fatality Rates', The Centre for Evidence-Based Medicine (7 October, 2020); and EuroMOMO Bulletin.

by the press and media. In fact, not only have official deaths from COVID-19 been hugely exaggerated as a result of the Government guidelines on subsuming all other contributing causes of death into this category, but the statistics on deaths in any other year where the underlying cause was respiratory disease are hugely underestimated.[31] In the UK, deaths in which the patient is infected with an influenza virus for which, following standard procedure, they haven't been tested are typically listed under a contributing and far more serious disease such as cancer or motor neurone disease, or simply as 'old age', even when the final illness was a respiratory infection. Even given the comparable mortality rates between COVID-19 and seasonal influenza, the changes to the taxonomy of this 'crisis' has skewed the figures towards raising the threat of the former. This can only have been done to serve a biopolitical agenda.

History teaches us that dictatorships don't arrive all at once and fully formed. They creep up, step by step, each one removing a little more of our rights and freedoms, until regulations we would have risen up against in outrage just a few months ago are meekly accepted — as the Government lawyers advising the Joint Committee on the Coronavirus Bill stated — as 'justified, proportionate and lawful'. This week, as anticipated, The Health Protection (Coronavirus, Restrictions) (England) Regulations 2020 were amended to extend the lockdown prohibitions as follows:

6.1. During the emergency period, no person may leave or be outside of the place where they are living without reasonable excuse.[32]

In the Explanatory Memorandum to this amendment provided for the MPs without the ability to read legislation on which they will not be called to vote 'by reason of urgency', the Secretary of State for Health and Social Care, Matt Hancock — a 41-year-old former computer software salesman with a background in the housing market but with no knowledge of either constitutional law or epidemiology — declared:

---

31. See John Lee, 'How deadly is the coronavirus? It's still far from clear', *The Spectator* (28 March, 2020).

32. UK Statutory Instruments, 'The Health Protection (Coronavirus, Restrictions) (England) (Amendment) Regulations 2020' (22 April, 2020), Regulation 2(4)(a).

5.1. In my view the provisions of The Health Protection (Coronavirus, Restrictions) (England) (Amendment) Regulations 2020 are compatible with the European Convention on Human Rights.[33]

Before we can talk about how to organise resistance to the State of Exception under which it now appears we will be living for the foreseeable future, we need to challenge the all but universal assumption that these dictatorial regulations and the surveillance state on which they are based — whether justifiably or not, whether proportionately or not, whether legally or not — have any basis in an increase in deaths caused by COVID-19 above or even equivalent to the usual rate of deaths from seasonal influenza.

It's for this reason that I continue to read these statistics, as others apparently are not, and try to show as clearly and patiently as I can why there is no basis for this assumption. Quite the opposite. What they show is that, despite the attempts to subject him to the biopolitics of COVID-19, Giorgio Agamben was not showing symptoms of paranoia, indulging in fantasies, raving, exhibiting signs of dementia, in a state of denial or indulging in conspiracy theories when he wrote, two months ago, that coronavirus is 'not too different from the normal influenzas that recur every year'. On the contrary, he was speaking what almost nobody is speaking any longer: the truth, not only about the virus but also, more importantly, about how it is being employed by our governments, by our media and by their corporate partners in the service of the biopolitics of what, in his most recent reflection, Agamben describes as a new totalitarianism:

From many sides the hypothesis is now being formulated that in reality we are experiencing the end of a world, that of bourgeois democracies, founded on rights, parliaments and the division of powers, which is giving way to a new despotism; that, as regards the pervasiveness of controls and the cessation of all political activity, it will be worse than the totalitarianisms that we have known so far. US political scientists call it the Security State, which is a state in which 'for security reasons' (in this case of 'public health'), any limit can be imposed to individual freedoms. . . . And the control that is exercised through video cameras

---

33. UK Statutory Instruments, 'Explanatory Memorandum to The Health Protection (Coronavirus, Restrictions) (England) Regulations 2020', p. 2.

and now, as has been proposed, through mobile phones, far exceeds any form of control exercised under totalitarian regimes such as fascism or Nazism.[34]

— 25 April, 2020

---

34. Giorgio Agamben, 'New Reflections', *Quodlibet* (22 April, 2020); collected in *Where Are We Now?*, pp. 42-43.

2. Manufacturing Consent: The Registering of COVID-19 Deaths

'If the truth is numerical, dry, factual, something that requires effort and study, then it is not truth for them, not something that can bewitch them. The truth must be said with calculation and listened to with calculation. And for us writers it is important whom we tell it to and who tells it to us. Many, proud that they have the courage to tell the truth, happy to have found it, perhaps tired from the work which it costs to put it in a serviceable form, waiting impatiently for those whose interests they are defending to take hold of it, do not consider it necessary on top of all of this to use especial cunning when spreading the truth. Thus the whole effect of their work often comes to nothing.'

— Bertolt Brecht, *Five Difficulties in Writing the Truth*, 1935

1. Five Difficulties in Writing the Truth

At the conclusion of the five articles on the coronavirus 'crisis' I published over the past two months since the 'pandemic' was declared this March, I promised that I would continue to read — as others apparently are not — the official statistics on deaths attributed to COVID-19 in order to show that they do not justify the dictatorial regulations and intrusive surveillance measures being imposed on us by the UK Government.[1]

This Tuesday, as on every Tuesday since 13 March this year, the Office for National Statistics (ONS) published its latest figures on deaths registered in England and Wales up to the week ending 17 April, 2020.[2] Although 11 days behind due to the time it takes to collate the data from various sources, the ONS figures have found general acceptance as the most authoritative record of the

---

1. See Simon Elmer, 'COVID-19 and Capitalism' (18 March, 2020), 'Sociology of a Disease: Age, Class and Mortality in the Coronavirus Pandemic' (24 March, 2020), 'Language is a Virus: SARS-CoV-2 and the Science of Political Control' (3 April, 2020), 'Coronazombies! Infection and Denial in the United Kingdom' (9 April, 2020), and 'Giorgio Agamben and the Biopolitics of COVID-19' (25 April, 2020), all published in *Architects for Social Housing*.

2. See Office for National Statistics, 'Deaths registered weekly in England and Wales, provisional: week ending 17 April 2020' (28 April, 2020).

extent and threat of COVID-19, and the official basis for the Government measures being taken to reduce both. As happened last Tuesday and the Tuesday before that, these figures have been quoted by our newspapers, media outlets and on social media as irrefutable proof of the seriousness of the coronavirus pandemic, and therefore as further evidence that the raft of regulations empowering the police, the unscrutinised and unapproved amendments to legislation, and the intrusions into our privacy and covert deals with tech companies the UK Government is pushing through during this *de facto* State of Emergency are justified, proportionate and legal.[3]

What my analysis of these statistics will show, to the contrary, is that they are nothing of the kind — not by challenging their veracity but by looking closely at the criteria by which the ONS, by their own account, has arrived at these figures, which are compiled from the Department of Health and Social Care, National Health Service England, Public Health Wales, and the Care Quality Commission. This article will follow how the Department of Health and Social Care has deliberately manipulated how a 'COVID-19 death' qualifies as such, and how the World Health Organization has issued directives on how such a death is certified, both of which have resulted in the gross exaggeration of the numbers of deaths attributed to the so-called 'coronavirus pandemic'.

In its rush to give credibility to the Government's enacting of these emergency powers, which have removed our human rights and civil liberties and replaced our political system of parliamentary democracy with the executive powers of a police state utilising all the technology of the surveillance industry, our media has not scrutinised these criteria — or, more accurately, it has deliberately closed its eyes to them. At this moment in time, therefore, looking closely at how COVID-19 deaths are registered as such in the UK is one of the ways in which we can begin to speak what almost nobody is speaking about this crisis-event: the truth.

As always, however, the truth isn't easy to speak, and still less to write, particularly in an era when written analysis and reasoned argument have been

---

3. See Sam Blanchard, Senior Health Reporter, and Stephen Matthews, Health Editor, 'Government pledges to publish REAL death totals including non-hospital deaths as Britain suffers 586 more coronavirus deaths after ONS suggest true total may now be 55% higher at more than 33,000', *Mail Online* (28 April, 2020); and Nick Triggle, Health Correspondent, 'Coronavirus: Care homes deaths up as hospital cases fall', *BBC* (28 April, 2020).

supplanted by the 140-character memes of Twitter and the easily consumed graphs being published by papers like the *Financial Times*.[4] In 1935, at a parallel moment in the rise of a dictatorship legally founded on a State of Emergency (the familiarly titled 'Decree for the Protection of People and State'), the German writer, Bertolt Brecht, published an article titled 'Five Difficulties in Writing the Truth'.[5] These were: 1) The courage to write the truth in the face of threats and censorship; 2) The ability to find the truth among the disinformation and lies with which we are inundated by mass media; 3) The skill to turn the truth into a weapon against the propaganda of Governments and their allies; 4) The judgement to identify in whose hands the truth can become effective; and 5) The cunning to disseminate the truth among as many of these people as possible. 85 years is a long time, though, so I want to add a contemporary gloss to these difficulties:

1. The courage to write the truth is, perhaps, for each of us to find within ourselves, but this is more often determined by the material disposition to do so that is dependent upon our independence from censorship by, for example, an employer. This is the case with those nurses and doctors who have been censored by the NHS from speaking about coronavirus on pain of losing their jobs.[6]

2. The ability to find the truth is determined not only by the education or training in how to first research and then understand the documents containing it, but also by the means and time to find them, both of which are often not available

---

4. See Chris Giles and Gill Plimmer, 'Coronavirus deaths more than twice hospital toll, data indicate', *Financial Times* (28 April, 2020).

5. See Bertolt Brecht, 'Five Difficulties in Writing the Truth', *Unsere Zeit*, no. 2-3 (April 1935); collected in *Brecht on Art and Politics*, edited by Tom Kuhn and Steve Giles, translated by Laura Bradley, Steve Giles and Tom Kuhn (Methuen Drama, 2003), pp. 141-157.

6. See Sarah Johnson, 'NHS staff forbidden from speaking out publicly about coronavirus', *The Guardian* (9 April, 2020). Although this article reports the gagging orders placed on NHS staff, the silenced words it relates are all about shortages of personal protective equipment to respond to the 'crisis', not about the lack of evidence for its existence in a month when NHS hospitals were empty. See Dave West, 'NHS hospitals have four times more empty beds than usual', *HSJ* (13 April, 2020). This is representative of the way the UK press is lending itself to disseminating lies and censoring the truth by purporting to report on its repression, in the practice of which *The Guardian* is perhaps the foremost exponent.

to those scraping a living under capitalism. In this, as in so many other ways, the educated middle classes from whom our intelligentsia is supposed to be drawn, but who instead spend their free time repeating and retweeting media propaganda without taking the trouble to verify its truth, have my complete contempt as the unthinking agents of the Government they unwittingly serve.

3. When users of Twitter and Facebook posters can reach far more people than the most powerful propagandists of Brecht's time, the ability to turn every bit of information into an ideological weapon is available to everyone. Unfortunately, with the size of their audience determined by the popularity of what they write rather than its truth, these weapons are being deployed overwhelmingly in the service of the Government, which has instructed users of social media not to disseminate anything that contradicts its narrative.[7] Whether any of us has the skill to make our dissenting voices heard above the white noise of online propaganda and the censorship of online platforms is a question this crisis-event will pose in the months and years to come.

4. With radicals, socialists, anarchists and communists that have disagreed on every social and political issue in the UK for the past 20 years all suddenly united in their eagerness to blame, chastise and demand of the Government that it increase its measures to stop the spread of SARS-CoV-2 and the impact of COVID-19 — even when few distinguish between the two — I admit that I lack the judgement to identify to whom I am writing, in whose hands the truth should best be placed, and what possible weapon can be made from it — not when there is such a small audience inclined to listen to the truth, let alone so few hands ready to wield it. More than the expected collusion of middle-class 'liberals' with the Government they elected to office, the collaboration in spreading the lies of this Government by the so-called political Left in this country is, perhaps, the clearest sign of how ripe we are for fascism.

5. Finally, while Brecht's article, written from exile in Denmark, was first published in Paris, Basel and Prague in the communist journal *Unsere Zeit*,

---

7. See HM Government, 'Take care with what you share using the SHARE checklist'.

and later smuggled into Nazi Germany as a pamphlet under the title *Practical Tips for First Aid*, it received little response at the time, and I don't expect a similar ruse to be any more effective 85 years later. But I will recall that, on the beam supporting the ceiling in Brecht's study in Svendborg he had written the words: 'Truth is concrete'.

The Office for National Statistics is fairly transparent about the criteria through which they arrive at the figures they are publishing on the official deaths attributed to Coronavirus Disease 2019 (COVID-19), the symptoms developed in a small percentage of people who have contracted Severe Acute Respiratory Syndrome Corona Virus 2 (SARS-CoV-2). In fact, so open have they been about these criteria that it's not impossible to suppose that the ONS is inviting a journalist or newspaper to expose just how open those criteria are to exaggerating the official number of deaths. If that's the case, they may be waiting a long time. Although the ONS is the executive office of the UK Statistics Authority, a non-ministerial department, and therefore has a degree of independence from the UK Government, it reports directly to Parliament, and therefore according to criteria set by UK legislation. With Parliament adjourned for four weeks and Members placed under the same regulations on social distancing as the rest of us by the Government's unilateral declaration of an 'emergency period', it is unclear exactly who has laid down the criteria by which someone dying in the UK is designated a 'COVID-19 death': possibly the Department of Health and Social Care (DHSC); possibly the World Health Organization (WHO). But to understand as clearly as possible what those criteria are, I am going to quote extensively from — and comment in detail on — four pages from the Office for National Statistics website: 1) the first recording deaths registered in England and Wales up to the week ending 17 April, 2020; 2) the second comparing weekly deaths in England and Wales up to the same date; 3) the third the website's user guide to mortality statistics; 4) and the fourth on the different uses of figures on deaths from COVID-19 published by the Department of Health and Social Care and the Office for National Statistics. Unfortunately, Brecht was right: the truth is concrete, and it takes a lot of hammering to release it from the lies in which it has been hidden.

2. Deaths Registered Weekly in England and Wales[8]

The following passages in smaller font size and indented from the left-hand margin are all quoted from the relevant webpages of the Office for National Statistics (abbreviated as ONS), with the section number and title given in bold for easy reference. My commentary on these passages is flush with the left-hand margin. The contents of the ONS webpages overlap with each other, so there is some repetition of points, though these deserve repeating.

2. Main points

- The provisional number of deaths registered in England and Wales in the week ending 17 April 2020 (Week 16) was 22,351; this represents an increase of 3,835 deaths registered compared with the previous week (Week 15) and 11,854 more than the five-year average; this is the highest weekly total recorded since comparable figures began in 1993.

Although limited to its remit of England and Wales and delayed by 10 days, the ONS record of overall deaths has become the accepted indicator of the severity of the coronavirus epidemic in the UK, from which newspapers such as the *Financial Times* have extrapolated that the actual number of deaths across the UK is more than double the ONS figures.[9] Accompanied by simplistic charts showing sharply rising mortality rates, it is these figures that have confirmed the warnings about the threat of COVID-19 and the proportionality of the Government's response.

However, if we look at the accompanying table published by the ONS, we can see that, in week 16 alone (ending 17 April, 2020), 5,157 of the recorded deaths in England and Wales were among those aged 90 years of age and older. Of the total deaths in week 16 leading to an increase of 11,854 over the average number of deaths over the last five years, 13,441 were over 80. With the average life expectancy in the UK 81.4 years old, is this really evidence of a deadly

---

8. See Office for National Statistics, 'Deaths registered weekly in England and Wales, provisional: week ending 17 April 2020' (28 April, 2020).

9. See Chris Giles, 'UK coronavirus deaths more than double official figure, according to FT study', *Financial Times* (22 April, 2020).

epidemic, or of elderly and sick people dying in a more concentrated period than usual? Neither the ONS, the NHS, the DHSC or the CQC has provided information about the presence of co-morbidities (pre-existing illnesses) that one would expect to find in so elderly a demographic of supposedly 'COVID-19 deaths'.

- Of the deaths registered in Week 16, 8,758 mentioned 'novel coronavirus (COVID-19)', which is 39.2% of all deaths; this compares with 6,213 (33.6% of all deaths) in Week 15.

Interestingly, this means that, even accepting the accuracy of 8,758 deaths being attributed to COVID-19 in the week ending 17 April, at least 3,096 of the 11,854 deaths in excess of the five-year average for this week were due to other causes. 1,776 of these are listed as 'deaths where the underlying cause was respiratory disease', but as the ONS chart clarifies: 'If a death had an underlying respiratory cause and a mention of COVID-19, then it would appear in both counts.' In other words, these 1,776 deaths are not in addition to the 8,757 in which COVID-19 'was mentioned on the death certificate', but overlap with the latter. How many the chart does not say; but between 1,320 and 3,096 deaths in excess of the five-year average for week 16 did not have COVID-19 even mentioned on the death certificate. So what caused this increase? The logical answer is the lockdown restrictions imposed on the UK — under which life-saving operations have been cancelled; under which staff from already under-staffed hospitals have been quarantined for testing positive for SARs-CoV-2, even if they display no or mild symptoms; under which vulnerable people of all ages have been either isolated in their homes away from their families and support networks for weeks on end, or forced to live in overcrowded homes, sometimes within violent households; under which people have been forced to watch the businesses and homes they have spent a lifetime building and paying for fall into bankruptcy and receivership; under which, offered nothing more than a future of infinitely extended social distancing, people have taken their own life. What of these deaths, which comprise maybe a quarter of the deaths in excess of the average for this week, and more than a third of the deaths attributed to COVID-19? Do these constitute mere collateral damage — as the US Military calls the civilian dead in its never-ending War on Terror — in our own war against the illusory threat of COVID-19?

- Of deaths involving COVID-19 registered up to Week 16, 77.4% (14,796 deaths) occurred in hospital with the remainder occurring in care homes, private homes and hospices.

I will return to this passage in more detail in Part 3 of this article, but many of the 3,835 additional death certificates that mention COVID-19 from the previous week are due to the 32.6 per cent of deaths that have occurred outside of hospital, and in particular in care homes, which have grabbed the press headlines and Twitter feeds recently. I'll come back to how and why these have been included in the Government's official death toll of COVID-19 deaths.

- The number of overall deaths in care homes for Week 16 was 7,316; this is 2,389 higher than Week 15, almost double the number in Week 14 and almost triple the number in Week 13.

Specifically, of the 11,854 additional overall deaths for the week ending 17 April over the five-year average for week 16 of the year, 7,316 of them, or 62 per cent, occurred in care homes. This, and not a sudden increase in deaths from COVID-19 across England and Wales, is the reason for the rise in overall deaths to the highest since records began in 1993. And these deaths, as we might expect in care homes, are among the very old, with 4,444 deaths in this week among those aged 85-89, and 5,157 deaths among those aged 90 and older.

3. Deaths registered by week

The number of deaths mentioning 'Influenza and Pneumonia' on the death certificate (without COVID-19) decreased from 2,003 in Week 15 to 1,931 in Week 16. There were 3,220 deaths in Week 16 that mentioned both 'Influenza and Pneumonia' and COVID-19 on the death certificate.

Number of deaths registered by week, England and Wales, 28 December 2019
to 17 April 2020

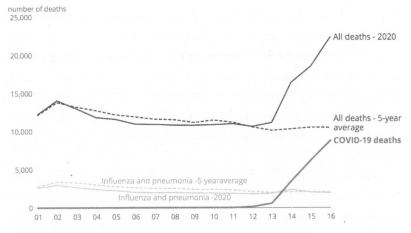

Source: Office for National Statistics — Deaths registered weekly in England and Wales

To recap, of the overall deaths in England and Wales in week 16 of this year, 1,776 were listed as 'deaths where the underlying cause was respiratory disease', 8,758 were deaths 'where COVID-19 was mentioned on the death certificate', and 3,220 mentioned both COVID-19 and influenza and pneumonia. It is worth asking, therefore, why, given the similarity of the symptoms of COVID-19 to other respiratory diseases such as influenza and pneumonia, and the sudden increase in deaths among those over 85 in care homes, the number of deaths mentioning influenza and pneumonia on the death certificate has decreased from week 15. This suggests a choice being made by the doctors or coroners filling out the death certificate, or the recorders of these deaths compiling these statistics, to identify COVID-19 as the cause of death over other respiratory diseases. In other words, the decrease in respiratory diseases as a cause of death in a week when overall deaths are rising is a product of the taxonomy of COVID-19 deaths.

In Week 16, 47.8% of all deaths mentioned 'Influenza and Pneumonia', COVID-19, or both. In comparison, for the five-year average, 19.4% of deaths mentioned 'Influenza and Pneumonia'. 'Influenza and Pneumonia' has been included for comparison, as a well-understood cause of death involving respiratory infection that is likely to have somewhat similar risk factors to COVID-19.

It is for this reason, I suspect, that the ONS has included these comparative figures for death certificates mentioning influenza and pneumonia: not only because of the similarity and familiarity of their symptomatology to COVID-19, but also because the identification of the presence of SARS-CoV-2 in the deceased under the current testing guidelines, which has never been conducted in the UK during previous epidemics of seasonal influenza, has established a causal connection that might not exist between potentially life-threatening symptoms such as pneumonia and testing positive for SARS-CoV-2, when numerous other, unidentified co-morbidities might be as or more responsible for the death of the deceased.

According to Dr. John Lee, a recently retired professor of pathology and a former NHS consultant pathologist, it is not the practice in the UK to test patients who have been admitted to hospital with a respiratory infection for a particular influenza virus, nor to list their deaths as caused by respiratory disease.[10] Instead, the cause of death is typically recorded as pneumonia, or attributed, where one is present, to a contributing and far more serious disease, such as cancer, or leukaemia, or diabetes, or other chronic diseases affecting the heart, lungs, kidneys or liver. That is until now. On 6 March, a Statutory Instrument was made into law by the Secretary of State for Health and Social Care, Matt Hancock, that added COVID-19 to the list of notifiable diseases, and SARs-CoV-2 to the list of notifiable causative agents.[11] This change in law was made by adding both to The Health Protection (Notification) Regulations 2010, and means that General Practitioners are now required as a statutory duty to report all suspected cases of COVID-19 to Public Health England.[12] Notifiable diseases include such extinct and rare conditions as botulism, smallpox, yellow fever and leprosy, and rare causative agents such as anthrax, cholera, plague and rabies, most of which most UK doctors will never see in their lives. The same day this change in law was made, the first death attributed to COVID-19 was officially recorded by Public

---

10. See John Lee, 'How deadly is the coronavirus? It's still far from clear', *The Spectator* (28 March, 2020).

11. See UK Statutory Instruments, 'The Health Protection (Notification) (Amendment) Regulations 2020' (6 March, 2020), Amendment 2.

12. See Department of Health and Social Care (now the UK Health Security Agency), 'Notifiable diseases and causative organisms: how to report' (1 May, 2010).

Health England.[13] As a result of this pivotal change in medical taxonomy, COVID-19 is now the official cause of 39.2 per cent of all deaths in England and Wales in the week ending 17 April, even when 60 per cent of the deceased were over 80, even when 62 per cent died in care homes. Did none of these people die of something other than COVID-19, something far more serious, that would have made them equally susceptible to seasonal influenza — which is not a notifiable disease — any other year?

4. Deaths registered by age group

In Week 16 (week ending 17 April 2020), there were no deaths registered involving the coronavirus (COVID-19) in the youngest age group (that is, those aged 1 year or under). The highest number (3,413) of COVID-19 deaths were among those aged 85 years and over, however, the highest proportion of deaths involving COVID-19 out of all causes was among those aged 65 to 74 years (42.7%).

Deaths by age group, England and Wales, week ending 17 April 2020

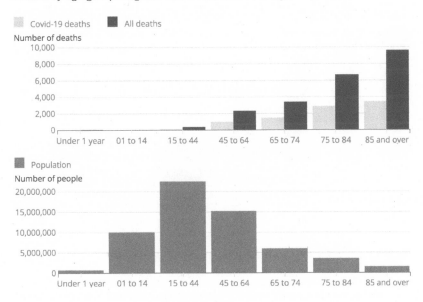

Source: Office for National Statistics — Deaths registered weekly in England and Wales

---

13. See Public Health England, 'Coronavirus data: Deaths in England'.

In fact, if we look at the far more detailed tables published by the ONS, we can see that, of the 1,768 people under the age of 60 who died in England and Wales in the week ending 17 April, 481 of them, or 27 per cent, had COVID-19 'mentioned' on their death certificate as a possible or contributing cause, or as a symptomatology similar to the deceased, or because they tested positive for SARS-CoV-2 at the time of death.

6. Deaths registered in the year-to-date, Week 1 to 16

Looking at the year-to-date (using the most up-to-date data we have available), the number of deaths is currently higher than the five-year average. The current number of deaths is 207,301, which is 22,085 more than the five-year average. Of the deaths registered by 17 April 2020, 19,112 mentioned the coronavirus (COVID-19) on the death certificate; this is 9.2% of all deaths.

Year-to-date analysis for deaths registered in England and Wales, 2020

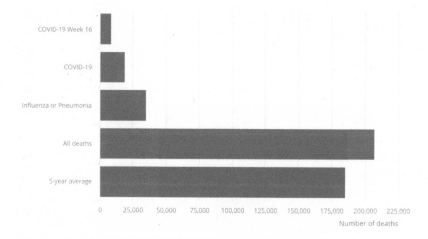

Source: Office for National Statistics — Deaths registered weekly in England and Wales

Averages, though, are not an accurate measure of what has gone before, even within the last five years. By week 16 of 2014, for example, following the influenza epidemic of that winter that was associated with 28,330 deaths in

England alone, there was a total of 191,261 deaths in England and Wales, 16,040 less than in 2020.[14] And in week 16 of 2018, after the 26,408 deaths associated with the influenza virus that season, there was a total of 198,943 deaths, just 8,358 less than in 2020. In the week ending 17 April of this year alone there were 5,157 deaths of people aged 90 years and over in England and Wales, 3,413 of them attributed to COVID-19. Yet it's on the basis of this increase of an average of 522 deaths per week this year out of a population of 56 million people in England and Wales that the Government has imposed the lockdown of the entire UK, the suspension of our civil liberties, and the removal of our legislature.

Given that 46,223 of the 217,311 deaths that have occurred so far this year in England and Wales — 21 per cent of all the deceased — have been people 90 years and older — some of whom, given the likely effect of co-morbidities on their state of health, might have died at some time during the year whether the coronavirus had spread to the UK or not — is it not reasonable to expect a reduction in deaths for the rest of the year once the coronavirus epidemic has tailed off, as it currently is doing, with the peak day for deaths on 10 April? It is even possible that, by the end of 2020, the total number of deaths might be lower than in 2018, during which few of us were even aware of an influenza 'epidemic' in the UK, let alone placed under restrictions on our movement, actions, rights, liberties, privacy and political system by the UK Government? Are these not questions we should be asking — ourselves as well as our Government — before accepting these prohibitions without question?

---

14. See Public Health England, 'Sources of UK flu data: influenza surveillance data in the UK' (7 January, 2014). On the Government webpage through which I accessed this information when I published this article in May 2020 it now says 'This guidance was withdrawn on 24 October 2022'. I'll leave it to the reader to ask what possible reasons the Government had for doing so.

3. Comparison of Weekly Deaths in England and Wales[15]

2. Main points

- A total of 19,112 deaths involving COVID-19 were registered in England and Wales between 28 December 2019 and 17 April 2020 (year to date).
- Including deaths that occurred up to 17 April but were registered up to 25 April, of those we have processed so far, the number involving COVID-19 was 21,284 for England and 1,016 for Wales.[16]

In fact, both these figures are contradicted by the ONS table recording a total of 19,093 deaths up to week 16 of 2020 'where COVID-19 was mentioned on the death certificate', and the 22,351 total deaths; but in my experience figures from different sources rarely match exactly, and the difference is only 19 in the former count and 51 in the latter. This does at least clarify the difference between deaths registered before 17 April and those that occurred up to 17 April but were registered afterwards, in this case up to 25 April. More important is the new addition of deaths occurring in care homes, described here as 'COVID-19 related':

This week we have included Care Quality Commission (CQC) data on notifications of COVID-19 related deaths explicitly stated as occurring in care home settings; from 10 April to 17 April, these total 1,968 deaths, which closely matches the 1,999 COVID-19 related deaths in care home settings that were registered in England over the same time period.

These 1,968 'COVID-19 related deaths' in care homes in the week ending 17 April constitute 27 per cent of the 7,316 total deaths in care homes over the same week that we looked at above; and 22 per cent of the 8,758 total deaths over the same week in which COVID-19 was 'mentioned on the death certificate'. It is important, therefore, in assessing the contribution of COVID-19 in raising overall

---

15. See Office for National Statistics, 'Comparison of weekly death occurrences in England and Wales: up to week ending 17 April 2020' (28 April, 2020).

16. See Office for National Statistics, 'Comparison of weekly death occurrences in England and Wales: up to week ending 17 April 2020' (28 April, 2020).

deaths to 'the highest weekly total recorded', to understand how deaths in care homes qualify as 'COVID-19 related'.

3. Comparisons

Difference between ONS, DHSC, NHS England and PHW figures

The difference between the NHS England and PHW figures and the ONS figures by date of death is because of the wider coverage of the ONS figures, including deaths outside of hospital and those where COVID-19 was reported on the death certificate but there was no positive test. Looking at the year to date, 22.6% of deaths in England and Wales registered by 17 April involving COVID-19 occurred outside hospital (4,316 deaths).

First of all, there is nothing new about how the ONS is recording deaths that occur outside of hospitals in which COVID-19 is mentioned or reported on the death certificate but there was no positive test for SARS-CoV-2. I continue to insist on this distinction, since COVID-19 is the disease, which manifests itself in mild or severe symptoms such as headache, sore throat, coughing, loss of taste or smell, shortness of breath and fever, while the so-called 'COVID-19 test' is for the coronavirus-2 that can cause it.[17] A swab testing positive for the latter does not mean a person has the former, as the elision of the two in everything I've read about testing and the numbers of cases encourages us to believe. Symptoms are the physical manifestation of the disease, which run from cold-like to life-threatening; infection means merely that someone has a virus that in 80 per cent or more of people will not develop into symptoms, or into only very mild symptoms requiring no more remedies than those for a common cold. This is important to remember always, but especially in assessing the identification of COVID-19 as a contributing or determining factor in deaths in care homes in which 'there was no positive test' for SARs-CoV-2.

---

17. See Milly Evans, 'COVID-19: Can I get tested for coronavirus?', *Patient* (6 April, 2020).

Deaths in care homes

The CQC is the independent regulator of health and social care in England. The data provided by the CQC are counts of deaths each day of care home residents who died in care homes, by date of notification. The data are from 10 April when CQC introduced a new way to understand whether COVID-19 was involved in the death. A death involving COVID-19 is based on the statement from the care home provider to the CQC: the assessment of whether COVID-19 was involved may or may not correspond to a medical diagnosis or test result or be reflected in the death certification.

Figure 3: The cumulative number of care home residence deaths in care homes involving COVID-19 in England

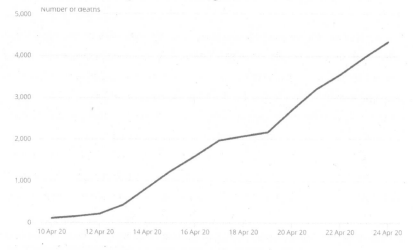

Source: Care Quality Commission data published by the Office for National Statistics

This bears repeating almost verbatim, so astonishing is it as criteria for establishing the cause of death during an epidemic that has justified the lockdown of the whole of the UK. In order to be added to the official tally of COVID-19 deaths, from 10 April the Care Quality Commission (CQC) can state that any death in care homes 'involved' COVID-19 without a medical diagnosis of the cause of death having been made, without a test for SARs-CoV-2 having been made, and without COVID-19 even being mentioned on the death certificate. One wonders on what basis such an involvement was inferred and by whom. Did the care home provider, which includes a range of private agencies such as Allied Healthcare and Bupa Home Healthcare, establish the involvement of COVID-19 in their client's death by observing symptoms that are so similar to pneumonia and other respiratory diseases that the ONS has included the deaths from the latter as a comparison?[18] Who conducted such an observation, and, if they were qualified to identify these symptoms, why did this observation not result in a medical diagnosis or even the mention of COVID-19 as a possible or contributing cause on the death certificate?

It beggars belief — even within the context of the diagnostic sloppiness with which the COVID-19 epidemic has been, and continues to be, recorded and reported — that deaths in care homes do not require any form of standard medical procedure in order to establish a medical diagnosis, in order to infer the meaningless statement that COVID-19 was 'involved' in the death of the deceased. Is it any wonder that, exactly a week later — and who can doubt that this 'new way to understand' COVID-19 was timed to increase these statistics exactly on 27 April? — 1,968 'COVID-related deaths' were added to the official count?

> An important difference between the two sources is that the ONS reports deaths where COVID-19 was mentioned on the death certificate, while CQC notifications rely on the statement of the care home provider that COVID-19 was suspected or confirmed.

A clarification on definitions. According to the Oxford *Dictionary of Epidemiology*, the mortality rate is an 'estimate of the portion of a population that dies during a specified period', while the case fatality rate (CFR) is 'the proportion of cases of a specified condition that are fatal within a specified time.'[19] Given the severity of the Government's response to COVID-19, what must we ask of a death count, published daily by the Department of Health and Social Care and disseminated without question by our media, that relies on 'mentions' on death

---

18. See National Health Service, 'National homecare providers' (last reviewed 1 September, 2021).

19. See Miquel Porta, *A Dictionary of Epidemiology*, 6th edition (Oxford University Press, 2014).

certificates and the 'suspicions' of private health companies to verify the impact of the coronavirus, and from this to extrapolate not even speculative, but purely fanciful, statistics about case fatality rates based on the unsubstantiated numbers of deaths actually caused by COVID-19 and the inadequate numbers of tests of SARS-CoV-2? This isn't the result of the degree of inaccuracy inherent in any attempt to assess and report on the degree of risk from a new virus as it is spreading; this is deliberate fearmongering in order to manufacture consensus to a response that is without medical justification, wildly disproportionate to the actual impact of the virus, and legal only because the Government, on the basis of these fanciful criteria, has declared an 'emergency period'.

Conclusion

The ONS and DHSC COVID-19 death numbers have different criteria. The DHSC count deaths where a person has been tested positive for COVID-19, and for England this is in hospitals only. The ONS counts deaths where COVID-19 (including suspected cases) was mentioned on the death certificate, regardless of location.

This is important in establishing that, in England, where the vast majority of the deaths attributed to COVID-19 are occurring in the UK, tests for SARS-CoV-2 are only carried out in hospitals. Even though this test in itself, as I have explained, does not mean that someone has symptoms of COVID-19, let alone died as a result of the disease, it does clarify that people who die outside of hospital, including those in care homes, do not have to have a positive test for the virus in order to be included in the ONS figures, which only requires that COVID-19 was 'suspected' as a possible or contributing cause of death.

5. Glossary

Coronavirus (COVID-19) deaths are those deaths registered in England and Wales in the stated week where COVID-19 was mentioned on the death certificate as 'deaths involving COVID-19'. A doctor can certify the involvement of COVID-19 based on symptoms and clinical findings — a positive test result is not required.

Again, in the glossary to these statistical tables and the webpages that accompany them, the ONS clarifies that, when a doctor fills out a death certificate, a positive test for SARs-CoV-2 is not required for COVID-19 to be mentioned as being 'involved' in the death and therefore, as a newly-categorised 'notifiable disease', to find its way into the official count of 'COVID-19 deaths'.

6. Measuring the data

Because of the coronavirus (COVID-19) pandemic, our regular weekly deaths release now provides a separate breakdown of the numbers of deaths involving COVID-19: that is, where COVID-19 or suspected COVID-19 was mentioned anywhere on the death certificate, including in combination with other health conditions. If a death certificate mentions COVID-19, it will not always be the main cause of death but may be a contributory factor.

And finally, even within these criteria of 'mentions' and 'suspicions' of 'involvement' — which sounds like the report of a police constable trying to blame a crime on a group of youths the local station has been looking for a reason to arrest — the ONS makes it clear that COVID-19 was present at the scene of the crime 'in combination with other health conditions' that may have had a far more severe and determining role on the death of the deceased. Even when COVID-19 may have contributed to someone's death — most obviously by weakening their immune system like any other influenza virus and therefore making them more susceptible to, for example, the pneumonia that kills them — it does not have to be the main cause of death to be recorded on the official list of COVID-19 deaths. And, importantly for measuring the impact of COVID-19, it will appear on this list without any pre-existing illnesses, even those that were the main cause of death, being mentioned as a contributing, let alone primary, cause of death.

4. User Guide to Mortality Statistics[20]

All of which brings us to how death certificates are filled out in the UK, and how they are turned into the mortality statistics by which the Government's official response to COVID-19 is justified.

2. Information collected at death registration

Mortality statistics are based on information recorded when deaths are certified and registered. Most deaths are certified by a medical practitioner, using the Medical Certificate of Cause of Death (MCCD). This certificate is taken to a registrar by an informant — usually a near relative of the deceased.

As we have seen, however, where the ONS requires the mention of COVID-19 on the death certificate to number the deceased among its record of COVID-19 deaths, deaths occurring outside of hospital do not require the mention of COVID-19 on the death certificate for them to be qualified as such by the Care Quality Commission, but only the statement by the care home provider that they 'suspect' COVID-19 was 'involved'. Both organisations, however, require a Medical Certificate of Cause of Death. So how do these certificates record the cause of death?

6. Certification of cause of death

When a death occurs, the attending doctor completes a Medical Certificate of Cause of Death (MCCD). This is normally taken to the local registrar of births and deaths in the district in which the death occurred.

Usually, the certifying doctor must have seen the deceased during the last two weeks of life to complete a MCCD. This is normally delivered to the registrar by the informant (often a relative of the deceased), within five days of the date of death, as required by law. The majority of deaths are registered in this way.

---

20. See Office for National Statistics, 'User guide to mortality statistics' (last revised 1 July, 2022).

To clarify, the Medical Certificate of Cause of Death (MCCD) is filled out by the medical practitioner, who must have seen the deceased at least two weeks before their death. The completed certificate is taken to the local registrar, who uses it to complete an entry form for registering deaths online.

9. Cause of Death Coding

Coding the underlying cause of death

The death certificate used in England and Wales is compatible with that recommended by WHO. It is set out in two parts. Part I gives the condition or sequence of conditions leading directly to death, while Part II gives details of any associated conditions that contributed to the death, but are not part of the causal sequence.

The MCCD lists three causes of death under Part I. a) 'Disease or condition directly leading to death'; b) 'Other disease or condition, if any, leading to (a)'; and c) 'Other disease or condition, if any, leading to (b)'. In addition to these causal diseases, under Part II the MCCD lists: 'Other significant conditions contributing to the death, but not related to the disease or condition causing it.' As laymen and not medical practitioners, it's important for us to understand that the disease or condition directly leading to death, 'does not mean the mode of dying, such as heart failure, asphyxia, asthenia, etc: it means the disease, injury or complication which caused death'.

The selection of the underlying cause of death is based on ICD rules and is made from the condition or conditions reported by the certifier, as recorded on the certificate. The underlying cause of death is defined by WHO as the disease or injury that initiated the train of events directly leading to death.

Finally, the certificate specifies that 'the condition thought to be the "Underlying Cause of Death" should appear in the lower completed line of Part I.' That is, where 'respiratory disease' was listed as the 'underlying cause of death' for the 28,404 people who had this written on their death certificate in England

41

and Wales up to 17 April, 2020, it would have appeared on the third line of Part I of the cause of death. However, there are exceptions to this rule.

Selection and modification rules

The selection of the underlying cause of death is generally made from the condition or conditions entered in the lowest completed line of Part I of the Medical Certificate of Cause of Death (MCCD). If the death certificate has not been completed correctly — for example, if there is more than one cause on a single line with no indication of sequence, or the conditions entered are not an acceptable causal sequence — it becomes necessary to apply one or more of the selection rules in the ICD-10.

ICD-10 is the tenth edition of the International Statistical Classification of Diseases and Related Health Problems. Approved by the World Health Organization (WHO), this was introduced in England and Wales in 2001, and was updated in 2010.

Even where the certificate has been completed properly, there are particular conditions, combinations or circumstances when modification rules have to be applied to select the correct underlying cause of death. On some death certificates, for example, when two or more causes are listed and then linked together, these may point to another cause. In other cases, the underlying cause of death can be selected from Part II of the MCCD.

In summary, the purpose behind the selection and modification rules is to derive the most useful information from the death certificate and to do it uniformly so that data will be comparable between places and times and each death certificate produces one, and only one, underlying cause of death.

These are the guidelines that have led to COVID-19 being identified not as the medical condition leading directly to death, which in most patients testing positive for SARS-CoV-2 is acute respiratory distress syndrome; or as the condition leading to this respiratory distress, which in most cases is pneumonia;

or even as a condition contributing to death but not related to the disease or condition that caused it, such as diseases affecting the heart, lungs, kidneys or liver; but as the 'underlying cause' of death. If this were any other seasonal influenza, COVID-19 would not be mentioned on the death certificate, but as a newly categorised 'notifiable disease' it now must be included, and the deceased therefore listed in the official record of COVID-19 deaths.

9.3 Final cause of death

In summary, further details on the causes of death can be obtained in one or other of the following ways.

Deaths certified by doctors may have their cause amended as a result of a post-mortem, or of tests initiated before death. The certifier sends this additional information directly to the cause coding team at ONS, where it is only used for statistical purposes and does not appear in the public record.

However, even when COVID-19 doesn't appear on the death certificate as an underlying, contributing, tributary or direct cause, a positive test for SARs-CoV-2, conducted pre- or post-mortem, whether or not the deceased showed any symptoms of COVID-19 while alive, is enough for their death to be recorded in the ONS figures, and therefore to make their way onto the Department of Health and Social Care's website publicising the official number of COVID-19 deaths. Given that the World Health Organization has identified hospitals and other health care facilities as the source of infections for 30 per cent of patients admitted to intensive care units even in high income countries like the UK, and that anyone admitted to an NHS hospital therefore has a high likelihood of contracting SARS-CoV-2 during this 'crisis', this further demonstrates the inaccuracy of these statistics in assessing the true impact of COVID-19.[21]

---

21. The original webpage containing these statistics has been removed by the WHO. But see World Health Organization, 'WHO launches first ever global report on infection prevention and control' (6 May, 2022).

10. ONS short list of cause of death

The Office for National Statistics (ONS) short list for cause of death is based on a standard tabulation list developed by ONS, in consultation with the Department of Health.

Each underlying cause of death has an ICD-10 code. For instance, J00-J99 are the codes for diseases of the respiratory system. These include J09, influenza due to certain identified influenza virus; J10-J11, influenza; J12-J18, pneumonia, J40-J44, bronchitis, emphysema and other chronic obstructive pulmonary disease; and J45-J46, asthma. However, a new addition to the ICD-10 codes used on the ONO statistical charts is U07.1 and U07.2. Since these are not included on the ONS shortlist of cause of death codes, it's not clear whether they are being used to code an underlying cause of death, as the other ICD-10 codes are, or whether they are code for a contributing, tributary or direct cause; but these are the codes used on a Medical Certificate of Cause of Death for 'deaths where COVID-19 was mentioned on the death certificate'.

According to the World Health Organization (WHO), which published these codes on their webpage titled 'Emergency use ICD codes for COVID-19 disease outbreak':

- An emergency ICD-10 code of 'U07.1 COVID-19, virus identified' is assigned to a disease diagnosis of COVID-19 confirmed by laboratory testing.
- An emergency ICD-10 code of 'U07.2 COVID-19, virus not identified' is assigned to a clinical or epidemiological diagnosis of COVID-19 where laboratory confirmation is inconclusive or not available.
- Both U07.1 and U07.2 may be used for mortality coding as cause of death.[22]

The WHO then directs the reader to the 'International Guidelines for Certification and Classification (Coding) of COVID-19 as Cause of Death', which it describes as 'very technical', and whose 'inexorable richness of medical

---

22. See World Health Organization, 'International Guidelines for Certification and Classification (Coding) of COVID-19 as Cause of Death', 2022.

language' is aimed at 'physicians'.[23] Presumably, this is meant to discourage laymen such as myself from reading these guidelines. This article is already long and technical enough, so I may return to them another day; but the guidelines specify that if COVID-19 is the 'suspected' or 'probable' or 'assumed' cause of death, it should be entered on the lowest line of Part 1 of the death certificate as the 'Underlying cause of death' (c), while co-morbidities such as diabetes or artery or pulmonary disease should be reported in Part 2 as a contributing cause.

Frame A: Medical data: Part 1 and 2				
1 Report disease or condition directly leading to death on line a			Cause of death	Time interval from onset to death
		a	Acute respiratory distress syndrome	2 days
Report chain of events in due to order (if applicable)		b	Due to: Pneumonia	10 days
State the underlying cause on the lowest used line		c	Due to: Suspected COVID-19	12 days
Underlying cause of death				
2 Other significant conditions contributing to death (time intervals can be included in brackets after the condition)			Coronary artery disease [5 years], Type 2 diabetes [14 Years], Chronic obstructive pulmonary disease [8 years]	

Manner of death:					
☒ Disease		☐ Assault		☐ Could not be determined	
☐ Accident		☐ Legal intervention		☐ Pending investigation	
☐ Intentional self harm		☐ War		☐ Unknown	

Source: World Health Organization

I'll draw this already overlong discussion on death certificates to a close with these lines from the WHO guidelines on coding for COVID-19, by which even the layman cannot fail to be astonished and appalled:

> Given the intense public health requirements for data, COVID-19 is not considered as due to, or as an obvious consequence of, anything else in analogy to the coding rules applied for influenza. Further to this, there is no provision in the classification to link COVID-19 to other causes. Always apply these instructions, whether they can be considered medically correct or not.

---

23. See World Health Organization, 'International Guidelines for Certification and Classification (Coding) of COVID-19 as Cause of Death' (20 April, 2020).

5. The Different Uses of Figures on Deaths from COVID-19[24]

This may be the last time I can analyse this data. On 28 April, 2020, Public Health England, the executive agency of the DHSC, decided to add every death in the UK to occur in a care home or otherwise outside a hospital since 2 March 2020 to its newly reconfigured website publishing the official count of COVID-19 deaths. At a single stroke, this decision — which supersedes the 'new way to understand whether COVID-19 was involved in the death' announced on 10 April, and whose flawed criteria I addressed above — added a further 4,240 deaths, raising the total UK deaths to over 26,000, surpassing the count in France and even Spain, and closing in on Italy. The same day, the Department of Health and Social Care announced that all such deaths will from now on be recorded as COVID-19 deaths. According to what the DHSC calls its 'official statement on the changes in reporting', which is published on the ONS webpage on 'Different uses of figures on deaths from COVID-19 published by DHSC and ONS':

> From 29 April 2020, DHSC are publishing as their daily announced figures on deaths from COVID-19 for the UK a new series that uses improved data for England produced by Public Health England (PHE). These figures provide a count of all deaths where a positive test for COVID-19 has been confirmed, wherever that death has taken place.

So let's look at what these latest changes to the registration of COVID-19 deaths are, and how they resulted in an additional 4,240 deaths being added to the official total.

Technical Definitions

The new data series produced by PHE is created by combining reports of deaths from three different sources in England. The three sources are:

---

24. See Office for National Statistics, 'Different uses of figures on deaths from COVID-19 published by DHSC and ONS' (31 March, 2020).

- deaths occurring in hospitals, notified to NHS England by NHS trusts using the COVID-19 Patient Notification System (CPNS) (previously the source of daily COVID-19 deaths in England);
- deaths notified to PHE Health Protection Teams during outbreak management (primarily in non-hospital settings) in people with a confirmed COVID-19 test and recorded in an electronic reporting system;
- all people with a laboratory confirmed COVID-19 test are reported to PHE through the Second Generation Surveillance System (a centralised repository of laboratory results from Public Health and NHS laboratories). This list is submitted on a daily basis to the Demographic Batch Service (DBS) to check NHS patient records for reports of individuals who died in the previous 24 hours. These reports include deaths in any setting.

Table 1: Definitions of COVID-19 deaths between different sources

	DHSC (published on GOV.UK) before 29 April	DHSC (published on GOV.UK) from 29 April	ONS COVID-19 deaths registered	ONS COVID-19 death occurrence (actual date of death)
Coverage	UK, but can be broken down for devolved administrations	UK, but can be broken down for devolved administrations	Registrations in England and Wales	Registrations in England and Wales
			Selected UK breakdowns are also published	Selected UK breakdowns are also published
Inclusion	Reported to only include deaths in hospitals, but figures from Scotland, Wales and Northern Ireland did include deaths in other settings	Includes any place of death, including care homes and community	Includes any place of death, including care homes and community	Includes any place of death, including care homes and community
	Only includes deaths where patient has for a laboratory confirmed COVID-19 test	Only includes deaths where patient has for a laboratory confirmed COVID-19 test	Contains deaths where COVID-19 has been mentioned on the death certificate	Contains deaths where COVID-19 has been mentioned on the death certificate

Source: Office for National Statistics

This requirement of a 'confirmed COVID-19 test' marks a significant revision to the criteria for recording care homes deaths attributed to COVID-19, so perhaps the Office for National Statistics is not as independent of political intervention as I (or they) hoped. But in a separate page titled 'Publication of statistics on deaths involving COVID-19 in care homes in England: transparency statement', published 'jointly' by the Office for National Statistics and the Care Quality Commission and also updated on 28 April, it has a very different definition of what constitutes a

COVID-19 death, one completely at odds with, and contradicting, the technical definitions in the DHSC statement:

> The information notified to CQC includes the date of death, place of death, and (from 10 April) whether the death was a result of confirmed or suspected coronavirus (COVID-19). The inclusion of a death in the published figures as being the result of COVID-19 is based on the statement of the care home provider, which may or may not correspond to a medical diagnosis or test result, or be reflected in the death certification.[25]

So, which is it? Does the sudden addition of thousands of deaths outside of hospitals require a positive test for SARS-CoV-2, or does it not? Both definitions have been published simultaneously, and both by the Office for National Statistics: one the 'official statement' by the Department of Health and Social Care, the other a 'joint statement of transparency' by the Office for National Statistics and the Care Quality Commission. Given the instructions from the World Health Organization to identify COVID-19 as the suspected, probable or assumed underlying cause of death whether this is 'medically correct or not', I'm guessing it's the latter. And this abandonment of medical diagnosis is not limited to deaths outside hospitals. The same day, 28 April, NHS England announced that it is now reporting patient deaths where there has been no positive test result for SARs-CoV-2, but where COVID-19 is documented as a 'direct or underlying cause of death' on either part 1 or part 2 of the death certificate.[26]

In a way it doesn't matter, because it now appears that the media boast that the UK will end up being the European country worst affected by the coronavirus will come true.[27] On 27 April, the day before these so-called 'changes in reporting' were made — which are in practice changes to the technical definition of what a COVID-19 death is — the Department of Health and Social Care's official death toll from COVID-19 was 338, the lowest since 29 March, and had been falling since its official peak of 980 on 10 April. Now these new official COVID-19 deaths

---

25. See Office for National Statistics, 'Publication of statistics on deaths involving COVID-19 in care homes in England: transparency statement' (28 April, 2020).

26. See NHS England, 'COVID-19 Deaths'.

27. See David Wood, 'Coronavirus: UK could be "worst affected country in Europe', *ITV News* (12 April, 2020).

outside of hospital — verified without the deceased even being tested for SARS-CoV-2, let alone COVID-19 being established as the actual cause of death — have been retrospectively added to the official count of daily deaths.

Daily number of COVID-19 associated UK deaths by date reported

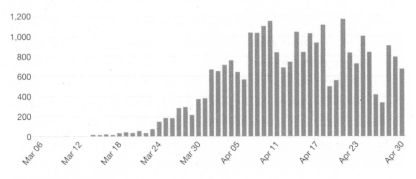

Source: Office for National Statistics

This means the new peak of 1,172 deaths has been brought forward to 21 April (*see above*) — 10 days ago now and 15 since the Government lockdown was extended by 3 weeks. It hardly seems likely that, when the lockdown is officially reviewed on 7 May, the Government that has deliberately increased the official figures for COVID-19 deaths won't extend the restrictions further, and possibly increase them. Flawed, inaccurate and undoubtedly exaggerated as they were as a measure of the threat and impact of this new coronavirus, the official figures recording COVID-19 deaths in the UK have now become completely meaningless. We have now passed from the realm of systemic distortion into the realm of make-believe. I want to end this article, therefore, by looking at what belief is and how it is made.

6. Irrational Belief and Political Responsibility

It's difficult to argue with irrational beliefs. I've always thought the attempts of the evolutionary biologist, Richard Dawkins, to convince Christians and other believers of the wrongness of their religious beliefs and the rightness of his scientific knowledge has always left him looking rather foolish. 5.7 billion people worldwide believe in a god not because they think the existence of a divine being or beings is a better explanation of the origins of the universe and the evolution of man than the theories of Einstein and Darwin — as Dawkins earnestly tries to argue — but because they were born or drawn into the ideologies of Christianity, Islam, Hinduism, Buddhism, Sikhism, Judaism and all the other religions with which our Governments control 84 per cent of the world's population.[28] Not only with these ideologies, of course, for capitalism is the most powerful ideology on this planet, and has been for some time. And science itself, as the Italian philosopher Giorgio Agamben has written in his recent commentary on our reaction to the coronavirus, has become the religion of our time.[29] There is little difference between the 46 per cent of US citizens who take prescription drugs on a regular basis and the 29 per cent who regularly attend church or synagogue, and neither group are made up of pharmacologists or theologists.[30] They pop pills and pray to their God because they believe it will make their lives better; or because they have been told to by the salesmen of religion and science; or because they need to believe in something bigger than themselves, whether capitalised Science or Religion; or because they were born into a family, community, culture or country that did the same; or perhaps, above all, because they're afraid of dying; and for a dozen other reasons why we think and act in irrational ways. So, although I might politely suggest to a friend that living day-to-day anaesthetised on prescription drugs might not be the best way to get through life, or that treating the world like the waiting-room for a future eternity blinds you to both the joys and duties of this life, I'm not going to argue the point with them rationally. Belief is not knowledge: it is historically determined, culturally contingent, emotively held, irrationally defended, and ideologically maintained by the vast reach and power over our lives of the myriad Christian churches, Islamic denominations, Hindu sects, Buddhist schools, Jewish movements, and the

---

28. See Harriet Sherwood, 'Religion: why faith is becoming more and more popular', *The Guardian* (27 August, 2018).

29. See Giorgio Agamben, 'Medicine as Religion', *Quodlibet* (2 May, 2020); collected in *Where Are We Now? The Epidemic as Politics*; second updated edition, translated by Valeria Dani (Eris, 2021), pp. 49-54.

30. See Shelly Hagan, 'Nearly One in Two Americans Takes Prescription Drugs: Survey', Bloomberg UK (8 May, 2019); and Statista, 'How often do you attend church or synagogue — at least once a week, almost every week, about once a month, seldom, or never?' (December 2021).

immense institutional, financial, judicial, military and government support they have.

What I will argue with, however, is what is done in the name of these beliefs, with the approval or agreement of these beliefs, on the justification or basis of these beliefs, with the consensus — by default or actively — attained by appealing to these beliefs. A believer is welcome to their history, culture, emotions and beliefs, no matter how irrational these are; but when those beliefs are used to govern societies, appoint leaders, legitimise social hierarchies, create inequality, sell commodities, start wars, accommodate dictators, justify genocide, enact racism, oppress women, shame difference, silence dissenters, abuse and kill those under their power, and all the other crimes of which religious institutions are guilty today — let alone in their blood-spattered past — then the irrationality of religion becomes not just a matter of personal belief but of political responsibility. 'Believers', as religions like to call their subordinates, are responsible for the words and deeds of the institutions to which they belong and to which they give financial backing, cultural legitimacy and political power.

Last month the *Economist* magazine published an article asking 'How deadly is the new coronavirus?'[31] The ground for posing this question was that, given the low level of testing for SARS-CoV-2 across the world — and particularly in the UK where, 4 months into an epidemic apparently warranting the lockdown of the state, about 1 in 50 of the population has been tested — the official case fatality rate of 3.6 per cent declared by the World Health Organization and repeated as a uniform percentage by Governments around the world is nothing more than speculation and will be shown to be far lower as testing for SARS-CoV-2 increases and the case fatality rate of COVID-19 inevitably drops. I couldn't read the whole article, since it was behind a firewall and I have no wish to subscribe to the *Economist*; yet this week, during a brief foray onto Twitter, I saw the article posted by someone who was clearly interested in the argument. The response, by members of the Twitterati — only a few of whom I'd imagine have a subscription and therefore could actually read the article — was several hundred comments, with nearly all of the ones I skimmed denouncing the article with varying degrees of fury, contempt, threats, sanctimony, sarcasm and all the other modes with which rational speech is drowned out and censored online. It reminded me of a

---

31. See 'How deadly is the new coronavirus?', *The Economist* (12 March, 2020).

TV documentary I saw years ago in which Richard Dawkins tried to convince Ted Haggard, the evangelical pastor of the New Life Church in Colorado Springs, USA, that creationism is irrational.[32] The pastor was, of course, a crook, but if the two of them were debating at the Oxford Union I would have to concede that the born-again evangelist and entrepreneur wiped the floor with the former Professor for Public Understanding of Science at Oxford University. Today I couldn't locate the Twitter post, which presumably has been removed by the tweeter under the weight of public approbation.

Which brings me to our collective response to the coronavirus 'crisis'. As a writer with an audience of maybe a thousand readers for a popular article, mostly writing about the housing 'crisis' but also about other social and political issues, I have to be very sure about my research and the conclusions I draw from it. Over the five years in which I've published over 200 articles, case studies, presentations and reports on the ASH website, not once has someone challenged me on either the accuracy of the data I've researched or the logic of my arguments. Instead, as happens to anyone who challenges the orthodoxies of mainstream media lies and social media hysteria, I've been subjected to plenty of abuse, smear campaigns and online threats, but no-one has ever challenged my conclusions with anything more than a vague suggestion that I am motivated by personal vendettas, political extremism or various psychological defects; and the same reaction has characterised the response to the six articles I have published about the coronavirus 'crisis', particularly from those who haven't read them but have recommended, for instance, reporting me to the police for 'endangering lives'.

Since these responses are based on nothing more than beliefs that have largely been placed there by the media, that allay the believer's fears, that feed their rising anxiety, that mirror the image they have of themselves, that accord with their cultural and religious backgrounds, that serve their class interests, that offer the comfort of a collectively held emotion, even when that emotion is panic, that allow them to indulge their fascination with death, that enable them to disguise that fascination with the most saccharine expressions of empathy with the deceased — that are, in other words, ideologically determined — these beliefs must be held with all the greater conviction. Anything that might shake that conviction through rational argument rather than irrational belief, through analysis

---

32. See Richard Dawkins, 'The Root of All Evil?', *Channel 4* (2006).

of empirical data rather than repetition of dogma, through logical deduction rather than emotional assumption, must not only be avoided but — as Christianity, Islam and Hinduism have done throughout their bloodstained histories — attacked, suppressed, destroyed, ridiculed, silenced, their authors denounced, censored, threatened and imprisoned. We are, as it were, entering into a new medievalism, in which, via the most advanced technologies of surveillance and control that have been welcomed into the space where we think our souls should be — or, more accurately, that penetrate and monitor our biological and political existences through our willing consumption of information technology — the media terrifies us into obedience to our rulers with threats to our society, threats to our wealth, threats to our future, threats to our safety, threats to our health, threats to our very lives. If science is the religion of our time, media platforms are our churches, their high priests the CEOs of the information technology companies with an oligopoly over the market of our souls: Apple, Microsoft, Alphabet, Amazon, Meta. It's at their altars that we pray, to their sermons that we listen, in their churches that we commune, by their precepts that we abide.

Individuals can be excused their inability to understand the complex and technical data I've analysed in this article, or their manipulation by the propaganda of our media, and perhaps even their refusal to question what is happening because of their fears and anxieties; but they cannot be excused their collective responsibility for the assumption of dictatorial powers by our Government, for the granting of greater powers of arrest and detention to our police and security forces, and for the further intrusion of technologies of surveillance and control into our collective and individual lives. Ignorance, stupidity, anxiety, fear, are not an excuse for what is being done with the compliance they have created. Watching what is happening in this country has made me realise that the universal excuse of the German people of the 1930s that they didn't know what was happening before it was too late doesn't describe how dictatorships arise from democratic societies. They can only do so with the consensus of the majority of the population. But that consent does not have to be active. It can be consent through default, consent through silence, consent through a refusal to question, consent through obedience to regulations. However, under a unified propaganda campaign implemented by the full spectrum of our media, increasing numbers of the UK population have already progressed to consent through the blind repetition of Government propaganda, consent through the policing of dissent, consent through the denunciation of disobedience, consent through collaboration with the State.

It is not yet too late to halt the creeping totalitarianism to which all of us, in different degrees, are giving our consent, whether passively or actively. But the time to do so is rapidly running out, and the most right-wing and authoritarian Government in modern British history, run by a bunch of crooks the like of which not even the Conservative Party has placed into power before, is not dragging its feet in building consent to ever more dictatorial limitations to our freedoms. Instead of sitting passively at home, justifying the latest restriction to our human rights and freedoms on the grounds that it may save lives, and waiting for permission to return to the 'New Normal' being prepared for us, we should be asking ourselves the following questions:

1. Do we have the courage to read, write, publish, speak, share and act on the truth about COVID-19?
2. Do we have the ability to recognise the truth beneath the media and government lies concealing it?
3. How do we turn the truth into a weapon?
4. Whose hands will wield the truth if not our own?
5. How do we spread this truth among as many people as possible, so that they too can arm themselves against our rapidly expanding consent to this indefinite State of Emergency as the political paradigm of our future Government?

Just as urgently, we must start acting on the answers we are prepared to give.

— 1 May, 2020

3. The State of Emergency as a Paradigm of Government: Coronavirus Legislation, Implementation and Enforcement

'It is evident that, beyond the emergency situation associated with a specific virus that will be replaced by another in the future, what is at stake is the design of a paradigm of governance whose effectiveness will far exceed that of all forms of governance known so far in the political history of the West. If, amidst the progressive decay of ideologies and political beliefs, security measures had already conditioned citizens to accept limitations on their freedom they were previously unwilling to accept, biosecurity has shown itself capable of presenting the absolute cessation of all political activity and all social relations as the highest form of civic participation.'

— Giorgio Agamben, *Biosecurity and Politics*, May 2020

1. The Registration of COVID-19 Deaths

In my recent article about the coronavirus 'crisis', 'Manufacturing Consensus', I followed in detail how the official death toll from COVID-19 in the UK is being exaggerated many times above the actual deaths that can be attributed to the disease with any medical certainty through the creation and implementation of the following definitions and guidelines:

- On 6 March, the Minister for Health and Social Care made The Health Protection (Notification) (Amendment) Regulations 2020 into law without a draft having been laid and approved by a resolution of each House of Parliament, and which added both COVID-19 and SARS-CoV-2 to the list of 'notifiable' diseases and causative agents that medical practitioners have a statutory duty to record on a death certificate, as they do not, for example, with pneumonia, the primary cause of death from respiratory diseases.[1]

---

1. See UK Statutory Instruments, 'The Health Protection (Notification) (Amendment) Regulations 2020' (6 March, 2020), Amendment 2.

- On 25 March, the World Health Organization created two new codes for COVID-19 deaths distinguishing whether the deceased had or had not tested positive for SARS-CoV-2, the virus that causes the coronavirus disease but whose case fatality rate it is impossible to establish until the entire population of the UK has been tested to establish the number of cases of infection.[2]

- On 31 March, the Office for National Statistics announced that, in order for a death to be included in its records of COVID-19 deaths, the disease merely has to be 'mentioned' anywhere on the death certificate, without it being 'the main cause of death'. This includes as a 'contributing' factor when 'combined with other health conditions', or when a doctor has diagnosed a 'possible' case of COVID-19 based on 'relevant symptoms' but with no test for SARS-CoV-2 having been conducted, or when the deceased tested positive for SARS-CoV-2 but a post mortem hasn't established the actual cause of death.[3]

- On 10 April, the Care Quality Commission introduced a 'new way' to understand whether COVID-19 was 'involved in the death' of someone in a care home. This merely requires a statement from the care home provider that COVID-19 was 'suspected', and which 'may or may not' correspond to a medical diagnosis, a positive test result for SARs-CoV-2, or even be reflected in the death certificate.[4]

- On 20 April, the World Health Organization issued guidelines to medical practitioners instructing them that, if COVID-19 is the 'suspected' or 'probable' or 'assumed' cause of death, it must always be recorded as the 'underlying cause' on death certificates, whether this 'can be considered medically correct or not.'[5]

- On 28 April, the National Health Service announced that it will include on its list of COVID-19 deaths all deaths where there has been no positive test for

---

2. See World Health Organization, 'International Guidelines for Certification and Classification (Coding) of COVID-19 as Cause of Death' (20 April, 2020).

3. See Office for National Statistics, 'Different uses of figures on deaths from COVID-19 published by DHSC and ONS' (31 March, 2020).

4. This webpage was subsequently withdrawn, but see Quality Care Commission, 'Care Quality Commission publishes data showing death notifications involving COVID-19 received from individual care homes' (21 July, 2021).

5. See World Health Organization, 'International Guidelines for Certification and Classification (Coding) of COVID-19 as Cause of Death' (20 April, 2020), p. 8.

SARs-CoV-2 but where COVID-19 has been entered on the death certificate as the 'underlying cause of death'.[6]

- On 28 April, the Office for National Statistics and the Care Quality Commission issued a joint transparency statement clarifying that their recording of a death as being the result of COVID-19 'may or may not correspond to a medical diagnosis or test result, or be reflected in the death certification.'[7]

- On 29 April, Public Health England announced that every death in the UK to occur in a care home or otherwise outside a hospital in which a positive test for SARs-CoV-2 has been made pre- or post-mortem will be added both retrospectively and in the future to the official number of COVID-19 deaths.[8]

If not evidence of a concerted effort by the World Health Organization, the UK Department of Health and Social Care, Public Health England, the National Health Service, the Care Quality Commission and the Office for National Statistics to conceal the true number of deaths that can be attributed with any medical accuracy or diagnostic certainty to COVID-19 and exaggerate that number many times over, this should at the very least raise questions about the deliberately inaccurate definitions, intentionally misleading guidelines and politically imposed changes to disease taxonomy through which the official figures on COVID-9 deaths the UK Government publishes every day have been calculated, and which are being unquestioningly disseminated by the media for consumption by a terrorised public.

One of the questions being asked of — or more accurately screamed at — those of us who argue that the causal agency of both SARS-CoV-2 and COVID-19 in the official death toll has been deliberately and grossly exaggerated is how the manufacture of a crisis that makes the Government of the UK look out of control and incompetent benefits that same Government? No less a thinker than the Slovenian philosopher, Zlavoj Žižek, raised exactly this question in response to the comment by the Italian philosopher, Giorgio Agamben, in one of a series of

---

6. See NHS England, 'COVID-19 Deaths'.

7. See Office for National Statistics, 'Publication of statistics on deaths involving COVID-19 in care homes in England: transparency statement' (28 April, 2020).

8. See Public Health England, 'Daily death reporting now includes all positive COVID-19 deaths' (29 April, 2020).

articles on the coronavirus 'crisis', that 'once terrorism was exhausted as a justification for exceptional measures, the invention of an epidemic could offer the ideal pretext for broadening such measures beyond any limitation'.[9] The question I address in this article, therefore, is to what ends this fabrication of COVID-19 deaths is being placed by the UK Government and its corporate clients. Under the cloak of the lockdown of the UK justified by this wildly inaccurate death toll, what s have been made into law, what Acts of Parliament have been passed without adequate scrutiny, what privatisation of public services have been implemented, what powers of surveillance and arrest have been extended to private security firms and police forces, what intrusions into our privacy and sharing of our personal data have been authorised without parliamentary approval? In other words, what has the most right-wing and authoritarian Government in modern British history been doing while Parliament has been suspended, the electorate under virtual house arrest, and the media has undergone the final stage in its transformation into the propaganda arm of the UK state? And, finally, what does this mean for our future?

2. The Health Protection (Coronavirus) Regulations 2020

On 10 February, the Secretary of State for Health and Social Care, exercising powers conferred by the Public Health (Control of Disease) Act 1984, but without an assessment of the impact of its regulations having been made, and without a draft being laid before or approved by resolution of either House of Parliament, employed a Statutory Instrument that made The Health Protection (Coronavirus) Regulations 2020 into law with immediate effect.[10] These Regulations:

1. By reason of urgency, came into force immediately after they were made.
2. Defines an 'infected area' as anywhere the Secretary of State has declared 'there is known, or thought, to be' sustained human-to-human transmission

---

9. See Zlavoj Žižek, 'Monitor and Punish? Yes, Please!', *The Philosophical Salon* (16 March, 2020); and Giorgio Agamben, 'The Invention of an Epidemic', *Il Manifesto* (26 February, 2020); collected in *Where Are We Now?*, pp. 11-13.

10. See UK Statutory Instruments, 'The Health Protection (Coronavirus) Regulations 2020' (10 February, 2020).

of the coronavirus; and that 'isolation' means at a person's home, in a hospital, or at a facility designated for the purpose by the Secretary of State.

3. Applies these Regulations until such time as the Health Secretary decides that the coronavirus no longer constitutes a 'serious and imminent threat to public health'.

4. Empowers the Secretary of State or a registered public health consultant to detain a person for the purposes of screening and assessing them on the grounds that 'they are, or may be', infected with coronavirus.

5. Empowers the Secretary of State or a registered public health consultant to impose restrictions and requirements necessary to assess whether a person 'presents, or could present,' a risk of infecting or contaminating others.

6. Compels a person to answer questions addressed to them by a registered public health consultant or officer about their health, travel history and other persons with whom they have been in contact; to produce any document requested relating to their health; to allow a biological sample to be taken by them, including of their blood and respiratory secretions; and to provide contact details for as long as the health consultant specifies.

7. Empowers the Secretary of State or a registered public health consultant to impose further unidentified and undefined restrictions and requirements at their discretion, in order to reduce or remove the risk of a person infecting or contaminating others.

8. Empowers the Secretary of State or a registered public health consultant to keep a person in isolation it there are reasonable grounds to believe that 'they are, or may be', infected or contaminated with coronavirus, and that it is necessary and proportionate to do so in order to reduce or remove the risk of them infecting or contaminating others.

9. Empowers the Secretary of State to compel a person so detained or kept in isolation, or subject to restrictions and requirements, to comply with screening requirements.

10. Empowers the Secretary of State or a registered public health consultant to impose said restrictions and requirements on groups of persons.

11. Extends the power of local authorities, under The Health Protection (Part 2A Orders) Regulations 2010, to obtain an order from a Justice of the Peace to

impose restrictions or requirements, to be made on application from a registered public health consultant or the Secretary of State.

12. Allows a person to appeal to a magistrates' court against the imposition of these Regulations.

13. Empowers police constables 'to use reasonable force' when taking a person into custody in order to enforce their detention or isolation.

14. Empowers police constables that have reasonable grounds to suspect that a person 'is, or may be' infected with coronavirus, or that there is a risk that a person might infect or contaminate others, or that it is necessary for the protection of other persons or for the maintenance of public safety, to direct a person to go to hospital or other place for screening, assessment or the imposition of other restrictions and requirements. For the purpose of which, a constable 'may enter any place', and 'use reasonable force' in the exercise of this Regulation. A person detained or isolated may be kept for up to 24 hours, at the end of which a police constable may authorise a further period of detention or isolation not exceeding 24 hours.

15. Makes it an 'offence' if a person fails to comply with a restriction or requirement, or absconds from detention or isolation, or obstructs anyone carrying out these Regulations, punishable on summary conviction by a fine not exceeding £1,000.

16. Issued notice that these Regulations will cease to have effect at the end of two years, which regulation does not affect the validity of 'anything' done in accordance with these Regulations.

On 16 March, five weeks after they came into force, Parliament approved the Health Protection (Coronavirus) Regulations 2020. It is not clear from these regulations on what grounds, and with what qualifications, a police constable — only 38 per cent of whom have a degree, and presumably not all in epidemiology or as a general medical practitioner — is qualified to suspect whether a person 'is, or may be' infected with SARS-CoV-2, or 'presents, or could present' a risk. Not only do at least 80 per cent and most likely far higher of those infected with the virus develop no symptoms, but the symptoms of COVID-19 identified by the Government (coughing and high temperature) are indistinguishable from the symptoms of influenza, the common cold, or any number of other illnesses not requiring the use of 'reasonable force' to detain and isolate the person coughing or sweating.[11] As legislation for new powers of arrest, these regulations were wide open to the widespread abuse with which they were duly enforced by the police across the UK.

3. The Guidance on Social Distancing

On the same day, 16 March, Public Health England, the executive agency of the Department of Health and Social Care, issued its 'Guidance on social distancing for everyone in the UK'.[12] These guidelines were that the population should:

1. Avoid contact with someone who is displaying symptoms of coronavirus (COVID-19), include high temperature and/or a new and continuous cough;
2. Avoid non-essential use of public transport when possible;
3. Work from home where possible;
4. Avoid large and small gatherings in public spaces;
5. Avoid gatherings with friends and family;
6. Use telephone or online services to contact a GP or other essential services.

This guidance compounded the lack of clarity in the Health Protection (Coronavirus) Regulations 2020 by issuing restrictions that went beyond what the police had the legal right to enforce, including the imposition of social distancing.

4. The COVID Support Force

On 19 March, the Ministry of Defence announced the formation of the COVID Support Force.[13] This comprised 20,000 British military personnel tasked with assisting with implementing the Government's response to the COVID-19 'crisis'. These forces were divided into Operation Broadshare, which was directed to defending British interests abroad, and Operation Rescript, which was directed to

---

11. See UK Health Security Agency, 'Stay at home: Guidance for households with possible or confirmed coronavirus (COVID-19) infection' (withdrawn on 24 February, 2022).

12. See Public Health England, 'Guidance on social distancing for everyone in the UK' (withdrawn on 1 May, 2020).

13. See Ministry of Defence, 'Ministry stands up COVID Support Force' (19 March, 2020).

maintain public order in the event of a breakdown of civil society in response to coronavirus-justified restrictions in the UK. On 2 April, a further 3,000 reservists joined the COVID Support Force.

These precautions indicate how unsure the Government was about the public's reaction to the lockdown of the UK it would announce within a few days, and its anticipation of widespread civil disobedience. In the event, it needn't have worried. The UK is almost unique in offering no opposition to, and no protest against, the removal of the rights and liberties of its people, the depression of its economy, the arbitrary policing of its public and private spaces. On the contrary, it has eagerly collaborated in implementing all the above, leaving the COVID Support Force free to build unused hospitals and transport equipment for private companies.

5. The Lockdown of the UK

On 23 March, in an address to the nation broadcast on the BBC, the Prime Minister announced the 'lockdown' of the UK. This restricted movement to 1) shopping for basic necessities, 2) one form of exercise per day, 3) receiving or delivering medical needs for yourself or a vulnerable person, and 4) travel to essential work when it is not possible to work from home. 'If you don't follow the rules,' the Prime Minister declared, 'the police will have power to enforce them, including through fines and dispersing gatherings.' To ensure compliance with the Government's instructions, all shops selling non-essential goods were immediately closed, as were libraries, playgrounds, outdoor gyms and places of worship; gatherings of more than two people in public were prohibited, as were all social events excluding funerals.

On 24 March, the National Chairman of the Police Federation of England and Wales, John Apter, who does not occupy an elected political office and has no authority over the creation or passing of UK legislation, warned the general public that: 'If you don't heed this Government's advice, then it is likely further steps may need to be taken; further laws and emergency legislation could be introduced to clamp down harder.'[14]

---

14. See John Apter, 'If you don't heed the government's advice steps could be taken to clamp down on selfishness', *The Telegraph* (24 March, 2020).

6. The Coronavirus Act 2020

On 25 March, the Coronavirus Act 2020 was made law.[15] Presented without debate or an impact assessment on 19 March, between the 2nd and 3rd reading and debate in the House of Commons and the 1st and only sitting of the scrutiny committee, both on 23 March, the 1st and 2nd reading in the House of Lords on 24 March, to the 1st and only sitting of the scrutiny committee, 3rd reading in the House of Lords and Royal Assent, all on 25 March, the 348 pages, 102 Provisions and 29 Schedules of the Coronavirus Bill had just 1 week of reading and 3 days of debate by Parliament before becoming law. Among this raft of legislation were the following numbered Provisions:

10. Modifies mental health and mental capacity legislation to allow the requirements for the detention and treatment of patients to be satisfied by the opinion of a single doctor. Extends the time for which a patient can be detained from 72 hours to 120 hours prior to sectioning. And reduces to 1 the number of doctors' opinions required to detain and move a person between court, prison and hospital. The Act claims that, by reducing the number of doctors required to enact these powers, 'undesireable delay' in sectioning those with coronavirus will be avoided.

19. Empowers a doctor who has not seen the deceased to certify the cause of death as COVID-19 without the death being referred to the coroner for certification before cremation of the deceased. Allows a person to register the death without attending the register office, and extends the list of people who can give the relevant information to the registrar to funeral directors, who require no medical training. The Act claims that, by allowing cremations to take place without a confirmatory medical certificate of death, it will free healthcare professionals to support the response to the coronavirus pandemic.

22. Empowers the Secretary of State to increase the number of Judicial Commissioners, and to vary the appointment process at the request of the Investigatory Powers Commissioner. This allows the Commissioner to directly appoint temporary Judicial Commissioners for a term of up to 6

---

15. See UK Public General Acts, 'The Coronavirus Act 2020' (25 March, 2020).

months, renewable to a maximum period of 12 months. The Act claims this provision is to over for a shortage of Judicial Commissioners as a result of the effects of COVID-19.

23. Empowers the Secretary of State by a Statutory Instrument to modify the time limits relevant to the issue, approval, duration, renewal and modification of warrants under the Investigatory Powers Act 2016. At the request of the Investigatory Powers Commissioner, the lifespan of a warrant can be extended from 5 days to up to 12 working days. The Act claims this is in order to mitigate the impact of the coronavirus pandemic, by protecting national security and prevent serious crime during 'a period of potential widespread upheaval.'

24. Empower the Secretary of State by regulations to extend the time limit for the statutory retention of biometric material such as fingerprints and DNA. The Act claims this is in anticipation of the impact of COVID-19 on the ability of Chief Officers to assess whether such material should be retained for the purposes of national security.

30. Since, under The Health Protection (Notification) (Amendment) Regulations 2020 made into law on 6 March, COVID-19 has been added to the list of notifiable diseases — according to which any inquest into a death for which the coroner suspects the cause was a notifiable disease must take place with a jury — this provision modifies the existing legislation to make COVID-19 not a notifiable disease. The Act claims this is to lessen coroner workload due to COVID-19 deaths. In other words, COVID-19 is considered sufficiently dangerous for the doctor to be obliged to notify Public Health England and identify its presence as the underlying cause of death on the death certificate if the doctor even suspects it as a possible or contributing cause or the deceased tested positive for SARS-CoV-2 at the time of death, but not dangerous enough for a jury to establish whether it is the actual cause of death.

37. Empowers the State to require or direct temporary closure of educational institutions and registered childcare premises; to specify directions in connection with their running; and to remove or vary existing requirements contained in education and childcare legislation.

51. Fills any gaps in existing powers to ensure the detention, screening and isolation of people who may be infected or contaminated with SARS-CoV-2. The linked Schedule 21 clarifies that a person is 'potentially infectious' if, at any time, they are, or may be, infected or contaminated with coronavirus, and there is a risk that they might infect or contaminate others with coronavirus, or the person has been in an infected area within the 14 days preceding that time. 'Infected area' means any country, territory or other area outside the UK where there is known, or thought to be, sustained human-to-human transmission of coronavirus, or from which there is a high risk that coronavirus will be transmitted to the United Kingdom. Under these powers, the Secretary of State or anyone designated by him for the purpose can:

- Use whatever force is necessary, including police constables, immigration officers or security personnel, to cover our face with a mask and remove us to a place of detention for 48 hours;
- Take a biological sample (blood, nasal swab or respiratory secretion) from us without our permission, against our will and without a lawyer being present;
- Compel us to answer questions about our movements and personal contacts, gain access to our health records, contacts details and whatever else they deem necessary for their assessment;
- Impose upon us, following their assessment, whatever restrictions and requirement upon our movements, actions and contacts they decide is necessary for an additional 14 days;
- And do so under the threat of our further detention, without time limit, together with the charge of a criminal offence and being taken into custody if we refuse or attempt to leave.

52. Empowers the Secretary of State to prohibit attendance at or impose restrictions on events and gatherings, prohibit or restrict entry into premises, to close premises, and to prohibit departure from premises, if he deems it necessary for the purpose of preventing, protecting against, delaying or otherwise controlling the incidence or transmission of coronavirus. Schedule 22 clarifies that 'premises' means any place, including any vehicle, train,

vessel, aircraft, tent or moveable structure; but does not define an 'event or gathering'. Any person designated to do so by the Secretary of State may take such action as is necessary to enforce compliance with any prohibition, direction or restriction in this provision, and any person who fails to comply with a prohibition, requirement or restriction imposed on the person commits an offence liable on summary conviction to a fine.

59. 60. 61. Empowers the Secretary of State, by regulations made by Statutory Instrument, to postpone elections and referendums due to be held in England in the period after 15 March, 2020; to postpone elections scheduled for 7 May, 2020; to postpone other elections and referendums (such as by-elections and local referendums) until 6 May 2021; with the Minister for the Cabinet Office to postpone a recall petition under the Recall of MPs Act 2015 until 21 April 2021; and to make supplementary provision to these regulations.

78. Empowers local authorities to relax requirements to hold local authority, committee or joint committee meeting, to change the times or places or frequency with which such meetings are held, the manner in which persons may attend, speak at, vote in or otherwise participate in them, the extent of public admission and access to them, and the places and manner in which documents relating to meetings are to be open to inspection or otherwise available to the public. The Act claims this is to lessen the anticipated increase in workload for local authorities as a result of the coronavirus 'crisis'.

89. Issued notice that the Act expires at the end of the period of 2 years beginning with the day on which it is passed, so on 25 March 2022. However, a Minister of the Crown may by regulations make transitional, transitory or saving provision in connection with the expiry of any provision of this Act.

90. Empowers a relevant national authority by regulations to alter the expiry date of any provision of this Act.

98. Requires a 6-month parliamentary review of the motion 'that the temporary provision of the Coronavirus Act 2020 should not yet expire'. Such a review must be held within a period 7 sitting days after 6 months from the day on which the Act is passed, and each subsequent period of 6 months. However, MPs will only be able to vote on the continuation of the powers conferred by

the Act if Parliament is sitting. If they are not able to vote, the powers will remain in force.

The explanatory notes explain that the Coronavirus Act is 'to enable the Government to respond to an emergency situation and manage the effects of the COVID-19 pandemic'; that these powers are 'extraordinary measures' that do not apply in normal circumstances; and that they are therefore time-limited to two years. The lifetime of the Act can be ended early if the 'best scientific evidence' supports a policy decision that these powers are no longer needed. However, with evidence supporting the opposite decision, the lifetime of the Act can also be extended 'for a further temporary period'.

According to a convention agreed to by the parliamentary Opposition, the Coronavirus Act 2020 was 'nodded through' by MPs, rather than approved by democratic vote. That same day, 25 March, the House of Commons and the House of Lords rose early for the Easter recess, with the agreement that they would return on 21 April, 15 days longer than the previous year.[16]

7. The Health Protection (Coronavirus, Restrictions) (England) Regulations 2020

On 26 March, the day after Parliament recessed, the Secretary of State for Health and Social Care, again exercising powers conferred by the Public Health (Control of Disease) Act 1984, made The Health Protection (Coronavirus, Restrictions) (England) Regulations 2020 into law.[17] Like their predecessors, these too were made without a draft having been laid before or approved by a resolution of each House of Parliament, and without an impact assessment having been made. These Regulations:

2. Replaced The Health Protection (Coronavirus) Regulations 2020, which continue in force, nonetheless, in relation to any offence committed under the first Regulations before these Regulations came into force.

---

16. See UK Parliament, 'Update from UK Parliament on coronavirus' (15 April, 2020).

17. See UK Statutory Instruments, 'The Health Protection (Coronavirus, Restrictions) (England) Regulations 2020 (the Regulations) 2020' (26 March, 2020).

3.   Initiated an 'emergency period' that will only end at a time specified by the Secretary of State, and will be reviewed every 21 days.

4.   Empowers the State to close premises and businesses in which food or drink are sold for consumption on the premises during the emergency period.

5.   Empowers the State to close premises offering goods for sale or hire, library services, holiday accommodation, a place of worship, community centre or burial ground.

6.   Empowers the State to restrict movement 'without reasonable excuse' during the emergency period.

7.   Empowers the State to prohibit public gatherings of more than two people not from the same household except where 'reasonably necessary' during the emergency period.

8.   Empowers a police constable, police community support officer or any person designated by a local authority or the Secretary of State to take such action as is necessary, and using 'reasonable force', to enforce a closure or restriction imposed by these Regulations; to direct a prohibited gathering to disperse; to direct or remove persons so gathering to the place they live; to take other such actions as is necessary to enforce the prohibitions; and to direct or remove any person outside of the place where they live without a reasonable excuse to the place where they live.

9.   Empowers the State to charge any person who fails to comply with or contravenes these Regulations with committing an offence punishable by a fine.

10. Empowers a police constable, community support office, or person designated by a local authority or the Secretary of State to impose by summary conviction a fixed-penalty notice of £60, doubling at each repeated offence up to £960 on any person who fails to comply with or contravenes these Regulations.

11. Empowers the State to bring proceedings by the Crown Prosecution Service against anyone who fails to comply with or contravenes these Regulations.

12. Issued notice that these Regulations will expire 6 months from the day on which they came into force, which regulation does not affect the validity of 'anything' done in accordance with these Regulations before they expire.

These Regulations made it clear that, without it being formally declared by the UK Government, the UK was now in a *de facto* State of Emergency, and its citizens under emergency powers. In this respect, the UK mirrors similar informally imposed powers in Austria, Belarus, Croatia, Denmark, France, Germany, Greece, Iceland, Ireland, Kosovo, Malta, Montenegro, Netherlands, Norway, Poland, Portugal, Slovenia and Sweden. In addition, either under Article 15 of the European Convention on Human Rights or in accordance with their country's constitutional provisions, a formal State of Emergency has been declared by the European governments of Albania, Belgium, Bosnia and Hercegovina, Bulgaria, Cyprus, the Czech Republic, Estonia, Finland, Hungary, Italy, Latvia, Lithuania, Luxembourg, North Macedonia, Romania, Serbia, Slovakia, Spain and Ukraine.[18] Not even the Third Reich, at the height of its dominance, held such dictatorial control over so many of the people of Europe. Article 15 of the European Convention on Human Rights states:

In time of war or other public emergency threatening the life of the nation, any High Contracting Party may take measures derogating from its obligations under [the] Convention to the extent strictly required by the exigencies of the situation, provided that such measures are not inconsistent with its other obligations under international law.[19]

Since the UK has been waging a 'War on Terror' for twenty years now, it may be some time before the Government identifies the exact location and bearer of this metonymic 'life of the nation' that is supposedly threatened by the coronavirus. But it is precisely this life, which is both individual and collective, that is the subject and object of a biopolitics in which, as Giorgio Agamben has argued, the distinction between politics and policing, the care of health and the fight against

---

18. See Alan Greene, 'State of emergency: how different countries are invoking extra powers to stop the coronavirus', *The Conversation* (30 March, 2020); and Karolina Zbytniewska, 'Coronavirus: Which European countries introduced the state of emergency?', *Euractiv* (6 May, 2020).

19. See European Court of Human Rights, 'Guide on Article 15 of the European Convention on Human Rights: Derogation in time of emergency' (updated on 31 August 2022).

the (invisible) enemy, disappears, as it has today in the UK.[20] However, having not evoked Article 15, and having withdrawn from the European Union on 31 January, 2020, the UK Government is not accountable to the 'other obligations under international law' that successive UK Governments have ignored for some time now, most notably in their treatment of Julian Assange, whose extra-legal imprisonment and torture has foreshadowed the use of these emergency powers.[21] Instead, these have been made by the present Government under the Public Health (Control of Disease) Act 1984, the amendments made in the Health and Social Care Act 2008, and potentially will be, in the future, under the Civil Contingencies Act 2004.

8. The Police State

On 30 March, in an interview on Radio 4, former Supreme Court Justice Jonathan Sumption, QC, said:

> The tradition of policing in this country is that policemen are citizens in uniform. They are not members of a disciplined hierarchy operating just at the government's command. Yet in some parts of the country, the police have been trying to stop people from doing things which are not contrary to the regulations, simply because ministers have said that they would prefer us not to. The police have no power to enforce ministers' preferences, but only legal regulations, which don't go anything like as far as the Government's Guidance. This is what a police

---

20. 'National Socialist biopolitics — and along with it, a good part of modern politics even outside the Third Reich — cannot be grasped if it is not understood as necessarily implying the disappearance of the difference between the two terms: the *police* now becomes *politics*, and the care of life coincides with the fight against the enemy. . . . Only a state essentially founded on the very life of the nation could identify its own principal vocation as the formation and care of the "body of the people".' Giorgio Agamben, *Homo Sacer: Sovereign Power and Bare Life*; translated by Daniel Heller-Roazen (Stanford University Press, 1998), pp. 147-148.

21. See Simon Elmer, 'The Persecution, Incarceration, Torture and Extra-territorial Extradition of Julian Assange: Template for a letter to your Member of Parliament', *Architects for Social Housing* (18 June, 2019); and Institute for Government, 'Government emergency powers and coronavirus' (updated 22 March, 2021).

state is like. It's a state in which the Government can issue orders or express preferences with no legal authority and the police will enforce ministers' wishes.[22]

On 30 March, the Cabinet Office announced measures to crackdown on the 'spread of false coronavirus information online'.[23] To this end, the Government's Rapid Response Unit is now working with social media companies to remove 'false and misleading narratives' that contradict their own. To help the public identify whether it should share or even read an article online, the Government has published a five-step Share Checklist.[24] Conflating such articles with the threat from the virus itself, the Government said this checklist will ensure the public has 'the right information to protect themselves and save lives'. By the same reasoning, anyone who contradicts the Government online can potentially be accused of endangering lives.

On 31 March, the National Police Chiefs' Council published 'COVID-19 — Policing brief in response to Coronavirus Government Legislation'. Together with the briefing from the College of Policing published five days earlier, this laid out the four-step escalation principles:

1. Engage: we police by consent. Officers will initially encourage voluntary compliance;
2. Explain: officers will stress the risks to public health and to the NHS, and educate people about the risks and the wider social factors;
3. Encourage: officers will encourage compliance and emphasise the benefits to the NHS by staying at home, how this can save lives and reduce risk for more vulnerable people in society; and
4. Enforce: if faced with non-compliance, officers will, if necessary and proportionate:
    a. direct those without a reasonable excuse to go home, using reasonable force if needed;

---

22. See Jonathan Sumption, 'Former Supreme Court Justice: "This is what a police state is like"', *The Spectator* (30 March, 2020).

23. See Department for Digital, Culture, Media and Sport, 'Government cracks down on spread of false coronavirus information online' (30 March, 2020).

24. See HM Government, 'Take care with what you share using the SHARE checklist'.

b. issue a penalty notice for disorder (PND) of £60, to discourage further non-compliance;

c. use prohibition notices to stop public gatherings; and

d. use existing licensing powers where businesses and organisations fail to comply.[25]

Despite these guidelines, police officers are patrolling armed with assault rifles, hand guns, taser guns and CS-gas sprays, and have been reported and recorded forcing entry into people's homes, using drones to order people to stop walking alone in the countryside, banning people from entering parks, chasing people off beaches, threatening people with pepper spray, assaulting people for non-compliance with directions, arresting people for refusing to give them their personal details, arresting people under the wrong powers, charging them with the wrong offences, prosecuting them for offences that don't exist, unlawfully issuing them with Fixed Penalty Notices, and numerous other abuses of their new powers.[26]

On 1 April, Devon and Cornwall Police released a statement saying that, regardless of the guidance from both the National Police Chiefs' Council and the College of Policing, it would not be changing its position on people travelling by car to a place for exercise.[27] 'Our interpretation is that it is not reasonable, for the majority, to drive miles to a specific place such as a beauty spot. It is also not within the spirit of what we are trying to achieve if you drive from Devon to the coast of Cornwall for surfing, regardless of whether that is "lawful" or not.' This last phrase was later removed from its website, but the Devon and Cornwall Police continue to enforce their own interpretation of the law.

The Metropolitan Police, the Thames Valley Police, the Greater Manchester Police, the West Yorkshire Police, the Lancashire Constabulary, the Avon and Somerset Police, the Staffordshire Police, the Kent Police, the Dyfed-Powys

---

25. Now withdrawn. See College of Policing, 'COVID-19 restrictions', 2022.

26. See NetPol undercover research group, 'Policing the corona state: a diary of security and surveillance during Britain's state of emergency'; and Pippa Woodrow and Kirsty Brimelow, QC, 'Guide to Coronavirus Offences: Help for the public, police and lawyers', Doughty Street Chambers (7 May, 2020).

27. See Chris Matthews, 'Devon and Cornwall police clarify travel to exercise guidance', *Cornwall Live* (2 April, 2020).

Police, the North Wales Police, have all set up webpages inviting members of the public to 'Tell us about a possible breach of coronavirus (COVID-19) measures'.[28] In response, by 30 April the National Police Chiefs' Council announced that it had received reports from public informants of more than 194,300 coronavirus-related incidents in England and Wales (at a rate of over 5,700 reports per day), and issued 9,176 fixed-penalty notices, in the little more than a month since The Health Protection (Coronavirus, Restrictions) Regulations had come into force on 26 March.[29]

9. The 5-Pillar Testing Strategy

On 2 April, the Secretary of State for Health and Social Care announced his 5-Pillar Testing Strategy: 1) Tests for SARs-CoV-2 in Public Health England laboratories and NHS hospitals; 2) Creation of 'brand new' testing capacity delivered by 'commercial partners' such as Amazon and Boots; 3) Antibody blood tests to establish immunity, to develop which the Government is working with 9 private companies; 4) Population surveillance programmes; and 5) Building a British diagnostics industry in collaboration with 'pharmaceutical giants'.[30] These include AstraZeneca, the British-Swedish multinational pharmaceutical and biopharmaceutical company that in 2010 agreed to pay £505 million to settle a UK tax dispute related to transfer mispricing; and GlaxoSmithKline, one of the largest, most predatory, most prosecuted and most fined of the so-called 'Big-Pharma' corporations, which specialises in respiratory products and vaccines, and is the company at which Patrick Vallance was President of Research and

---

28. See Thames Valley Police, 'Tell us about a possible breach of coronavirus (Covid-19) measures'; Greater Manchester Police, 'Tell us about a possible breach of coronavirus (Covid-19) measures'; West Yorkshire Police, 'Report a breach of coronavirus (COVID-19) Restrictions'; Lancashire Constabulary, 'Report a COVID-19 incident'; Staffordshire Police, 'Tell us about a possible breach of coronavirus (Covid-19) measures'. The equivalent webpages for the other police forces have since been removed.

29. See Lizzie Dearden, 'Coronavirus: Police issue almost 9,000 fines for lockdown breaches in England', *The Independent* (30 April, 2020).

30. See Matt Hancock, 'Health and Social Care Secretary's statement on coronavirus (COVID-19): 2 April 2020' (published 30 April, 2020); and Department of Health and Social Care, 'Coronavirus (COVID-19): Scaling up our testing programmes' (4 April, 2020).

Development for 6 years until, in March 2018, he was appointed Chief Scientific Advisor to the Government.[31]

On 3 April, the Secretary of State for Health and Social Care clarified of the social distancing prohibitions: 'This advice is not a request. It is an instruction. Stay at home.'[32]

On 5 April, the Secretary of State for Health and Social Care warned: 'I say this to the small minority of people who are breaking the rules or pushing the boundaries. You are risking your own life, and the lives of others.' He went on to announce the latest technology, a coronavirus status checker, saying that 'the smart use of data like this and digital technologies is one the strongest bulwarks we have against coronavirus'.[33]

On 10 April, the Secretary of State for Health and Social Care announced that AstraZeneca and GlaxoSmithKline, 'two of the biggest pharmaceutical companies in the world', had opened a 'mega-lab' in Cambridge. He thanked Burberry, Rolls-Royce, McLaren, Ineos and Diageo for their production of personal protective equipment, and invited other companies to help meet the department's PPE plan.[34]

On 12 April, the Secretary of State for Health and Social Care announced a new NHS 'app' for contact tracing that, in the event of the users showing 'the symptoms of coronavirus', will send an alert to other app users with whom the user has been in contact. He assured us that 'All data will be handled according to the highest ethical and security standards and would only be used for NHS care and research and we won't hold it any longer than it's needed.' Without identifying who they are, the Secretary further assured us that: 'We're working closely with the world's leading tech companies and renowned experts in clinical safety and digital ethics so that we can get this right.'[35]

---

31. See Kristin Compton, 'Big Pharma and Medical Device Manufacturers', *Drug Watch* (last modified 8 September, 2022).

32. See Matt Hancock, 'Health and Social Care Secretary's statement on coronavirus (COVID-19): 3 April 2020' (published 30 April, 2020).

33. See Matt Hancock, 'Health and Social Care Secretary's statement on coronavirus (COVID-19): 5 April 2020' (published 30 April, 2020).

34. See Matt Hancock, 'Health and Social Care Secretary's statement on coronavirus (COVID-19): 10 April 2020' (published 30 April, 2020).

35. See Matt Hancock, 'Health and Social Care Secretary's statement on coronavirus (COVID-19): 12 April 2020' (published 30 April, 2020).

10. The Five Conditions for Lifting the Lockdown of the UK

On 16 April, the Secretary of State for Foreign and Commonwealth Affairs announced that the Government-imposed lockdown of the UK would only be lifted when five conditions are met.[36] 1) The NHS is able to provide sufficient critical care and specialist treatment; 2) There is a sustained and consistent fall in the daily death rates from coronavirus; 3) The Scientific Advisory Group for Emergencies (SAGE) shows that the rate of infection is decreasing to manageable levels across the board; 4) The supply of testing capacity and personal protection equipment is able to meet future demand; and 5) Removing the lockdown does not risk a second peak of infections that overwhelms the NHS.

These conditions for lifting the lockdown of the UK have been imposed despite the fact that:

1. Far from being overwhelmed, only 41 per cent of NHS acute care beds were in use as of the weekend before the First Secretary made this statement, nearly four times the normal amount of free acute beds at this time of year.[37] And of the 4,000 beds in the Nightingale hospital built in 9 days in East London, only 60 were in use by 29 April, while the Nightingale hospital in the East Midlands had yet to admit any patients. Of the 7 Nightingale hospitals that will provide over 12,000 beds, 6 have so far opened.[38]

2. There are no records of how many people have died as a result of coronavirus disease in the UK, only of how many have had COVID-19 attributed to their deaths as a suspected, possible, contributing, or underlying cause, with or without a positive test for SARS-CoV-2 or COVID-19 being mentioned on the death certificate. And the First Secretary didn't clarify what fall in the number of deaths he considered to be 'consistent and sustained'.

3. The rate of infection (R0), which estimates the average number of people who will contract a disease from one person with that disease, is highly speculative and currently determined by the level of testing, which to date is

---

36. See Dominic Raab, 'Foreign Secretary's statement on coronavirus (COVID-19): 16 April 2020' (published on 16 April, 2020).

37. See Dave West, 'NHS hospitals have four times more empty beds than normal', *HSJ* (13 April, 2020).

38. See Verity Bowman, 'Why do so any NHS Nightingale hospitals remain empty?', *The Telegraph* (29 April, 2020).

1 in 46 of the UK population.[39] And once again, the First Secretary did not specify what rate of infection is 'manageable'.

4.   Future demands on testing capacity and personal protective equipment are also unknown, and just as the former capacity has no bearing on the safety of the population from COVID-19, so demands on the latter provide no justification for the lockdown of the roughly 80 per cent of the population for which the coronavirus virus presents little or no threat. The NHS has reported that, as of 5 May, only 238 people in England under the age of 60 and without pre-existing medical conditions have died even testing positive for SARS-CoV-2, let alone dying as a result of COVID-19.

5.   There is no evidence that the lockdown has done anything to lessen the rate of infection with SARS-CoV-2, particularly when countries that have not imposed lockdowns, such as Iceland (1,800 cases), Sweden (27,200), South Korea (10,900) and Japan (15,850), have a far lower number of cases of infection than the UK (226,500); while there is, to the contrary, considerable evidence to show the lockdown has increased the rate of excess deaths not attributed to COVID-19, with 13,237 recorded in England and Wales between 20 March, when deaths first began to exceed the average over the last five years, and 1 March, the most recent date for which we have figures from the Office for National Statistics. These unexplained deaths comprise 28 per cent of all excess deaths since the lockdown.[40]

Despite these serious flaws in their criteria, these five conditions have been repeated since by every Government Minister in their press briefings, including by the Business Secretary, the Education Secretary, the Transport Secretary, the Environment Secretary, the Health and Social Care Secretary, the Home Secretary, the Chancellor of the Exchequer and the Prime Minister.

On 19 April, in an interview with CNN, the CEO of YouTube, Susan Wojcicki, announced that, following new policy changes, any video that 'goes against' the

39. See Dr. Waqar Rashid, 'Is the R number a flawed measure?', *The Spectator* (14 May, 2020).

40. See Paul Nuki, 'Two new waves of deaths are about to break over the NHS, new analysis warns', *The Telegraph* (25 April, 2020); and Office for National Statistics, 'Deaths registered weekly in England and Wales, provisional'.

World Health Organization recommendations on the COVID-19 'crisis' will be deleted, so that users get 'the right information'.[41]

Following these policy changes, a video interview with Professor Knut Wittkowski, an internationally renowned epidemiologist who for 20 years was head of the Department of Biostatistics, Epidemiology and Research Design at the Rockefeller University in New York City, and who has been modelling epidemics for 35 years, was removed 'for violating YouTube's terms and conditions'.[42] This is just one example of many of the censorship of critical or dissenting voices.

11. The Virtual Parliament

On 21 April, the returned House of Commons, without a vote being held, approved a motion facilitating 'hybrid proceedings' that, under the 'social distancing' prohibitions imposed by the Prime Minister, allow a maximum of 50 MPs to be present in the Chamber at any one time, with 120 MPs able to participate remotely online.[43] MPs wishing to participate in the hybrid proceedings, which have been reduced from 8 hours to approximately 2 hours, must notify the House Service in advance, and all questions are published in advance. There are 650 seats in the House of Commons with 639 votes.

These arrangements have been dubbed the 'virtual Parliament', and mean that, although the Government can be asked a limited number of questions about its actions by the parliamentary opposition, no vote can be held on any legislation it makes, effectively handing the legislative functions of Parliament to the executive, and with it the conditions for a parliamentary democracy. But in fact, the existing legislation required to implement and maintain the lockdown of the UK, including a virtual Parliament, was made law on the 25 and 26 of March.

---

41. See 'Inside YouTube's "numerous policy changes" during the pandemic', *CNN Business* (19 April, 2020).

42. See John Kirby, Libby Handros and Lee Davis, 'Perspectives on the Pandemic II: A Conversation with Dr. Knut Wittowski', *Ratical* (1-2 April, 2020).

43. The webpages to these decisions have since been removed from the UK Parliament website.

12. The Track and Trace Mission

On the same day, 21 April, the Secretary of State for Health and Social Care made an Amendment to The Health protection (Coronavirus, Restrictions) (England) Regulations 2020, without a draft having been laid before, or a resolution approved, by Parliament, extended the lockdown prohibitions to leaving or staying outside a place where a person is living 'without reasonable excuse'.[44]

On the same day, the Secretary of State for Health and Social Care announced that 'In the long run, the best way to defeat coronavirus is through a vaccine.'

On the same day, The Investigatory Powers (Communications Data) (Relevant Public Authorities and Designated Senior Officers) Regulations 2020, without an impact assessment having been made, extended the power to obtain communications data under the Investigatory Powers Act 2016, or so-called 'snooper's charter', to five additional public bodies.[45]

On 23 April, the Secretary of State for Health and Social Care took the opportunity to 'applaud' the private companies involved in producing testing for SARs-CoV-2.[46] These include Amazon, the US multinational conglomerate technology company that in July 2019 was awarded a contract by the UK Government that gives it free access to information about healthcare published by the NHS; Boots, the UK pharmacy retailer that in February 2018 was criticised for charging excessive prices for low-value products supplied to the NHS; ThermoFisher, the US provisioner of scientific instrumentation, reagents, consumables, software and services to healthcare, life science and other laboratories that supplied DNA sequencing equipment to police in China's Xinjiang region in support of a mandatory biometric collection and surveillance program; Randox, a UK company in the *in vitro* diagnostics industry that in February 2017 faced charges against two employees arrested on suspicion of

---

44. See UK Statutory Instruments, 'The Health Protection (Coronavirus, Restrictions) (England) (Amendment) Regulations 2020' (21 April, 2020).

45. See UK Statutory Instruments, 'The Investigatory Powers (Communications Data) (Relevant Public Authorities and Designated Senior Officers) Regulations 2020' (21 April, 2020).

46. See Matt Hancock, 'Health and Social Care Secretary's statement on coronavirus (COVID-19): 23 April 2020' (published 30 April, 2020).

perverting the course of justice amid allegations of data tampering within its testing services used by police in England and Wales; Roche, the Swiss multinational healthcare company that in 1999 pleaded guilty to participating with its competitors to raise and fix prices for vitamins sold globally; Oxford Nanopore, the UK company developing and selling nanopore sequencing products (including the portable DNA sequencer MinION); and, once again, AstraZeneca and GlaxoSmithKline. He then appealed for people to 'take part' in virus infection and antibody trials, and announced that the government is putting in place the infrastructure necessary to 'roll out contact tracing on a large scale'. Restating the necessity of our obedience to the Health Protection Regulations, he ended by saying: 'We have travelled together too far to go backwards now.'

On 28 April, Matthew Gould, the Chief Executive of NHSX, the unit that sets national policy and best practice for the NHS on digital technology, including data sharing and transparency, told the Parliamentary Science and Technology Committee that the NHSX is exploring the creation of Immunity Passports as part of the UK's exit strategy from the lockdown. These will signal whether a person has immunity to SARS-CoV-2, and will require an artificial intelligence facial recognition check that matches a Government-approved ID to confirm a person's health status via a Quick Response (QR) code when entering any public space using the bio-security system. The CEO told the Committee that he had been approached by any number of private companies to provide the technology, including from biometric and digital identification company Onfido. In its proposal to NHSX, Onfido wrote: 'Our aim is to collaboratively build a solution that helps establish a "new normal" in which individuals can start to move more freely and safely.' In its final considerations on whether the programme should be voluntary or mandatory, Onfido concluded: 'If a programme is mandatory, privacy by design and default becomes ever more critical as participation should be possible without further intrusion on a person's civil liberties and freedoms'.[47]

On 29 April, a letter addressed to the Government and signed by 170 UK Professors, Doctors, researchers and scientists working in information security and privacy voiced their concerns that the NHS app does not become 'a tool that

---

47. See Onfido, 'The role of Digital Identity in Immunity Passports', UK Parliament Committees (April 2020).

enables data collection on the population, or on targeted sections of society, for surveillance.'[48]

On 1 May, the Secretary of State for Health and Social Care announced that by mid-May the Government will have 18,000 contact tracers in place.[49] 'The combination of contact tracers and new technology, through our new COVID-19 NHS app, will help tell us where the virus is spreading and help everyone to control new infections'. A member of the public that has diagnosed themselves as having the symptoms of coronavirus will declare their status in the app on their smartphone. The software will then send a yellow alert, supposedly anonymously, to other users of the app that have been in contact with them. This will be established through GPS location data and Bluetooth signals in their smartphones — the latter of which can pass through walls and therefore doesn't establish possibility of infection or contagion — supplemented by QR codes posted to public amenities. The person will be sent a home test, and if the result confirms their infection with SARS-CoV-2 a red alert will be sent, informing the other users to go into quarantine. The Secretary of State added: 'Tracking and tracing will allow us . . . to lift lockdown measures.' This occasioned a brief meditation on how the Government's new mission to 'track and trace' will impose a new relation between freedom and safety:

> In recent weeks, we have had to impinge on historic liberties to protect our NHS and our loved ones, and yet our goal must be freedom. Freedom from the virus, yes — and we will not lift measures until it is safe to do so. But also we care about the restoration of social freedom and economic freedom too. Each citizen's right to do as they please. For now, we are working together to stay home. We are impinging on the freedom of all, for the safety of all. With this next mission, of track and trace, I am seeking a solution that allows us — by each of us participating — to target the measures that are needed with much more precision, and so to reassert as much as is safely possible the liberty of us all. That is our next mission.

---

48. See Professor Martin Albrecht, *et al.*, 'Joint Statement' (29 April, 2020).

49. See Matt Hancock, 'Health and Social Care Secretary's statement on coronavirus (COVID-19): 1 May 2020' (published 1 May, 2020).

On the same day, 1 May, the Cabinet Office issued guidance on 'Staying at home and away from others (social distancing)'.[50] Superseding that issued on 16 March, this summarised some of the effects of the legislation made over the intervening 6 weeks, and was divided into 1) Staying at home, 2) Closing certain businesses and venues, 3) Stopping public gatherings, 4) Going to work, 5) Enforcing the law, and 6) Clinically vulnerable people.

13. The Exploitation of the Coronavirus Crisis

On 5 May, the Secretary of State for Foreign and Commonwealth Affairs brought our attention to the news that 'there will always be some who seek to exploit a crisis for their own criminal and hostile ends'. This apparently takes the form of 'cyber-attacks' from criminal gangs, hackers, hostile states, and what in the cyber security world are known as 'advanced persistent attack groups' targeting national and international organisations responding to the COVID-19 pandemic. 'There are various objectives and motivations that lie behind these attacks', the First Secretary explained, 'from fraud on the one hand to espionage. But they tend to be designed to steal bulk personal data, intellectual property and wider information that supports those aims.'[51]

That same day, the *Guardian* newspaper reported that the Government is using the coronavirus pandemic to accelerate the transfer of key public health duties from the NHS and other state bodies into the private sector.[52] Ministers have used special powers to bypass normal tendering processes and award a string of contracts to private companies and management consultants. These include Amazon; Archus, an advisory, investment and development partner with a focus on health and social care infrastructure; AstraZeneca; Boots; Clipper Logistics; Deloitte, the largest professional services network in the world that in 2016 failed to protect itself against a cyberattack that breached the confidentiality of its clients and 244,000 staff, allowing the attackers to access usernames,

---

50. See Cabinet Office, 'Staying at home and away from others (social distancing)' (1 May, 2020)

51. See Dominic Raab, 'Foreign Secretary's statement on coronavirus (COVID-19): 5 May 2020' (published 5 May, 2020).

52. See Juliette Garside and Rupert Neate, 'UK government "using pandemic to transfer NHS duties to private sector"', *The Guardian* (4 May, 2020).

passwords, IP addresses and health information; G4S, the UK's largest security services company that has been accused of using immigrant-detainee labour in prisons, extreme misconduct in child custodial institutions in the UK and the US, and of collaborating in police telephone data manipulation; GlaxoSmithKline, which in 2012 was fined $3 billion after admitting bribing US doctors and encouraging the prescription of unsuitable anti-depressants to children; Interserve, the multinational group of support services and construction companies that last year went into administration; KPMG, the multinational professions service network that in 2004 admitted criminal wrongdoing in creating fraudulent tax shelters to help wealthy clients avoid $2.5 billion in taxes between 1996 and 2002, and subsequently agreed to pay $456 million in penalties to avoid indictment; Mitie, the UK strategic outsourcing company with businesses in everything from property management and cleaning to home care, immigration detention and deportation, prisons and custodial health services; Mott MacDonald, the UK multidisciplinary consultancy that in 2017 was suspended from bidding for Government contracts in Hong Kong when it was found to have disclosed confidential population and employment data to outsiders; Palantir, the US software company that provides tracking and surveillance infrastructure to the US military, Immigration Customs and Enforcement and local police departments; Serco, the UK provider of public services in health, education, housing, transport, prisons, border security, military defence and information technology that last year was fined £19.2m by the Serious Fraud Office; and Sodexo, the French food services and facilities management company and one of the world's largest multinational corporations, whose subsidiary, Sodexo Justice Services, was criticised by the UK Ministry of Justice in February 2019 for failing to prevent repeated and systemic breaches of the human rights of inmates at HMP Peterborough. All these companies of questionable probity and competence have been awarded taxpayer-funded commissions to manage COVID-19 test centres, run test laboratories, carry out contact tracing, purchase PPE, recruit hospital staff and build the 7 empty Nightingale hospitals.[53] The NHS has subsequently been told by Ministers that it can only order key equipment through a centralised procurement team.

---

53. See Anoosh Chakelian, 'Interserve, and the other companies running Britain that you've never heard of', *The New Statesman* (11 March, 2019).

Also on the same day, the *Guardian* reported that over the past 18 months the Government has awarded at least seven contracts worth almost £1 million to Faculty, a start-up employed by Dominic Cummings, the senior advisor to the Prime Minister, with the Brexit campaign; that last year was tasked with finding ways to apply artificial intelligence across Government; in which Theodore Agnew, the Cabinet Office Minister in charge of the Office for Artificial Intelligence and Government Digital Service, has £90,000 of shares; and whose CEO, Marc Warner, has attended the Government's Scientific Advisory Group on Emergencies (SAGE), which is chaired by Patrick Vallance, the former President of Research and Development at GlaxoSmithKline, one of the pharmaceutical companies contracted by the Government.[54]

There are various objectives and motivations that lie behind these untendered Government contracts, from the privatisation of public services to the surveillance and control of the UK population through technology utilising artificial intelligence managed by multinational corporations. But they tend to be designed to steal the biometric data, digital records and personal information that supports those aims.

14. The COVID Alert System

On 10 May, in an address to the nation broadcast on the BBC, the Prime Minister announced what he called the 'sketch of a roadmap for reopening society'.[55] Beginning with the assertion that the efficacy of the lockdown was a 'fact', when in fact there is no evidence for that and plenty to the contrary, he went on to claim that without the lockdown half a million people in the UK would have died of COVID-19.

This figure is based on the by now famous report published on 16 March by Imperial College London that had been commissioned by the Government, that wasn't peer reviewed before publication, whose estimates of case fatality rate were far higher than those in a report published by the same team only a week

---

54. See Rob Evans and David Pegg, 'Vote Leave AI firm wins seven government contracts in 18 months', *The Guardian* (4 May, 2020).

55. See Boris Johnson, 'Prime Minister's statement on coronavirus (COVID-19): 10 May 2020' (published 10 May, 2020).

earlier, that has been challenged by other virus modellers, and whose numbers were retracted nine days later by the head of the team that modelled them, Professor Niall Ferguson, who has a record of extravagant claims that have subsequently and repeatedly been proven untrue by many orders of magnitude.[56] In 2001, as a result of Professor Ferguson's modelling of the spread of Foot and Mouth Disease, 12 million farm animals were slaughtered in the UK, with a cost to the UK economy estimated at £10 billion. In 2002, he predicted that up to 50,000 people would die from BSE (Mad Cow Disease), increasing to 150,000 if the epidemic expanded to include sheep. Since 1990 a total of 178 people in the UK have died from the disease. In 2005 he claimed that up to 200 million people worldwide would be killed by bird-flu. Between 2003 and 2009 only 282 people died from the disease. And in 2009 Professor Ferguson and his team at Imperial College advised the Government that swine flu would probably kill 65,000 people in the UK. Swine flu eventually killed just 457 people.[57] On 5 May, five days before the Prime Minister's address, Professor Ferguson had resigned from his position on the Government's Scientific Advisory Group for Emergencies.

The Prime Minister reiterated that this was a conditional plan, that has to meet the five conditions for lifting the lockdown of the UK already introduced by the First Secretary on 16 April, all of which, as we have seen, are based on inaccurate assessments of the present, meaningless criteria, impossible to make assessments, factors irrelevant to the decision, or some combination of them all.

The Prime Minister then introduced the new COVID Alert System, whose 5 levels run from 5) the overwhelming of the NHS; 4) the situation in which we have supposedly been during the lockdown; 3) where we're supposed to be going next; 2) didn't get a mention; and 1) when the coronavirus is no longer present in the UK. These alert levels will be determined by the rate of infection (R0) of SARS-CoV-2, which he claimed is currently between 0.5 and 0.9.

---

56. See Neil Ferguson, et al., 'Report 9: Impact of non-pharmaceutical interventions (NPIs) to reduce COVID-19 mortality and healthcare demand', Imperial College COVID-19 Response Team (16 March, 2020); Paul Taylor, 'Susceptible, Infectious, Recovered', *London Review of Books* (7 May, 2020); Nic Lewis, 'Imperial College UK COVID-19 numbers don't seem to add up', *Climate Etc.* (1 April, 2020); and David Adam, 'UK has enough intensive care units for coronavirus, expert predicts', *New Scientist* (25 March, 2020).

57. See Steerpike, 'Six questions that Neil Ferguson should be asked', *The Spectator* (16 April, 2020).

In fact, until the entire population of the UK has been tested (and at the time of writing only 1,460,517 people had been tested out of a population of 67,886,000), this is speculation, and will remain so until the other 66,425,000 people are tested. Even at the target rate of 100,000 tests per day the Government has consistently failed to meet, this would take a further 664 days, or around the time it will take to develop a vaccine. As a criterion for setting an alert level or as a condition of lifting the lockdown of the UK, this too is meaningless.

To keep this purely speculative rate of infection down, the Prime Minister said we would need to 1) reverse the epidemic in care homes and the NHS; and 2) 'control the virus' by a system of testing possible victims and tracing their contacts.

He said no more about the tracking and tracing system the NHSX has been developing with Onfido and other tech companies; but the measures to implement this were filled out in more detail in the 50-page document that was presented to the virtual Parliament the next day. As for the idea of 'controlling' a virus, that is more meaningless bravado presumably to justify eventually making the uploading of the Track and Trace app and other surveillance technology such as the Immunity Passport mandatory. The Prime Minister then laid out three steps in his roadmap:

1. Those who can't work from home should be actively encouraged to return to work, but social distancing both on public transport and at work 'must and will be maintained'. In addition, people are now allowed unlimited exercise; but those who disobey the prohibitions on social distancing will now be issued with increased fines, with fixed notice penalties of £100 rising to a maximum of £3,200.

2. By 1 June at the earliest, there will be the phased opening of schools, with primary schools first; and the opening of some shops.

3. By 4 July at the earliest, some businesses in the hospitality industry will be allowed to open, together with other public places. However, social distancing will still be imposed.

Finally, without saying when it would come into effect, the Prime Minister added that people arriving in the UK by plane would now be quarantined. It later emerged that this wouldn't include people coming from France, according to a reciprocal agreement between Prime Minister Boris Johnson and President Emmanuel Macron.[58] Since Britain and France have, respectively, the first and third highest number of deaths in Europe officially attributed to COVID-19, one can only presume that a large number of Government officials and their corporate backers have their weekend homes in the South of France. It also emerged that social distancing wouldn't apply to cleaners and nannies, which MPs presumably consider essential to keeping their London, constituency and second homes tidy, and looking after their kids for them while they're busy not attending Parliament. Whatever the case, these exceptions to the rules blatantly biased towards the needs of the middle classes revealed the contingency of measures supposedly based on the 'best scientific evidence'.

What this roadmap didn't contain is any indication of when social distancing prohibitions will be lifted, except by the meaningless criterion of reaching level 1 on the New COVID Alert System. This most obviously parallels the five levels in the UK Terror Threat Levels that were introduced by the Government in 2006 for much the same purpose, and on which we have never dropped below Level 3: Substantial, indicating that 'an attack is a strong possibility'.[59] On this possibility, the Government imposition of social distancing looks to be the 'New Normal' for the foreseeable future.

15. The State of Emergency as a Paradigm of Government

So many new regulations and laws have been made, so many civil liberties and human rights contravened, and so many public services privatised and outsourced to corporate clients during this Government-imposed State of Emergency that there is a point at which any commentary on everything done under the aegis of the coronavirus 'crisis' has to choose what to report. But let's stop here and look at what can be done, and what is likely to be done, under the current legislation. Specifically, I want to look at the Government's 'Track and Trace' mission, and how it is likely to be used and extended in the future by

---

58. See 'No quarantine in UK for travellers from France, Macron and Johnson agree', *The Local* (10 May, 2020).

59. See Security Service MI5, 'Threat Levels'.

amendments to legislation justified by the apparent necessity of preventing infection and contamination with SARS-CoV-2.

At present, both the Chief Executive of NHSX and the Secretary of State for Health and Social Care have avoided answering the question of whether use of biometric technology like the Track and Trace programme and the Immunity Passport will be voluntary or mandatory. However, it has been suggested that unless a significant proportion of the population downloads the app containing this technology — with the figure of 60 per cent being advanced — it won't fulfil its function. After a voluntary stage, therefore, in which the relevant app is uploaded by tech consumers and those terrified by the media, we can anticipate its employment being a condition of entering public places for which there are or can be security guards, such as a supermarket, park, gym, library, cinema, pub, restaurant, hotel, gallery, museum, concert hall, football ground or place of worship; or of using public services, such as buses, trains, planes, post offices, clinics, hospitals, housing offices, homeless hostels, job centres, benefit-claimant or immigration offices; and above all as a condition of entering a place of work or study, whether factory, warehouse, work site, call centre, office, lecture hall or classroom. Doing so will require proof of immunity to the coronavirus. Finally, when its use has become the 'New Normal', the uploading of the app, the submission of the biometric data and the creation of the digital identity it requires will be made mandatory on the basis that the number of people using the app is insufficient to safeguard the public against infection. This will then be rolled out with yet more regulations or amendments to legislation imposing increased fines and further prosecution for any person failing to comply, along with the police powers necessary to enforce compliance.

Not only will a person's access to work, to entertainment, to public life, to other people, their freedoms of movement, assembly and association, be determined and controlled by their ongoing submission of their biological data to a testing and tracking device that monitors their every move and interaction through every moment of their lives, but any deviation from the instructions they receive from the monitors of these devices, any failure to update further technology or upload additional data — or any other deviation from Government directives, including political protest, dissenting speech or refusal to obey or implement any biosecurity or anti-terrorist measures — can be punished by the simple recourse of removing their access to all public places and services, their place of employment, even their place of accommodation. US property technology companies are already using the supposed threat of COVID-19 to implement biometric access controls and facial recognition entry systems to screen tenants in restricted access buildings, the surveillance of gated communities, and to compile and extend data bases on the population.[60] With very little change to existing technology and legislation in the UK, any dissenting person could effectively be made an 'unperson', to use George Orwell's prophetic term, as well as potentially charged with, for example, 'endangering the lives of others'. We shouldn't forget that coughing at key workers or members of the public by someone claiming to have coronavirus is now categorised by the Crown Prosecution Service as assault punishable by up to 12 months in prison.[61] It's a small step from there to prosecuting someone for refusing to confirm whether they have coronavirus. Indeed, under existing powers, a police constable, community support officer, or anyone designated by a local authority or the Secretary of State, can compel a person they suspect 'has, or may have' coronavirus to be tested, so the legislation to make the use of this app mandatory is already in place.

The commonly heard response from liberals concerned at the raft of legislation and regulations made by the Government under the lockdown of the UK is that it 'sets a disturbing precedent for the future'. It doesn't. As should be clear to anyone reading this article and the legislation it summarises, that future is now. This is already happening — has happened, the consequences of which are unfolding before us every day. When I started this article, I intended to end by speculating on how this legislation will be employed in the immediate future, but it's already too late: that future has overtaken us and is now our present.

Here's how Onfido described how an Immunity Passport will work when their technology is loaded onto the NHSX track and trace app and a user wants to return to work — a situation in which millions of UK citizens now find themselves:

---

60. See Erin McElroy, Meredith Whittaker and Genevieve Fried, 'COVID-19 Crisis Capitalism Comes to Real Estate', *Boston Review* (7 May, 2020).

61. See Crown Prosecution Service, 'Coronavirus coughs' at key workers will be charged as assault, CPS warns' (26 March, 2020).

Alice works for a consultancy firm and has been working from home during the lockdown period. She now wants to go back to work from the office and must prove her immunity from COVID-19 in order to do so:

1. She signs up for an immunity test with the NHS. She is asked to register and verify her identity ahead of her appointment. She can do this via her smartphone or computer, using the in-built camera on either device to take a picture of her face and associate it with her registration.

2. She goes to an NHS centre to be tested. Her picture is taken via a hands-free camera and is compared to the image of her face taken during registration, to prove that she is the same person who originally signed up for the test. The images match, and the test is administered.

3. When complete, the immunity certificate is created and connected to her digital identity.

4. She uses this digital identity, now associated with her immunity certificate, as a passport to access her office.[62]

When considering the possibility of such measures being enacted, we should ask ourselves why, given the legislative ability to do so, the Government wouldn't do so? What Government in modern British history has ever not enacted to their full extent its powers to monitor and control the population of the UK? In the light of this question, the scenarios I have drawn from the current legislation, let alone that which will be made in the future (and the 10 anti-terrorist Acts passed in the past 20 years is an indicator of what's in store for us), is not a possibility or even a probability, but a likelihood that we should expect and, if we still have the mind and will to do so, plan to resist. Although there has been some limited concern about this legislation from lawyers, the organisations that might be expected to organise such resistance are too busy collaborating, intentionally or unwittingly, in creating and maintaining the illusion of a threat on which this legislation has been made by Government, nodded through by Parliament and accepted by the population of the UK. It would be inaccurate to call what we are living under fascism, as fascism was a historical moment at a different stage in the

---

62. See Onfido, 'The role of Digital Identity in Immunity Passports', UK Parliament Committees (April 2020).

development of capitalism; but we are, without a shadow of a doubt, living under
— or rather with, in the sense that we are its willing collaborators and
implementors — legislation and technologies of surveillance and control about
which the totalitarian states of the Twentieth Century could only dream.

It's a quirk of history that it always appears to happen to somebody else, in
some other country, and always in the past. The German citizens photographed
sunbathing on Berlin's most popular beach in the summer of 1933 didn't realise
they had just entered 12 years of totalitarian dictatorship. Yet, just like us, they
had obeyed the emergency decree suspending their freedoms and rights on the
justification of a fabricated threat to national safety; read the Enabling Act passing
legislative power to the government; listened half-believing to their leader
describe the threat from an almost invisible enemy; and observed with growing
anxiety the actions of their police and paramilitary forces in controlling it. Hitler
had to overcome the requirement of forming a majority coalition Government, the
parliamentary opposition of the Social Democrats, and the largest and best
organised Communist Party in Europe both in and outside the Reichstag. In
comparison, the Government of Boris Johnson has a free ride, with the largest
parliamentary majority for the Conservative Party in 32 years, the complete
collaboration of the parliamentary opposition, and a political left with no
representation either in Parliament or on the street competing on social media to
see who can demand the sternest response to a non-existent threat.

In his 2003 study of the historical, political and juridical contexts for the *State
of Exception*, the Italian philosopher, Giorgio Agamben, reminds us that — from
its origin in the 'state of siege' decreed by the French Constituent Assembly in
1791, its introduction as the conditions under which the French constitution could
be suspended in 1799, its enactment in the 'Decree for the Protection of People
and State' issued by President von Hindenburg in 1933, through to its application
to the 'military order' issued by President Bush in November 2001 that authorised
the indefinite detention of enemy combatants deprived of legal status in
Guantanamo Bay prison camp (and, by extension, the extra-legal imprisonment
and torture of Julian Assange by successive UK Governments) — it has been
within the democratic tradition, and not an absolutist one, that the state of
exception has emerged as what he calls 'the dominant paradigm of government

in contemporary politics'.[63] In a passage quoted by Agamben from *Constitutional Government and Democracy* (1941), the political theorist Carl J. Friedrich wrote:

> The quasi-dictatorial provisions of modern constitutional systems, be they martial rule, state of siege, or constitutional emergency powers, fail to conform to any exacting standard of effective limitations upon a temporary concentration of powers. Consequently, all these systems are liable to be transformed into totalitarian schemes if conditions become favourable to it.

I ask again: under our current conditions, within the new legislative powers, and given the public mood created by the media, why would the UK Government not enact the scenario I have described above? And when it does, what will you do in response? Acquiesce passively, as if nothing had changed except to increase our safety? Collaborate actively and willingly in implementing the 'New Normal' the Government has prepared for us? Resist, to the extent that is still possible to do so under these conditions of surveillance and control? Or flee the country while you still can? The choices are as stark as they were facing the citizens of Germany 87 years ago. The collective consequences of those individual choices will fall upon us all.

16. The Foreseeable Future

On 11 May, the day before this article was published, the Prime Minister presented to the virtual Parliament 'Our plan to rebuild: The UK Government's COVID-19 recovery strategy'.[64] This 50-page document would take an article in itself to summarise and critique; but as a coda to this article, excerpted below are some of the key indications of what the Government plans to implement with the consensus it has manufactured in the UK public over the past three months. As always with such documents, the plan is short on details, but it is extraordinarily — almost brazenly — open about the society the Government is preparing for us.

---

63. See Giorgio Agamben, *State of Exception*, Homo Sacer II, 1; translated by Kevin Attell (University of Chicago Press, 2005).

64. See HM Government, 'Our plan to rebuild: The UK Government's COVID-19 recovery strategy' (May 2020).

And for once, the word that describes this society is accurate, proportional and fully warranted: totalitarian.

Foreword. This document sets out a plan to rebuild the UK for a world with COVID-19. It is not a quick return to 'normality'. It is clear that the only feasible long-term solution lies with a vaccine or drug-based treatment. A mass vaccine or treatment may be more than a year away. Indeed, in a worst-case scenario, we may never find a vaccine. So our plan must countenance a situation where we are in this, together, for the long haul. We must acknowledge that life will be different, at least for the foreseeable future. That will require a widespread system of testing, of tracing and monitoring the spread of the disease . . . and of re-designing workplaces and public spaces to make them 'COVID-19 Secure'. Then, as vaccines and treatment become available, we will move to another new phase, where we will learn to live with COVID-19 for the longer term without it dominating our lives.

The challenges ahead. 1) This is not a short-term crisis. It is likely that COVID-19 will circulate in the human population long-term, possibly causing periodic epidemics. In the near future, large epidemic waves cannot be excluded without continuing some measures. 2) In the near term, we cannot afford to make drastic changes. 3) There is no easy or quick solution. Only the development of a vaccine or effective drugs can reliably control this epidemic and reduce mortality without some form of social distancing or contact tracing in place. 6) The virus' spread is difficult to detect. Some people carry the disease asymptomatically, which may mean that they can spread the virus without knowing that they are infectious. Even those who are not at risk of significant harm themselves may pose a real risk of inadvertently infecting others. This is why a significant part of the next phase of the Government's response will be to improve its monitoring of and response to new infections. 8) The plan depends on continued widespread compliance.

Overarching principles. 1) Informed by the science. 2) Fairness. 3) Proportionality, 4) Privacy. The Government will always seek to protect personal privacy and be transparent with people when enacting measures that, barring this once-in-a-century event, would never normally be considered. 5) Transparency. Balancing the different considerations will involve some difficult choices. For example, the Government will face a choice between the extent and speed of the freedoms enjoyed by some lower-risk people and the risk to others: if all people at lower personal risk were allowed to resume their lives exactly as before the outbreak, this would increase the level of risk to those that are more vulnerable.

Joint Biosecurity Centre (JBC). The success of any strategy based on releasing the current social restrictions while maintaining the epidemic at a manageable level will depend on the Government's ability to monitor the pandemic accurately. To achieve this, the Government is establishing a new biosecurity monitoring system, led by a new Joint Biosecurity Centre now being established. The Government's new approach to biosecurity will bring together the UK's world-leading epidemiological expertise and fuse it with the best analytical capability from across Government in an integrated approach. It will work closely with local partners and businesses to collect a wide range of data to build a picture of COVID-19 infection rates across the country — from testing, environmental and workplace data to local infrastructure testing (e.g. swab tests). The Centre will also have a response function that will identify specific actions to address local spikes in infections, in partnership with local agencies — for example, advising Ministers, businesses and local partners to close schools or workplaces. The JBC will be responsible for setting the new COVID-19 Alert level. Over time the Government will consider whether the JBC should form part of an extended infrastructure to address biosecurity threats to the UK, and whether the COVID-19 alert level system should be expanded to other potential infectious diseases.

Testing and tracing. The COVID-19 Test and Trace Taskforce . . . programme will ensure that, when someone develops COVID-19-like symptoms, they can rapidly have a test to find out if they have the virus — and people who they've had recent close contact with can be alerted and provided with advice. This will identify who is infected more precisely, to reduce the number of people who are self-isolating with symptoms but who are not actually infected, and to ensure those who are infected continue to take stringent self-isolation measures; and ensure those who have been in recent close contact with an infected person receive rapid advice and, if necessary, self-isolate, quickly breaking the transmission chain. For such a system to work, several systems need to be built and successfully integrated. These include automated, app-based contact-tracing through the new NHS COVID-19 app to (anonymously) alert users when they have been in close contact with someone identified as having been infected. Whilst the measures above will involve an unprecedented degree of data-collection, as many Asian countries implemented after the SARS and MERS outbreaks, the Government will enact robust safety measures. Part of the tracing effort will include a voluntary NHS contact tracing application for smartphones; this will help increase the speed and effectiveness of the tracing effort. Information collected through the Test and Trace programme, together with wider data from sources such as 111 online, will form part of a core national COVID-19 dataset. The creators of a number of independent apps and websites which have already launched to collect similar data have agreed to work openly with the NHS and have aligned their products and data as part of this central, national effort.

Economic and social support to maintain livelihoods and restore the economy. These measures are extraordinarily costly and cannot be sustained for a prolonged period of time. The Office for Budget Responsibility has estimated that the direct cost to the Government of the response to COVID-19 could rise above £100bn in 2020-21. In addition to this, support of approximately £330bn (equivalent to 15% of GDP) in the form of guarantees and loans has been made available to business. So as the UK adjusts the current restrictions, the Government will also need to wind down the economic support measures while people are eased back to work. The world will not return to "normal" after COVID-19; much of the global economy is likely to change significantly. The UK will need to be agile in adapting to and shaping this new world.

Public communication, understanding and enforcement. As the UK moves into the next phase, where the Government will need to trust people to comply with more subtle social restrictions, the Government will also need to ensure robust enforcement measures to deter and reduce the threat from the small minority who elect not to act responsibly.

Sustainable government structures. COVID-19 has been perhaps the biggest test of governments worldwide since the 1940s. As the Government navigates towards recovery, it must ensure it learns the right lessons from this crisis and acts now to ensure that governmental structures are fit to cope with a future epidemic. This will require a rapid re-engineering of government's structures and institutions to deal with this historic emergency. COVID-19 will not be the last major disease that endangers us. The Government must prepare and build now for diseases that could threaten us in the future.

How you can help. The UK now needs to prepare for an extended period of living with and managing the threat from the virus; this will continue to require everyone's support and adherence.

On 12 May, the day I publish this article, the Office for National Statistics released its latest statistics for overall deaths this year.[65] This showed that, as of 1 May, the 18th week of 2020, there have been 247,261 deaths in England and Wales. In comparison, in 2018, following the seasonal influenza virus of 2017-18, 219,402 people had died by the end of week 18. That's 27,859 less than this year, or, over 18 weeks, an additional 1,547 people dying per week. The average number of deaths per week in the first 18 weeks of 2018 was 12,149, or 1,741 per day. In other words, 18 weeks into 2020 we have had the equivalent of an additional 16 days at the average daily death rate over the same period in 2018. This, however, doesn't take into account the 13,237 excess deaths recorded in England and Wales in the 7 weeks to 24 April that haven't been attributed to COVID-19. Deduct these excess deaths, which must at least in part be attributable to the lethal effects of the lockdown of the UK, and the increase in overall deaths this year attributed to COVID-19 over overall deaths in 2018 at the same stage is 14,622. Given that 52 per cent of the deaths attributed to COVID-19 in England as of 5 May were of people over 80 years of age, by the end of the year the overall deaths in 2020 could equal or even drop below those in 2018.

But leaving these unexplained deaths aside for the moment — or attributing them to some other deadly disease yet to be discovered by the Joint Biosecurity Centre and monitored by the Test and Trace programme — it's on the justification of this 12 per cent increase in mortality over a year in which not a single emergency measure was even contemplated by Parliament that the Government has locked down the country for the past two months, and is planning to subject the 67,886,000 citizens of the UK to a totalitarian programme of surveillance and control for the foreseeable future. And, to answer Žižek's question, the more the Government appears to be out of control, incompetent, panicking, to be placing

---

65. See Office for National Statistics, 'Deaths registered weekly in England and Wales, provisional'.

the lives of the populace at risk, the more that populace clamours for the extension of the lockdown, for stronger measures, more intrusive solutions, for better protection from the invisible threat. Whether this 'crisis' has been manufactured by the Government and its corporate clients and to what purpose should no longer be questions except for those who refuse to read the data and legislation I have presented and analysed in my last two articles: the question we must answer is how to oppose the totalitarian measures this 'crisis' has ushered in.

— 12 May, 2020

4. Lockdown: Collateral Damage in the War on COVID-19

'At issue is an entire conception of the destinies of human society from a perspective that, in many ways, seems to have adopted the apocalyptic idea of the end of the world from religions whose suns are now setting. Having superseded politics, even the economy, in order to govern, must now be integrated into the new paradigm of biosecurity, to which all other needs will have to be sacrificed. It is legitimate to ask whether such a society can still be defined as human, or whether the loss of sensible relations, of the face, of friendship, of love, can truly be compensated for by an abstract and presumably completely fictitious health security.'

— Giorgio Agamben, *Biosecurity and Politics*, May 2020

One of the things to have been revealed by the 'crisis' caused by the global response to the coronavirus is that the overwhelming majority of people, and certainly in liberal democracies, would rather believe a lie to which we've been told how to react — in this case a civilisation-threatening viral pandemic that can be combatted through standing two metres apart, increasing the powers of police to arrest us and biometrically tracking our every move — than believe a truth to which we don't have a clue how to respond. Confronted with the accelerated totalitarianisation of the UK being implemented under a *de facto* State of Emergency, we have chosen to listen to the lies of the Government and its media telling us exactly what to do and for how long, rather than hear a truth on which we will have to think and act for ourselves.

If you're one of the former, as 99.9 per cent of people in the UK appear to be, then you won't have read even this far, and will most likely have already dismissed me as a 'coronavirus denier' — that new favoured safe-word of liberals. But if you're one of the 0.1 per cent that is still thinking, questioning and interested in resisting, this article is an attempt to estimate the collateral damage caused by the so-called 'lockdown' of the UK imposed by the Government on 23 March, 2020. In little more than two months, this decision, which has been enacted with varying degrees of severity by nearly 150 countries around the world, has changed the country we lived in for the foreseeable future.[1] My last two articles looked at, respectively, the manufacturing of consensus for this decision and the regulations, legislation and deals made by the Government with this consensus. This article, my ninth on the coronavirus 'crisis', will look at the ongoing costs of this decision, which has been made not only by the Government of the UK but by us, its people, who have acquiesced without question or protest to every measure imposed upon us. Part of that acquiescence has been our collective refusal to look at the collateral costs of the lockdown, both now and in the future. This article is my contribution to beginning that act of looking.

1. Four Anecdotes

I want to start with some anecdotes. I wouldn't usually when discussing a nationwide, and now worldwide, 'pandemic'; but anecdote has been raised to the status of holy writ in the debates about the actions of the UK Government in response to the coronavirus 'crisis'. Logic of argument, citation of facts, proof of statistics, authority of sources: all have fallen beneath the mighty weight of personal anecdote. 'Tell that to the families of the dead', runs the often-repeated rejoinder to the incontrovertible fact that COVID-19 is a threat almost exclusively to those over 65 years of age with one or more pre-existing chronic illnesses, as if the writer had personal access to the feelings of everyone in the UK who knows someone that has died. 'My sister is a nurse, and she's been traumatised by this experience . . . ' begins the response to the information that, far from being overwhelmed by the vast numbers of COVID-19 deaths during this unprecedented epidemic, our hospitals are in fact empty. And the newly knighted (but still underpaid) heroes of our 'frontline' in this war against an invisible enemy haven't been shy about coming forward. 'I woke from sleep after my night-shift to find the beaches and parks filled with people. Why do I bother?' comes the plaintive cry on Twitter, retweeted thousands of times over, of any number of medical practitioners turned social media gurus. All it has taken to justify the latest regulation, a new measure, the turning of a guidance into an instruction, or the

---

1. See Daniel Dunford, Becky Dale, Nassos Stylianou, Ed Lowther, Maryam Ahmed and Irene de la Torre Arenas, 'Coronavirus: The world in lockdown in maps and charts', *BBC* (7 April, 2020).

roll-out of a biosecurity system out of the dystopian nightmares of our future, is the report of the death of a single mini-cab driver, bus driver, construction worker, cleaner or other (until very recently) unskilled worker uncritically and unquestioningly attributed to COVID-19. So before I move into more reasoned arguments, let me begin with a few personal anecdotes of my own. All are about people I know personally, but to protect their identities I won't reveal here either how I know them or their real names.

P. owns and works in a Chinese take-away restaurant. He's in his late 70s, has a background in construction and is on his feet most of the day, so looks fit for his age. Before the coronavirus 'crisis' he had been waiting over a year for an operation there was a small percentage chance that he wouldn't survive. He had recently been contacted by the hospital at the last minute and offered a brief window of opportunity, but at such short notice he declined. The last time I asked him about whether he'd heard something he placed his heavy hand on mine and gently told me he wished everyone would stop asking him, as it was making the waiting worse. I swore I wouldn't ask him again. When the virus officially reached these shores, he told me that he intended to keep on working as usual, and that a positive frame of mind was the key to good health. The next time I went for a takeaway P. had some news. He'd gone in for a preliminary check-up, and the hospital had discovered he had cancer. It was so advanced that he was operated on within 24 hours, had been in bed for a week, but was now looking surprisingly hale. I saw him once more in the pub after that, and the news was good: it looked like they'd caught the cancer in time. The following week, social distancing was enforced, and shortly after that the lockdown of the UK was imposed. The restaurant is still serving takeaway, and every time I go I ask after P. He's well, but, as someone of his age who has recently had an operation, he is quite reasonably in isolation in the family home. He's an independent man, and after a day on his feet likes a late-night pint. I can imagine how being locked inside is making him feel, but he's one of the lucky ones. He has family around him to keep his spirits up, and, even more fortunately, the operation that saved his life was conducted the week before the NHS began to prepare for COVID-19. If it wasn't, would he have been invited into the hospital for a check-up? If he had been, would he have gone with all the fearmongering in the media? And if he was invited and had gone and they had found the cancer, would they have performed the operation?

The second anecdote is about R. A retired barrister, he too is in his late 70s, but has a history of respiratory disease. Unlike P., he lives on his own in a private housing estate. That means the one bench in the estate's communal garden hasn't been covered with tape by the council, but fear has been enough to keep his neighbours from stopping for a chat. I have watched young women who share his entrance hall flee him like a leper in their haste to get inside their flats. Before social distancing, R. had a social life composed of classical concerts, singing groups, and recently even the local church. Now that's all gone. We visit him once a week, where we stand or sit outside his flat or in the communal garden, careful not to cough in his direction but otherwise behaving normally. But the real danger to him isn't infection with the virus but the lockdown itself. Maybe 6 months before the coronavirus 'crisis' reached the UK, R. began to show the first signs of dementia. A juggler of words with a dry sense of humour, he began to struggle to find the right one. While his memory of the past remained extraordinary (on the cusp of social distancing we spent an evening with him recalling past legal cases from the 1970s), he has recently and rapidly declined into more than memory loss. I say dementia, but it could also be Alzheimer's disease, or even be the result of head trauma. Before lockdown, he too had been waiting for an appointment: not for an operation, but to assess the cause of his memory loss and, through that assessment, to qualify for some form of home care and, possibly, care home. Although he goes for long walks in the middle of the night when the police won't stop him, living alone in his apartment and seeing maybe two people a week for an hour at a time, has rapidly accelerated his inability to function. The array of technology and gadgets that allow us not only to stay in touch with the outside world and our friends but also to live alone have turned into an incomprehensible puzzle for him. We advised him to stop using social media, which was increasing his anxiety. His laptop and phone have become a malign gremlin in his home. Now he no longer knows how to use the oven. He needs either home care to visit him or to move into a care home. But seeing R. on a weekly basis over the past few months, it is clear that his condition has been worsened and accelerated by the lockdown.

My third anecdote is about M., whom I know less well. I'd guess in his mid-40s, he and his wife run an Italian restaurant. For the past five years they've worked hard to build a clientele for authentic Italian dishes in an area where takeaway pizza is the more usual association with their country's cuisine. Their *spaghetti al nero* is a thing of delectation. As COVID-19 was scything through the disproportionately elderly population of Italy, we visited their restaurant. The local vicar sat at one end of the room, M. at the other. He looked worried, not only by the stories of what was happening in his homeland printed in lurid detail on the front covers of our press, but at the thought of what would happen to his business when the virus reached the UK. Since the lockdown started they too have been providing takeaway food. The squid ink pasta is off the menu, but we have done our best to support them financially, not only by ordering takeaway meals but also buying our pasta from their dwindling stock. But the last time we met, M.'s wife told us they are broke. All their savings from five years of work have gone keeping the shop afloat during the imposed suspension of trading under lockdown. Now they will have to sell up for what they can get and return to Italy. She was furious, and wasn't shy about expressing her view that the whole coronavirus 'crisis' had been grossly exaggerated, both in Italy and in the UK. My neighbourhood will be much the poorer for their departure.

My fourth and last anecdote is about D. In his late-20s, D. works as a forklift driver in Derby for Holland and Barrett, the UK health-food retailer that three years ago was purchased for £1.8 billion by Russian Billionaire Mikhail Fridman. When social distancing came into effect, D. was told H&B are an essential business and he continued to work in the company's warehouses, in close proximity to his fellow workers. When the lockdown of the UK's businesses was announced, Holland and Barrett was exempt and D. was not offered furlough. Instead, workers from a local warehouse that was closed down were drafted in, increasing the density of workers. D. has a healthy suspicion of anything the Government tells us, but even he began to worry about his health under the barrage of daily scaremongering in the media. Then, a fortnight ago, an employee in Burton tested positive for SARs-Cov-2. In response, Holland and Barrett told the *Derby Telegraph* that all its staff had been tested, that social distancing is strictly enforced in the workplace, and that all workers have Personal Protective

Equipment.[2] In reality, neither D. nor any of his fellow employees had been tested, and they only found out about the story on social media. D. made this point online in a comment on a *Burton Mail* post linked to the *Telegraph* article, and the next day he was sacked. As an agency worker with no unionisation, D. has no employment rights, so his only recourse now is to try to find new employment in a collapsing job market, without a recommendation from his previous employer, and most likely having been blacklisted in the industry — or to apply for Universal Credit. Even as a skilled forklift driver he made £8.82 per hour, so he has no savings, and is facing at least a month without pay, at the end of which he will have to find the money for his next month's rent for his private landlord. Unsurprisingly, D.'s last Facebook post reported that his anxiety levels were 'through the roof'.[3]

2. Two Metaphors

These, and the millions like them, are the people I want to talk about in this article: the 'collateral damage', as the US Military likes to call its unintended victims, of what has from the very start been characterised and conducted in this country as a 'war' on the coronavirus epidemic, with its 'frontline' workers, its medical 'heroes', and the daily reports of the fallen dead. Like the victims of collateral damage, these will eventually far outnumber those who have died on the field of battle, for the real casualties of war take years after the battles have ended to accumulate their gruesome numbers. And like all collateral damage, the casualties are not limited to loss of life, but include the infrastructure of our society, from the small businesses struggling to survive the enforced suspension of trade to the national institutions — most obviously the NHS — whose privatisation is being accelerated and expanded under the cloak of this manufactured 'crisis'. For just like every warzone, it is under the cloak of media lies and the protection of martial law, through terrorised civilians and a society in ruins, that the multinational

---

2. See Ben Waldron, 'Holland and Barrett worker in Burton tests positive for coronavirus', *Derby Telegraph* (29 May, 2020).

3. I followed up on what happened to these friends and acquaintances in an article not included in this collection. See Simon Elmer, 'Five Stories Under Lockdown', *Architects for Social Housing* (1 December, 2020).

corporations funding the war enter with their irresistible plans to save a defeated people.

I owe it to Peter Hitchens, the *Mail on Sunday* columnist, for reminding me that the term 'lockdown', which has slipped so easily into our vocabulary, is a term used within the gulag of the US prison system to describe the confinement of inmates to their cells when there is a perceived risk of an uprising. Indeed — although Hitchens will not thank me for pointing it out — it is this solitary confinement that the UK Government has imposed on Julian Assange since his extra-legal incarceration and torture in Belmarsh Prison. It shouldn't surprise us, then, that the always obedient British poodle to the constantly barking US watchdog has so readily adopted this terminology for the emergency measures it has imposed on the UK public under the aegis of the coronavirus 'crisis'.

There are two metaphors, then, that have been deployed to justify the suspension of our civil liberties, human rights and political agency for the foreseeable future: 1) the prison metaphor, in which UK citizens have first been isolated from each other and, under the new Test and Trace programme, are now being subjected to a digital panopticism in order to avoid and monitor contagion; 2) and the war metaphor, in which collateral damage from the lockdown has been justified as a necessary evil whose consideration, let alone publication, is bad for the 'morale of the nation', as our would-be Churchillian Prime Minister would no doubt argue. It's a characteristic of contemporary warfare that it is conducted with an almost complete absence of scrutiny of its human and financial costs by the people in whose name it is being perpetrated and whose taxes pay for it, and the war on COVID-19 has been no different. That this is a civil war, waged against an invisible enemy whose host is ourselves, has only increased the opportunities for exaggerated figures, groundless analogies and fictitious narratives of threats to our biosecurity.

3. Unexplained Deaths

So let's start with the most measurable effect of the lockdown. According to the Office for National Statistics, the 11th week of 2020, ending 13 March, was when the first deaths in England and Wales officially attributed to COVID-19 were registered.[4] It was only in the following week, however, ending 20 March, that the total number of weekly deaths exceeded the average deaths for the corresponding week over the previous 5 years. It wasn't the first time this had happened in 2020. In the first two weeks of the year, ending respectively on 3 and 10 January, the 12,254 and 14,058 deaths exceeded the average for that week by 79 and 236, the latter due to the 2,477 deaths that week whose underlying cause was a respiratory disease, around 300 higher than the preceding or following week. From then, though, 2020 has been consistently lower in the overall deaths in England and Wales than the average for the preceding five years. This is not surprising, given the seasonal influenza epidemics of 2017-18, when there were 26,400 excess deaths attributed to influenza-related diseases in England alone, and of 2014-15, when there were over 28,300 excess deaths.[5]

However, from week 12 of 2020, ending 20 March, to week 21, ending 22 May, the last for which we have data, the total weekly deaths in England and Wales has been consistently higher than the average over the previous 5 years. This doesn't tell us that much, as in many weeks in 2015 and 2018 there was as high or a higher number of deaths than in all but the highest number of deaths between weeks 12 and 18 of 2020; but it does give us an average from which we can extrapolate so-called 'excess deaths'. It has been on the number of overall deaths above this average that the 'lockdown' of the UK has been justified by the UK Government, so it seems fair to use the same measure to arrive at the number of excess deaths caused by that lockdown.

Between weeks 12 and 18 of 2020 there were a total of 118,990 deaths in England and Wales. This is 46,566 more than the average number of deaths in these seven weeks over the past five years. Of these excess deaths, 33,360 have been attributed to COVID-19; but this figure leaves 13,206 unexplained deaths in excess of the average for the same 7 weeks of this year. The following week, the 3,930 deaths attributed to COVID-19 outstripped the 3,081 excess deaths; but in the week after that, ending 15 May, the 3,810 deaths attributed to COVID-19 left

---

4. See Office for National Statistics, 'Deaths registered weekly in England and Wales, provisional (2020 edition of this dataset up to week ending 1 January 2021)'.

5. See Public Health England, 'Surveillance of influenza and other respiratory viruses in the United Kingdom: Winter 2014 to 2015', *The National Archives* (May 2015) and 'Surveillance of influenza and other respiratory viruses in the UK: Winter 2017 to 2018', *The National Archives* (May 2018).

575 of the 4,385 excess deaths that week unexplained. In week 21 the excess deaths again fell below the deaths attributed to COVID-19; making a total of 13,781 unexplained deaths between weeks 12 and 21. This represents nearly 25 per cent of all 56,380 excess deaths in this 10-week period.

Age-standardised mortality rate for the five leading causes of death, per 100,000 people, England and Wales, occurring in March 2020

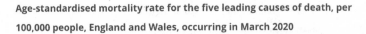

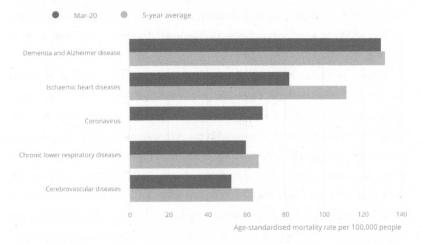

Source: Office for National Statistics — Analysis of deaths involving COVID-19

In reality, though, given the extraordinarily lax criteria for attributing a death to COVID-19, which I analysed in detail in 'Manufacturing Consensus: The Registering of COVID-19 Deaths', the actual number of excess deaths not caused by COVID-19 is undoubtedly far higher. Analysis by the Office for National Statistics has found that 14 per cent of death certificates 'mentioning' COVID-19 in March did not list the disease itself as the 'underlying cause of death'.[6] Not only that, but of the deaths that month in which COVID-19 was mentioned somewhere on the certificate, there was at least one pre-existing medical condition in 91 per cent of cases, with an average of 2.7 co-morbidities. These included influenza and pneumonia, dementia and Alzheimer's disease, and chronic obstructive pulmonary disease. The most common of these pre-existing conditions, however,

---

6. See Office for National Statistics, 'Deaths involving COVID-19, England and Wales: deaths occurring in March 2020' (16 April, 2020).

was ischaemic heart disease, which was listed as a co-morbidity on 14 per cent of deaths in which COVID-19 appeared on the death certificate. Significantly, the mortality rate from ischaemic heart disease — usually one of the biggest killers in the UK — was 29.5 per cent below the 5-year average for the month, and lower for the other leading causes of death, dementia and Alzheimer's disease, chronic lower respiratory disease and cerebrovascular disease. This could mean that COVID-19 accelerated the demise of some people who were already close to death, but it could also mean that some deaths from heart disease and other health conditions were being incorrectly attributed to COVID-19, as NHS doctors are finally coming forward to admit.[7]

The only figure I'm aware of indicating what the actual number of deaths caused by COVID-19 might be is that calculated by Professor Walter Ricciardi, President of the National Institute of Health in Italy and scientific adviser to the Italian Minister for Health. Back in March, following a re-evaluation of death certificates 'mentioning' COVID-19, he announced that only 12 per cent showed a direct causality from the coronavirus.[8] If we were to extrapolate from this percentage and apply it to the 43,689 deaths attributed to COVID-19 between 20 March and 22 May, according to which only 5,242 would show a direct causality to the disease, the remaining 38,446 deaths, added to the 13,781 unexplained deaths over these 10 weeks, would push that figure up to 52,227 deaths in excess of the average for this period over the past five years, and which cannot be explained or do not have a direct causality from COVID-19.

To make such a calculation, of course, would be to make an over projection, and I'm certainly not claiming it as accurate; but it at least points towards the numbers we're discussing when trying, in the absence of official figures, to estimate the collateral damage since the imposition of social distancing as Government guidance on 16 March and the official 'lockdown' of the UK imposed on 23 March by The Health Protection (Coronavirus, Business Closure) (England) Regulations 2020, the exact week when deaths in England and Wales began to

---

7. The article publishing UK doctors testifying about misdiagnoses was published by RT UK, which in March 2022 has banned by Ofcom as part of Western sanctions against the Russian Federation.

8. See Sarah Newey, 'Why have so many coronavirus patients died in Italy?', *The Telegraph* (23 March, 2020).

rise above the average over the past five years.[9] But whether it's 52,227 excess deaths without direct causality from COVID-19 or 13,781 deaths unattributed to COVID-19, these deaths need to be accounted for, explained and justified with more than the easy dismissal as 'collateral damage' with which they have been largely buried by the UK media.

4. Causes of Excess Deaths

One attempt to try to explain these unexplained deaths, usefully summarised by *Full Fact*, has been to attribute them to deaths from COVID-19 in care homes or at the home of the deceased where, either because the doctor wasn't certain or because a test for SARs-CoV-2 wasn't available, the disease wasn't mentioned on the death certificate.[10] This has supported the claim, gleefully pounced upon by the fearmongers in the media, that the number of COVID-19 deaths is in fact far higher than the already exaggerated official total.

However, while this failure to identity possible cases of COVID-19 may have been the case up until 10 April, when the Office for National Statistics began including figures on 'COVID-related deaths' in care homes that require nothing more than a statement from the care home provider to the Care Quality Commission that they 'suspect' the 'involvement' of COVID-19 — whether or not this corresponds to a medical diagnosis or positive test for SARs-CoV-2 or is otherwise reflected in the death certification — it has not been in the weeks since.

Moreover, if deaths in care homes accounted for the unexplained excess deaths, we would expect to see a sudden narrowing of this gap between excess deaths and deaths attributed to COVID-19 after 10 April. But in fact, while the previous week there had been a gap of 1,754 unexplained deaths, in the following week, ending 17 April, although the number of deaths attributed to COVID-19 under the new rules rose from 6,242 to 8,791, the number of unexplained deaths rose to 3,063; in the week ending 24 April there was a gap of 3,298, and in the week ending 1 May there was a gap of 1,976. Only in the week after that, ending 8 May, did the deaths attributed to COVID-19 exceed the excess deaths; but the

---

9. See UK Statutory Instruments, 'The Health Protection (Coronavirus, Business Closure) (England) Regulations 2020' (21 March, 2020).

10. See Leo Benedictus, 'What we know, and what we don't, about the true coronavirus death toll', *Full Fact* (1 May, 2020).

following week, ending 15 May, the gap had returned with 575 unexplained deaths. So the care home hypothesis doesn't bear examination by the facts.

Speaking about the ONS data last week at the Science Media Centre, Professor David Spiegelhalter, Chair of the Winton Centre for Risk and Evidence Communication at the University of Cambridge, calculated that, over the seven weeks to 15 May, 8,800 fewer non-COVID-19 deaths than normal had occurred in hospitals.[11] Since only a few care home residents normally die in hospitals, he argued that these deaths had not been 'exported' to care homes. By his own calculations, only 1,800 of the roughly 12,000 extra deaths were attributed to COVID-19, leaving 10,500 unexplained excess deaths. Spiegelhalter concluded:

> If up to 8,800 of these deaths would normally have occurred in hospitals, this would leave at least 1,700 unexplained non-COVID deaths at home. This is a vital issue if we are to understand the consequences of the actions taken.

Another explanation might come from a recent study published on 28 April titled 'Excess mortality in people with cancer and multimorbidity during the COVID-19 emergency'.[12] This has found that, due to the emergency, there has been a 45-66 per cent reduction in admissions to chemotherapy, and a 70-89 per cent reduction in referrals for early cancer diagnosis. As a result, the study estimates that deaths of newly-diagnosed patients with cancer in England over the next year, previously estimated at 31,354, could increase by 20 per cent to an additional 6,270 patients, the underlying cause of whose deaths may be cancer, COVID-19 or co-morbidities. Moreover, if people currently living with cancer are included, this figure could rise to 17,991 excess deaths.

The question is, what constitutes this 'emergency'? The reduction in cancer services necessitated by what the Government told us is an overwhelmed National Health Service? Or the huge reduction in care for newly-diagnosed and existing cancer patients by hospitals that, in the month this study was published, had only 41 per cent of acute care beds occupied, nearly four times the normal

---

11. See Shaun Griffin, 'Covid-19: "Huge rise" in deaths at home is not fully explained by virus, say experts', *British Medical Journal* (27 May, 2020).

12. See Alvina Lai, Amitava Banerjee, Laura Pasea and Spiros Denaxas, 'Estimating excess mortality in people with cancer and multimorbidity in the COVID-19 emergency', *Research Gate* (28 April 2020).

amount of free acute beds at that time of year?[13] In other words, was the lockdown of the UK, which included the radical reprioritising of the National Health Service on 17 March, and which led to the discharge of up to 25,000 hospital patients without being tested for SARS-CoV-2 into care homes, also responsible for these nearly 18,000 anticipated deaths, which have not yet appeared on any record of increased overall mortality?[14]

The number of deaths of care home residents, England and Wales, from 28 December 2019 to 1 May 2020, registered up to 9 May 2020

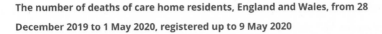

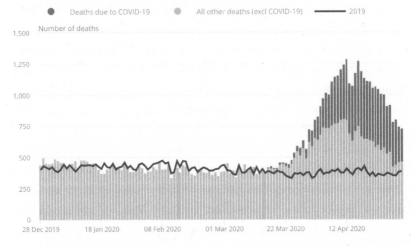

Source: Office for National Statistics

A further explanation comes from the Office for National Statistics, which in its report on 'Deaths involving COVID-19 in the care sector, England and Wales', published on 15 May, revealed that there were 83 per cent more deaths from dementia than usual in April this year, with charities reporting that a reduction in

---

13. See Dave West, 'NHS hospitals have four times more empty beds than usual', *HSJ* (13 April, 2020).

14. See the letter dated 17 March, 2020, sent by Sir Simon Stevens, NHS Chief Executive, and Amanda Pritchard, NHS Chief Operating Officer, to Chief executives of all NHS trusts and foundation trusts, CCG Accountable Officers, GP practices and Primary Care Networks Providers of community health services; and Samuel Lovett, 'Coronavirus: 25,000 patients discharged into care homes without being tested, report finds', *The Independent* (12 June, 2020).

essential medical care and family visits are responsible.[15] A survey of 128 care homes by the Alzheimer's Society corroborated this, reporting that 79 per cent said a lack of social contact is causing a deterioration in the health and well-being of residents with dementia, and with three-quarters of care homes reporting that General Practitioners have been reluctant to visit residents.[16] Not only did a quarter of those whose deaths were attributed to COVID-19 have dementia — making it the most common pre-existing disease in such deaths — but in April there were a further 9,429 deaths from dementia and Alzheimer's disease alone in England and 462 in Wales, 83 per cent higher than usual in England, and 54 per cent higher in Wales.

Finally, another explanation is that, after months of fearmongering backed by daily reports of mounting deaths out of all context or definition designed to terrorise the British public into acquiescence to the lockdown, those at most risk from COVID-19 have been too terrified to go to hospital when they should have for fear of catching the virus, with visits to Accident and Emergency wards in April down by 50 per cent.[17]

A measure of this is the increase in anxiety under the lockdown. In the most recent survey by the Office of National Statistics of the social impact of the coronavirus 'crisis', conducted between 14 and 17 May 2020, 72 per cent of adults in Great Britain were 'concerned' about the effect the coronavirus 'crisis' was having on their life.[18] This included concerns about our lack of freedom and independence, about our inability to make plans, about our ability or otherwise to work, and about our health, well-being and access to medical care. This rose to 73 per cent of those over the age of 70, and 82 per cent of those with underlying health conditions. Extraordinarily, 41 per cent of adults said they felt 'unsafe' or 'very unsafe' when leaving their home because of COVID-19; while for those with

---

15. See Office for National Statistics, 'Deaths involving COVID-19 in the care sector, England and Wales: deaths occurring up to 1 May 2020 and registered up to 9 May 2020 (provisional)' (15 May, 2020).

16. See Hannah Devlin, 'Extra 10,000 dementia deaths in England and Wales in April, *The Guardian* (5 June, 2020).

17. See Sarah Marsh, 'Fears that seriously ill people are avoiding A&E as numbers drop', *The Guardian* (27 March, 2020); and Kate Ng, 'Coronavirus: NHS urges people to go to hospital for emergencies as A&E visits fall by 50 per cent', *The Independent* (25 April, 2020).

18. See Office for National Statistics, 'Coronavirus and the social impacts on Great Britain: 22 May 2020' (22 May, 2020).

an underlying health condition this rose to 54 per cent. As a result, 1 in 7 people surveyed said they had not left home for any reason in the previous week, rising to 1 in 3 of those aged over 70 or with underlying health conditions. 91 per cent of adults said they are avoiding contact with older or vulnerable adults, with 11 per cent saying the people they are avoiding are those to whom they provide care. 43 per cent of people felt their well-being was being affected, rising to 55 per cent of those with underlying health conditions. Over 32 per cent of adults said they were experiencing high levels of anxiety, and 23 per cent reported they felt alone. Once again, these effects are increasing among those over 70 years of age or with underlying health conditions.

This fear, too, and the consequences it is having on mortality rates, is a product of the lockdown, for which the UK Government and the British media — the latter of which have behaved like vultures around the COVID-19 carcass — must bear full responsibility (which they will undoubtedly shirk).

Since first publishing this article on 2 June, a study titled 'An Improved Measure of Deaths Due to COVID-19 in England and Wales', published on 25 June, has found that the actual number of deaths caused by COVID-19 during the period studied (from the week ending 17 or 24 April to the week ending 8 May) were between 4,670 and 4,727 fewer deaths per week (54-63 per cent lower) than the official figures for excess deaths.[19] The authors conclude that, primarily due to the reduction in provision of and access to cancer and cardiac treatments, compounded by reduced attendance at and admission to Accident and Emergency wards, lockdown 'resulted in more, not less, deaths'.

More recently, on 15 July, the Office for National Statistics published its report titled 'Direct and Indirect Impacts of COVID-19 on Excess Deaths and Morbidity'.[20] This estimates the following number of excess deaths due to changes to health and social care implemented in response to the coronavirus:

---

19. See Karligash Glass, Professor of Financial Economics at the University of Loughborough, Anthony Glass, Professor of Managerial Economics at the University of Sheffield, Sam Williams, founder and Director of Economic Insight, and Alasdair Crookes, Consultant at Economic Insight, 'An Improved Measure of Deaths Due to COVID-19 in England and Wales', *Social Science Research Network* (posted 2 July, 2020).

20. See Office for National Statistics, 'Direct and Indirect Impacts of COVID-19 on Excess Deaths and Morbidity: Executive Summary for the Department of Health and Social Care, the Government's Actuary Department and Home Office,' (15 July 2020).

- *Changes to emergency care:* 6,000 existing excess deaths in March and April 2020, with an additional 10,000 excess deaths if emergency care in hospitals continues to be reduced this year.
- *Changes to adult social care:* 10,000 non-COVID-19 excess deaths of care home residents in March and April 2020, with an additional 16,000 excess deaths over the whole year.
- *Changes to elective care:* could equate to 12,500 excess deaths over 5 years, with many non-urgent elective treatments having been postponed or cancelled by the NHS.
- *Changes to primary and community care:* could result in 1,400 excess deaths, with cancer diagnoses, GP referrals and emergency representations stopped or reduced.
- *Medium-term impact of a lockdown-induced recession:* 18,000 excess deaths occurring between 2-5 years following the lockdown due to increased heart disease and mental health problems.
- *Long-term impact of a lockdown-induced recession:* 15,000 excess deaths for younger people entering the labour market a few years before, during, and within a few years after the recession.

This adds up to a potential 88,900 excess deaths resulting from the UK Government's ongoing response to the coronavirus. In addition, the ONS estimates 17,000 excess deaths per year for as long as GDP remains at a low level indexed to multiple deprivation.

5. Collateral Damage

But an increase in mortality rate is not the only measure of the effects of this lockdown. Just as the excess deaths from cancelled operations, stopped treatment, the effects of increased anxiety and isolation on elderly people living alone or in care homes with serious illnesses, suicide in the face of withdrawn help and collapsed futures, and people too terrified to visit Accident and Emergency wards, will far outstrip the current number of deaths in the months and years to come, so the full impact of the lockdown of the UK will only be felt in the 'New Normal' the Government has prepared for us.

The document titled 'Our plan to rebuild: The UK Government's COVID-19 recovery strategy', published on 5 May, revealed that the Office for Budget Responsibility has estimated that the direct cost to the Government of the lockdown could rise above £100 billion in 2020-21.[21] Under the Government's Coronavirus Job Retention Scheme, 28 per cent of workers have been furloughed across all industries. Paying 80 per cent of the normal wages of 10 million workers up to £2,500 per month is currently costing the Government an estimated £14 billion per month. Running the scheme until the end of July will cost £63 billion, with the extension till the end of October announced by the Chancellor adding another £31 billion. Finally, the Self-employed Income Support Scheme has so far added a further £10.5 billion. In addition to these sums, support of approximately £330 billion in the form of guarantees and loans, equivalent to 15 per cent of GDP, has been made available to UK businesses. In April alone, the UK public sector borrowed £62.1 billion, almost as much as the £62.7 billion it borrowed in the whole of the last financial year. By the end of April, UK public sector debt was just under £1.9 trillion, equivalent to nearly 98 per cent of Gross Domestic Product.

In its latest bulletin on 'Coronavirus and the latest indicators for the UK economy and society', published on 28 May, the Office for National Statistics reported that 18 per cent of businesses had paused trading.[22] 79 per cent of businesses in the UK had applied to the Coronavirus Job Retention Scheme. 42 per cent of businesses had less than 6 months of cash reserves, rising to 58 per cent of those who has paused trading, while around 4 per cent of businesses who had not permanently ceased trading said they had no cash reserves.

The record fall in retail sales has continued, with volumes dropping by 18.1 per cent in April compared with 5.2 per cent the previous month. Clothing sales declined by 50.2 per cent, having already fallen by 34.9 per cent the previous month. Sales at food stores also declined by 4.1 per cent as lockdown measures were introduced. 72 per cent of exporting businesses in the UK said they are exporting less than normal, while 59 per cent of importers report that imports are lower than normal, with, respectively, 81 per cent and 80 per cent reporting a reduction in trade. In line with Government guidance, industries employing 11 per

---

21. See HM Government, 'Our plan to rebuild: The UK Government's COVID-19 recovery strategy' (May 2020).

22. See Office for National Statistics, 'Coronavirus and the latest indicators for the UK economy and society' (28 May, 2020).

cent of the UK workforce have largely shut down. Between 6 and 19 April, 23 per cent of businesses had paused operations, and 47 per cent of workers were working remotely.

As a result of these measures, from January to March 2020 the total number of hours worked dropped by 12.4 million hours (1.2 per cent) compared with the previous year. This was the largest annual fall in a decade. This fall in hours worked occurred as lockdown measures were introduced, with average hours around 25 per cent below usual levels in the final week of March. There was also a 1.2 per cent annual decline in the number of paid employees; with 637,000 job vacancies between February and April, 170,000 fewer than in the three months to January 2020, and 210,000 fewer than a year earlier. The total job vacancies are the lowest since the first quarter of 2014, and the quarterly fall is a series record since 2001.

In its 'Monetary Policy Report' for May 2020, the Bank of England forecast that the UK's GDP would be close to 30 per cent lower in the second quarter of 2020 than it was at the end of 2019, that the economy would shrink by 25 per cent in the second quarter of the year, and could fall by 14 per cent in 2020.[23] That's more than twice the 6 per cent by which the UK economy shrunk in the 2008 recession during the Global Financial Crisis.[24] The Bank also forecast that unemployment is expected to more than double, from 4 per cent to a 26-year high of 9 per cent in 2021.

The latest claimant figures from the Office for National Statistics show almost 2.1 million people claimed unemployment benefit in April 2020, an increase of 856,500 from March 2020.[25] Figures from the Department for Work and Pensions show 1.5 million claims for Universal Credit were made between 13 March and 9 April 2020, six times more than were made in the same period last year, and the most in a single month since its introduction in April 2013.[26] This led to 1.2 million starts on Universal Credit. Despite the 300,000 denied claims, the overall number

---

23. See Bank of England, 'Monetary Policy Report' (May 2020).

24. See Office for National Statistics, 'The 2008 recession ten years on' (30 April, 2018).

25. See Office for National Statistics, 'Claimant Count : K02000001 UK : People : SA : Thousands' (19 May, 2020).

26. See Department for Work and Pensions, 'Universal Credit: 29 April 2013 to 9 April 2020' (19 May, 2020).

of people on Universal Credit increased in April by 40 per cent over the previous month to 4.2 million.

Perhaps the last word on the economic consequences of the Government imposed lockdown should go to the *Financial Times*, which reported that this year will experience the 'fastest and deepest' recession in the UK since the Great Frost of 1709, when Europe experienced the coldest winter for the past 500 years.[27]

6. The Worst-Case Scenario

The response to all this, of course, is that if the UK Government hadn't imposed, and the UK public hadn't observed, the lockdown of the UK, the deaths from COVID-19 would be worse — many times worse, even — and perhaps reaching the figures published on 16 March by the now discredited Professor Neil Ferguson of Imperial College London, whose report on the 'Impact of non-pharmaceutical interventions (NPIs) to reduce COVID-19 mortality and healthcare demand' predicted 550,000 deaths in the UK if we did nothing, 250,000 if we isolated the vulnerable and quarantined the infected, and 20,000 if the Government that commissioned his estimates locked down the country.[28]

This is an argument based on speculative predictions of the worst-case scenario based on computer simulations in which every minor change in input produces huge numerical changes in outcome. As an example of which, Ferguson's estimation that 30 per cent of all those hospitalised with COVID-19 would require critical care was reportedly based on nothing more than a personal communication from a clinician who had been in China at the outbreak of the virus.[29] On such back-of-the-envelope estimates were the Government's fears of an overwhelmed NHS based. Indeed, even Ferguson's report concluded that 'No public health intervention with such disruptive effects on society has been

---

27. Chris Giles, 'BoE warns UK set to enter worst recession for 300 years', *Financial Times* (7 May, 2020).

28. See Neil Ferguson, et al., 'Report 9. Impact of non-pharmaceutical interventions (NPIs) to reduce COVID-19 mortality and healthcare demand', Imperial College London (16 March, 2020); and David Richards and Konstantin Boudnik, 'Neil Ferguson's Imperial model could be the most devastating software mistake of all time', *The Telegraph* (16 May, 2020).

29. See Paul Taylor, 'Susceptible, Infectious, Recovered', *London Review of Books* (7 May, 2020).

previously attempted for such a long duration of time. How populations and societies will respond remains unclear.'

But although there is no way of knowing whether the number of deaths caused by COVID-19 and not merely with it mentioned on the death certificate would have increased if the UK wasn't under lockdown, or whether, to the contrary, the overall mortality rate, including the unexplained excess deaths, would be less than it has been, let alone will be in the future, there are, nonetheless, two ways to estimate what may have happened. First, we can ask what effect the lockdown has had on the number of deaths in the UK from respiratory diseases other than COVID-19 that might be expected to have dropped due to the prohibition on leaving our homes without a 'reasonable excuse' and the social distancing measures imposed on us when we do. And, second, we can ask what has happened in other countries that have not imposed a lockdown of the severity of that in the UK.

The answer to the first of these questions is the easiest. The lockdown of the UK was imposed by the Government on 23 March. According to the Office for National Statistics, since the week ending 3 April, when we might expect the first deaths caused by a virus contracted since the lockdown to be registered, and 22 May, the last week for which we have data, there have been 11,403 deaths in England and Wales where the underlying cause was respiratory disease (ICD-10 J00-J99).[30] Over the same 8-week period last year there were 11,006 deaths with the same underlying cause; in 2018 there were 11,650 deaths; in 2017 there were 10,455 deaths; in 2016 there were 12,057; and in 2015 there were 11,646. Over the previous five years, between 2015 and 2019, the average number of deaths between weeks 14 and 21 of the year in which the underlying cause was respiratory disease was 11,362. The obvious question in response to these figures is, if the lockdown of the UK has been successful at saving lives threatened by an infectious and contagious virus, why are there 41 more deaths this year in which the underlying cause was respiratory disease?

Now, one answer to that is that on some death certificates both respiratory disease and COVID-19 is written; and that the large number of deaths attributed to COVID-19 will therefore mean an increase in death certificates mentioning

---

30. See Office for National Statistics, 'Deaths registered weekly in England and Wales, provisional (2020 edition of this dataset up to week ending 1 January 2021)'.

respiratory disease. However, this would be the wrong answer. The ONS makes it clear that, while COVID-19 (ICD-10 U07.1 and U07.2) merely has to be mentioned on the death certificate in order to appear in its breakdown of overall deaths, respiratory disease must be included as the 'underlying cause' to appear on the same. While the presence of COVID-19 deaths in the increase in overall mortality has clearly been hugely exaggerated by this method of calculation — which is a direct result of changes to disease taxonomy by the Department of Health and Social Care and official guidelines from the World Health Organization on filling out death certificates — the number of deaths in which respiratory disease is the underlying cause has not. COVID-19 can appear on the death certificate of someone in whose death respiratory disease was the underlying cause, but COVID-19 can't increase the number of deaths in which the underlying cause was respiratory disease.

The only logical conclusion that can be drawn from this is that the lockdown has had no effect on lessening the mortality rate from influenza, pneumonia, bronchitis, emphysema, asthma and other chronic obstructive pulmonary diseases included under this taxonomy. It is equally logical to deduce from this that the lockdown has had no effect on the rate of infection or contagion of non-COVID-19 respiratory diseases spread by social contact, such as seasonal influenza and pneumonia. It is, therefore, logical to conclude that, despite the Prime Minister claiming that the lockdown has saved 'half a million people' in the UK from COVID-19, there is absolutely no evidence to support this claim. There is, however, plenty of evidence to support the counter accusation that the lockdown has already directly or indirectly killed many thousands of British citizens and is likely to kill thousands more in the future.

7. Comparative Government Responses

Answering the second question is a little more complex. The gap between total excess deaths and deaths attributed to COVID-19 is not confined to the UK, but has appeared in other countries under similarly severe lockdowns. According to a regularly updated article in *The Economist* titled 'Tracking covid-19 excess deaths across countries', as of 27 May, Britain had 13,802 unexplained deaths in excess of those officially attributed to COVID-19 (23 per cent of the total), Italy had 11,853 (an extraordinary 49 per cent of excess deaths), Netherlands 3,745 (40 per cent), Spain 3,142 (10 per cent), and France 1,237 (5 per cent); while outside of Europe, New York City alone had 3,365 (14 per cent).[31]

Helpfully for us, the Oxford COVID-19 Government Response Tracker (OxCGRT) systematically collects information on several different common policy responses that governments have taken, records the stringency of each policy on a scale to reflect the extent of government action, and aggregates these scores into 17 policy indices.[32] These are divided into the following three categories: containment and closure policies; economic policies; and health system policies. This data has been used to produce interactive global maps tracking 'Policy Responses to the Coronavirus Pandemic', which are available on the website *Our World in Data*.[33] These chart nine metrics of where and when the following policies of 'lockdown' were implemented: 1) school closures, 2) workplaces closures, 3) cancellation of public events, 4) restrictions on public gatherings, 5) public information campaigns, 6) stay-at-home restrictions, 7) public transport closures, 8) restrictions on internal movement, and 9) international travel controls. Together, these policies produce a Government Response Stringency Index ranging from 0 to 100, with 100 being the most stringent.

On 16 March, when the Government imposed Social Distancing measures, the UK registered 20.37 on this Stringency Index. On 21 March the index rose to 29.63, and the following day it rose again to 35.19. Then, on 23 March, the lockdown was implemented, and the index doubled to 70.37. Three days later, on 26 March, The Health Protection (Coronavirus, Restrictions) (England) Regulations 2020 were made law, and the index rose to 75.93, where it stayed until 12 May, after which the Government's 'sketch of a roadmap for reopening society' came into effect.[34] From 13 May, when workers were encouraged by the Government to

31. See 'Tracking covid-19 excess deaths across countries', *The Economist* (last published 20 October, 2021).

32. See University of Oxford, Blavatnik School of Government, 'COVID-19 Government Response Tracker' (March 2020-December 2022).

33. See Edouard Mathieu, Hannah Ritchie, Lucas Rodés-Guirao, Cameron Appel, Daniel Gavrilov, Charlie Giattino, Joe Hasell, Bobbie Macdonald, Saloni Dattani, Diana Beltekian, Esteban Ortiz-Ospina and Max Roser, 'Policy Responses to the Coronavirus Pandemic', *Our World in Data*.

34. See UK Statutory Instruments, 'The Health Protection (Coronavirus, Restrictions) (England) Regulations 2020' (26 March, 2020); and Boris Johnson, 'Prime Minister's statement on coronavirus (COVID-19): 10 May 2020' (published 10 May, 2020).

return to work and UK citizens were permitted to leave home, the index dropped to 66.67, where it has remained since. It was over these 7 weeks of lockdown, when the stringency index of the UK Government's response to the coronavirus 'crisis' was at its highest, that the UK economy was forced into the worse depression in over 300 years, and 12,394 unexplained excess deaths and perhaps 35,688 excess deaths without established causality from COVID-19 occurred.

How equivalent lockdown measures affected the economies of other countries is beyond the scope of this article; but we can compare countries with a similar index rating and look at their official death toll from COVID-19. As I concluded in my article on 'Manufacturing Consensus', in the UK, at least, the calculation of these deaths has become almost meaningless, so loose is the criteria for counting them; so comparing the wildly inaccurate figures in the UK with the possibly as inaccurate figures in other countries is never going to arrive at any accurate calculation. However, so conclusive is the evidence from countries with a far lower stringency index than the UK that the huge degree of inaccuracy in how the UK Government calculates and reports so-called 'COVID-19 deaths' doesn't matter.

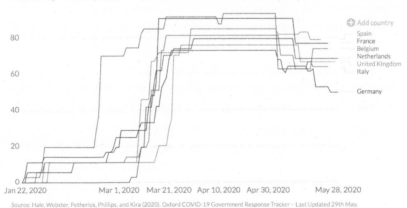

COVID-19: Government Response Stringency Index, Jan 22, 2020 to May 28, 2020

The Government Response Stringency Index is a composite measure based on nine response indicators including school closures, workplace closures, and travel bans, rescaled to a value from 0 to 100 (100 = strictest response).

Source: Hale, Webster, Petherick, Phillips, and Kira (2020). Oxford COVID-19 Government Response Tracker – Last Updated 29th May.

Source: Oxford COVID-19 Government Response Tracker, University of Oxford

Let's start with European countries with a similar Government Response Stringency Index to the UK and similar levels of infrastructure and health services. Between 17 March and 10 May France had an index rating of 90.74, even higher than the UK, since when it has dropped to 76.85. Italy, which on 4 March rose to 74.54, comparable to UK under lockdown, by 12 April had risen to 93.52, where it remained until 4 May. Spain, which on 17 March had an index of 71.76, by 30 March had hit 85.19, where it remained until 4 May, when it dropped to 81.94, and currently sits on 79.17. Finally, on 22 March Germany had an index rating of 73.15, remaining there until 4 May, when it dropped to 68.06. It has since dropped to an even 50.00. All these European countries, therefore, have been under as severe or more stringent lockdown measures for as long as or longer than the UK. The exception is Germany, which has a slightly less high stringency index than the UK, but for almost the exact same period of time.

Most people in the UK will be familiar by now with how these measures have fared in their respective countries. I won't mention here the number of so-called 'cases', which refer not to people with COVID-19 but to those infected with SARS-CoV-2, and which is a measure almost entirely dictated by the number of tests conducted, which varies hugely from country to country. However, according to the official figures, as of today, 2 June, the countries with the highest number of deaths attributed to COVID-19 are, in order, the UK with 39,045; Italy with 33,475; France with 28,833; and Spain with 27,127.[35] These are, of course, the European countries with the largest populations, so we might expect them to have the highest number of deaths; but they also have the highest number of deaths per capita, with Spain on 580 deaths per million of the population, the UK on 575, Italy 554 and France 442. Only Belgium, a far smaller country with 9,505 official COVID-19 deaths, exceeds these proportions with 820 deaths per million; and between March 20 and 4 May Belgium had an index rating of 81.48, and currently sits on 74.07, so lockdown doesn't appear to have done it any good either. While the Netherlands, with 5,967 deaths attributed to COVID-19 at 348 per million of the population, on 23 March had an index rating of 74.07, rising to 79.63 between 31 March and 3 May, and currently sits on 68.52. So lockdown also doesn't appear to have done it any good; but it has done a lot of harm, with 3,745 unexplained excess deaths as of 27 May.

---

35. See Worldometer, 'COVID-19 Coronavirus Pandemic'.

The exception, again, is Germany, which with the highest population in Europe has an official toll of 8,618 'COVID-19 deaths' at 103 deaths per million people. But far from proving the effectiveness of lockdown, Germany's record suggests that SARS-CoV-2 is nothing like as virulent as the governments of the UK, Italy, France and Spain are claiming, and that the increased overall mortality rate in the countries supposedly worst-hit by COVID-19 have other causes, which Germany — with nearly 3 times as many hospital beds per 100,000 people compared to the UK and 4 times as many intensive care beds per 100,000 people as the NHS — has managed to negate.[36] In the complete and unexplained absence of accurate figures establishing the actual cause of deaths officially attributed to COVID-19 in these countries, it's impossible to be certain; but taken together, what these figures strongly suggest is not only that lockdown across these countries, the worst affected in Europe, did nothing to slow the rate of infection from SARS-CoV-2, but that these measures most likely increased the case fatality rate from COVID-19. It undoubtedly increased the overall mortality rate in these countries.

8. Alternatives to Lockdown

But what of the countries that have not imposed lockdowns, or not to the same degree of severity as the UK? What do they have to tell us about the negative and unnecessary effects of the Government's decision?

Further evidence in support of the ineffectiveness of lockdown comes, of course, from Sweden. Despite immense pressure from the international community (which is to say, the USA) and the World Health Organization, Sweden's Government Response Stringency Index has never risen above 40.74, which it only reached on 24 April. This was in response to a sudden increase in mortality on the 21 and 22 of April, when the deaths of 357 people were attributed to COVID-19. For the three weeks prior to that, starting from 4 April, it was 37.96; and before that 32.41. With a population of just over 10 million, Sweden has an official total of 4,468 'COVID-19 deaths' as of 2 June, at 433 deaths per million of the population. Despite being below Spain, the UK, Italy and France, so hysterical

---

36. See Fred Roeder, 'What the NHS can learn from Germany's Hospital System', *Comment Central* (8 April, 2020).

have been the arguments for the benefits of lockdown that the Swedish Government was accused of 'playing Russian roulette' with the lives of its citizens for leaving bars, restaurants and schools open but limiting public gatherings to 50 people, advising citizens to avoid non-essential travel on public transport, and encouraging the sick and elderly to stay at home, but not shutting down the economy.[37] In response to this accusation, Anders Tegnell, the State Epidemiologist of the Public Health Agency of Sweden to whose advice the Government has listened, responded that, to the contrary, it was the UK and other nations imposing lockdowns that were indulging in an experiment that had no precedent in national responses to previous viral epidemics.[38] Where Sweden has admitted failing is in not protecting the elderly and sick in care homes where, up to 14 May, 48.9 per cent of all deaths attributed to COVID-19 were resident. In this it shares something with England and Wales, where 11,650 of the 41,220 deaths attributed to COVID-19 by 15 May, 28.2 per cent of the total, occurred in care homes.

What this comparison suggests is that the less restrictive guidelines issued by the Swedish Government and the severe lockdown imposed by the UK Government both failed to protect those most at risk from COVID-19. However, the far higher mortality rate in the UK outside of care homes compared to Sweden also suggests, once again, that the lockdown caused more deaths than it saved. In an article titled 'The Invisible Pandemic', published on 5 May in the medical journal *The Lancet*, Johan Giesecke, the Swedish physician and Professor Emeritus at the Karolinska Institute in Stockholm, and the former Swedish State Epidemiologist, wrote:

> It has become clear that a hard lockdown does not protect old and frail people living in care homes — a population the lockdown was designed to protect. Neither does it decrease mortality from COVID-19, which is evident when comparing the UK's experience with that of other European countries.

---

37. See Jon Henley, 'Swedish PM warned over "Russian roulette-style" Covid-19 strategy', *The Guardian* (23 March, 2020).

38. See Richard Orange, 'Will Sweden's herd immunity experiment pay off?', *Prospect* (1 May, 2020).

PCR testing and some straightforward assumptions indicate that, as of April 29, 2020, more than half a million people in Stockholm county, Sweden, which is about 20–25% of the population, have been infected. 98–99% of these people are probably unaware or uncertain of having had the infection; they either had symptoms that were severe, but not severe enough for them to go to a hospital and get tested, or no symptoms at all.

These facts have led me to the following conclusions. Everyone will be exposed to severe acute respiratory syndrome coronavirus 2, and most people will become infected. There is very little we can do to prevent this spread: a lockdown might delay severe cases for a while, but once restrictions are eased, cases will reappear. I expect that, when we count the number of deaths from COVID-19 in each country in 1 year from now, the figures will be similar, regardless of measures taken.[39]

The most important difference between Sweden and the UK, however, is neither the increase in overall mortality nor the number of deaths officially attributed to COVID-19, but the respective state of their economies. All the evidence points to the conclusion that, higher as the percentage of deaths already is in the UK (575 per million of the population) compared to Sweden (443 per million), the UK will continue to ruin and lose lives to the negative economic effects of the lockdown for years to come, while Sweden's economy has suffered far less in comparison. Undoubtedly, as a high-export economy, Sweden will feel the effects of the rest of Europe's panic; but the country's statistics office has just reported adjusted GDP growth of 0.4 per cent for the first quarter of 2020.[40] And while the National Institute for Economic Research has predicted a 7 per cent reduction in Sweden's economy this year, this is half the 14 per cent the Bank of England has predicted for the UK.[41] What is certain is that the UK, for all the opprobrium our arrogant and fearmongering media has flung at Sweden, has nothing to say to anyone about how they should or shouldn't respond to the coronavirus.

---

39. Johan Giesecke, 'The Invisible Pandemic', *The Lancet* (5 May, 2020).

40. See Statistics Sweden, 'GDP largely unchanged in the first quarter of 2020' (29 May, 2020).

41. See Sam Meredith, 'Sweden's economy actually grew in the first quarter after it opted against a full virus lockdown', *CNBC* (29 May, 2020).

Even more damaging to the claims for the efficacy of lockdown are the examples of Japan and Taiwan.[42] The former, with a population of 126.5 million, 45 per cent of which live in three densely populated cities, has attributed just 892 deaths to COVID-19 at a rate of 7 deaths per million of the population; while the latter, with a population of 23.8 million, has attributed just 7 deaths to COVID-19 at a rate of 0.3 per million. Yet both these countries, situated off the coast of China and therefore among the first countries to report cases of infection (respectively, on 16 and 21 January), have employed some of the lightest measures in the world, barely warranting the term 'lockdown'. Rising by steady increments to 43.52 on 2 March, Japan's Government Response Stringency Index took until 16 April to rise to 47.22, at a time when the UK's was at 75.93. Social distancing was encouraged but not imposed by emergency regulations, and music venues and gyms were closed; but bars and restaurants stayed open, although not as late, and people still went to work. On 25 May, after 10 days at an index rating lowered still further to 40.74, Japan's Prime Minister announced the end of its State of Emergency, without a lockdown ever having been imposed.

The Taiwanese Government has been even less severe. After an initial rise to 30.56 on 2 February, its index rating had dropped to 19.44 by 25 February, rose again on 19 March to 27.78, where it stayed until 8 May, when it dropped down to where it remains now at 22.22. Throughout these months its citizens kept working and its economy kept working. This isn't to say that Taiwan hasn't introduced programmes to track and trace its citizens via their mobile phones, used monitors to test their temperatures when entering public buildings, offices and schools, and issued severe fines for non-compliance; but none of these intrusive measures, which our Government is in the course of introducing in the UK, will have done anything to stop the spread of the virus or reduce the infection fatality rate from SARS-CoV-2.[43] Quarantining was imposed, and with just 443 official 'cases' this appears to have been the key decision in slowing the rate of infection; but this was done early, and without a lockdown being imposed. In the UK, by comparison, we are imposing the same measures but in reverse, first forcing the economy into an unnecessary depression that will be felt for a

---

42. See Philip Patrick, 'Japan's COVID success is a mystery', *The Spectator* (27 May, 2020).

43. See Cindy Sui, 'In Taiwan, the coronavirus pandemic is playing out very differently. What does life without a lockdown look like?', *NBC News* (23 April, 2020).

generation, then ostensibly attempting to trace and contain a highly infectious virus that has been in the country for at least 5 months.

COVID-19: Government Response Stringency Index, Jan 21, 2020 to May 27, 2020

The Government Response Stringency Index is a composite measure based on nine response indicators including school closures, workplace closures, and travel bans, rescaled to a value from 0 to 100 (100 = strictest response).

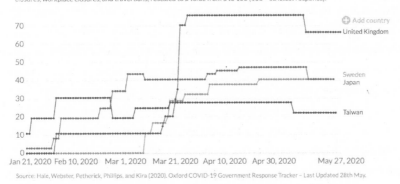

Source: Hale, Webster, Petherick, Phillips, and Kira (2020). Oxford COVID-19 Government Response Tracker – Last Updated 28th May.

Source: Oxford COVID-19 Government Response Tracker, University of Oxford

It's important to remember, too, that the Government Response Stringency Index is an indication of policies, not of their implementation or effectiveness. In India, where 1.3 billion people have officially been under a lockdown with an index rating of 100 — the highest possible — since 22 March, marginally dropping to 96.3 on 20 April and currently on 79.17, 78 million people live in slums and tenements, 18 million children live on the streets, 13.7 million households live in informal settlements, and 1.7 million people don't have a home of any sort in which to be confined. Despite these conditions, which severely restrict the imposition of a lockdown, there have been only 5,612 deaths officially attributed to COVID-19 at a rate of 4 deaths per million of the population, since the first official death on March 12. And out of the 101,487 'cases' of infection that have had an outcome so far, 95,875 — 94 per cent — have recovered.

Is this really the outcome of a deadly virus sweeping for 3 months through a country in which 640 million people live in poverty and 69 per cent of all Indian houses have only one or two rooms, making quarantining measures impossible?[44]

44. See Ritwika Mitra, 'Over 1.7 million homeless residents across India struggle to fight coronavirus', *The New Indian Express* (23 March, 2020).

Africa, a similarly impoverished continent, which Bill Gates recently described falling into disaster with a '2 per cent overall death rate', has rather inconveniently reported just 4,344 deaths attributed to COVID-19 out of a population of 1.34 billion (or 0.0003 per cent).[45] Is this evidence of a civilisation-threatening virus? Or is it, to the contrary, further proof of what the Centers for Disease Control and Prevention in the US are belatedly establishing is an overall infection fatality rate between 0.2 percent and 0.3 percent, compared to the 0.9 per cent assumed by Professor Neil Ferguson in the report justifying the lockdown of the UK?[46]

Proclaimed a 'mystery' by the British press otherwise insistent on imposing 'the best scientific opinion' on the British people whatever the cost, it is impossible for the coronavirus to be anything like as virulent as we have been led by the nose to believe and leave Japan, Taiwan, India and Africa almost untouched relative to their overall mortality rate.[47] It's a principle of science that the natural world behaves in repetitive ways which, studied for long enough, reveal its mysteries, but only to the observer who doesn't come to the microscope, so to speak, with their head full of preconceptions, and above all when they're not blinded by propaganda serving the political ends of the Government. We've been lied to — a lie that may one day kill as many people as the lie that has led to the death of hundreds of thousands of Iraqis as the result of an equally fictitious reason to go to war against an enemy that did not threaten the UK, but whose defeat would make the perpetrators of the war richer and more powerful. I want to end, therefore, by looking at who is getting rich and who is gaining power at whose expense from the coronavirus lie.

9. Spreading Inequality

None of what I've written above is to say that the coronavirus 'crisis', which is a product of government reactions to SARS-CoV-2, won't negatively impact the

---

45. See Bill Gates, 'Transcript: Bill Gates speaks to the FT about the global fight against coronavirus', *Financial Times* (9 April, 2020); and Abdur Rahman Alfa Shaban, 'Africa COVID-19 stats: 874,036 cases; 18,498 deaths; 524,557 recoveries', *Africa News* (29 July, 2020).

46. See Jacob Sullum, 'The CDC's New "Best Estimate" Implies a COVID-19 Infection Fatality Rate Below 0.3%', *Reason* (24 May, 2020).

47. See Soutik Biswas, 'India coronavirus: The "mystery" of low Covid-19 death rates', *BBC News* (28 April, 2020).

poorest and most vulnerable members of society. The 'collateral damage' from the so-called war on COVID-19, in both lives lost and economic impact, has not been suffered evenly. Despite the Government's worn-out mantra — dutifully repeated by an obedient public — that 'we're all in this together', the negative effects of the lockdown have been, and will continue to be, borne by the poorest members of the UK. Coronavirus is named after the crown-like spikes that bind to the host cell, and parasitical aristocrats, landowners and landlords continue to receive rents on their land and properties from households, businesses and workers prohibited by the Government from making a living on them. But the exacerbation of economic inequality goes farther than a rentier society. While many capitalists will lose fortunes to this unprecedented and extended cessation of global trade, we can expect them to recuperate those losses, just as they did after the financial crisis of 2008, from the poorest and most vulnerable members of UK society through policies of fiscal austerity that will make the last 12 years look like an orgy of public expenditure. Indeed, since I published this article on 2 June, it has been reported that UK-registered billionaires have seen their wealth grow by 20 per cent during the lockdown, with the 45 richest individuals increasing their wealth from £121.57 billion to £146.61 billion in just three months, all while claiming hundreds of millions of pounds of public money for the bailout of their businesses and the furlough of thousands of workers facing the sack when that funding is withdrawn.[48]

The Resolution Foundation, an independent think-tank focused on improving living standards for workers on low to middle incomes, has produced reports on both 'The effects of the coronavirus crisis on workers', published on 16 May, and 'Coping with housing costs during the coronavirus crisis', published on 30 May.[49] This is not my research, so I will only report its findings; but these show that — bad as the forecasts for 'the nation' are, and eagerly as the Government's package of fiscal support has been greeted by liberals as the return of 'socialism' — the economic costs of the lockdown are already being distributed unequally across the classes.

---

48. See Martin Williams, 'UK billionaires see personal wealth grow by £25bn during pandemic lockdown', *The Herald Scotland* (14 June, 2020).

49. See Laura Gardiner and Hannah Slaughter, 'The effects of the coronavirus crisis on workers', *The Resolution Foundation* (16 May, 2020); and Lindsay Judge, 'Coping with housing costs during the coronavirus crisis', *The Resolution Foundation* (30 May, 2020).

From online interviews with over 6,000 employees aged 18-65, plus fieldwork undertaken between 6-11 May, the first report found that 30 per cent of the lowest-earning fifth of employees have either been furloughed or lost their jobs, and 22 per cent of the next lowest-earning fifth, compared to 9 per cent of the top-earning fifth of employees. This discrepancy gets greater for different types of work. 38 per cent of unsalaried workers, 32 per cent of workers with variable hours, 28 per cent of workers on zero-hour contracts, and 22 per cent of agency workers, have been furloughed or lost their jobs under the lockdown, with a huge 19 per cent of workers on a temporary contract losing their jobs outright. And while, respectively, just 23, 17 and 25 per cent of furloughed workers in the bottom three fifths of earners are receiving 100 per cent of their pay, in the second highest-earning fifth that figure jumps to 31 per cent.

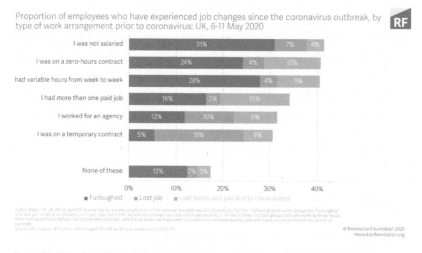

Source: Resolution Foundation analysis of YouGov, Adults aged 18 to 65 and the coronavirus (COVID-19)

Things are even worse for the self-employed, with only 39 per cent having applied or planning to apply to the Self-employed Income Support Scheme. By comparison, 83 per cent in the highest-earning fifth of employees were currently working some or all of the time from home last month, and 60 per cent expect to work from home more after the lockdown than they did before. Unsurprisingly, expectations of the future are low, with 13 per cent of all those currently working thinking it fairly or very likely or almost certain that they will lose their job over the next 3 months, 15 per cent have similar expectations of being furloughed, and 23 per cent expect their hours to be reduced.

As for the effects of the lockdown on housing, the inequality being spread by the Government's measures is even greater, as one would expect of a country in which so much of the national wealth is invested in property, and the single largest monthly or weekly expenditure for most households is on their housing costs. 24 per cent of social renters and 20 per cent of private renters have either been furloughed or lost their job, compared to 14 per cent of mortgagors. But the effects of tenure type become more apparent when looking at the ability to cover housing costs. Only 8 per cent of home owners with a mortgage have failed to cover their housing costs under lockdown, compared to 13 per cent of private renters; while 17 per cent of social renters have fallen into rent arrears, twice the rate of mortgaged home owners.

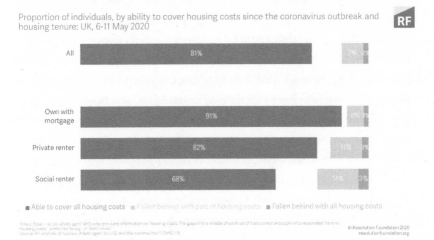

Proportion of individuals, by ability to cover housing costs since the coronavirus outbreak and housing tenure: UK, 6-11 May 2020

Source: Resolution Foundation analysis of YouGov, Adults aged 18 to 65 and the coronavirus (COVID-19)

There are various reasons for this huge difference in the ability of households to meet housing costs. One reason is because home-owners entered the lockdown with lower housing costs relative to their incomes (an average of 13 per cent) compared to social renters (18 per cent) and private renters (a massive 32 per cent). Another reason is because home-owners are in general wealthier, with only 13 per cent holding no savings before the lockdown, compared with 23 per cent of private renters and 47 per cent of social renters. But there is a third reason, which is that homeowners have received greater support from the Government.

13 per cent of mortgaged home owners have applied for a mortgage holiday in recent weeks, with 92 per cent being granted relief from their repayments for three months. In stark contrast, while 10 per cent of private renters have tried to lower their housing costs under the lockdown, either through negotiating a lower rent with their landlord or being granted a rent holiday, only 50 per cent have been successful. The even lower 4 per cent of social renters who have attempted to renegotiate their rent with local authorities or housing associations have had the same rate of success. Admittedly, the Government instructing a handful of lenders to grant a holiday to mortgagors is easier to impose through policy than compelling thousands of landlords to do the same for private renters, and under current legislation private renters and, increasingly, social renters have little or no rights. But this is a failure not only of existing housing legislation but also of the Government's indifference to the financial plight of renters under lockdown.

As a result of this protection of UK residential property values over and above ensuring the ability of UK citizens to afford to live in those properties, 37 per cent of renters who have made a claim for Universal Credit since the lockdown began are currently unable to meet their housing costs. Again, as a result of this failure of the benefit system to compensate households financially for being refused the right to support themselves financially, 24 per cent of private renters and 19 per cent of social renters are cutting down on other items in order to afford their rent, with 12 per cent of all renters experiencing material deprivation as a result. In comparison, 16 per cent of mortgaged home-owners have cut expenditure to afford housing costs, with only 4 per cent experiencing deprivation.

The consequences of all this are becoming apparent. 20.56 million people in England alone, 36 per cent of all households, rent from a private or social landlord, and they've been thrown to the wolves by the Government.[50] Despite the extension of the notice period for evictions of private and social renters from 2 to 3 months under the Coronavirus Act 2020 (something the Secretary of State for Housing, Communities and Local Government dishonestly tried to pass off as a 3-month 'ban'), and which ends on 25 June, tens — and perhaps hundreds — of

---

50. See Ministry of Housing, Communities and Local Government, 'English Housing Survey: Headline Report, 2018-19' (January 2020).

thousands of renters are currently living with the threat of eviction: either under Section 21 of the Housing Act 1988, which empowers landlords to evict tenants without reason on two months' notice, or under a Section 8 notice, which allows a landlord to evict through possession proceedings on the grounds of non-payment if a tenant hasn't paid rent for 8 weeks.[51]

So far, just as the ridiculously underfunded 'Everyone In' programme to get rough sleepers off the street at the height of the coronavirus 'crisis' appears to have been abandoned by the Government like the public relations stunt it was, so too the Government has resisted all calls either to ban evictions of renters or to raise housing benefits sufficient to afford rents.[52]

10. Outsourcing the State

That the poor are getting shafted by a Government that has first removed their ability to work then told them that a 20 per cent wage cut or life on Universal Credit is sustainable for millions of workers that were 'just about managing' on their previous salaries shouldn't surprise anyone who has observed the steady dismantling of the welfare state over the past decade. But the greed and opportunism with which the rich are profiting from the coronavirus 'crisis' may surprise those who have chosen to believe the Government's lies about us coming together during this 'period of national emergency'. But surprising or not, things are very different at the other end of the economic scale.

Under new procurement policy published on 18 March and justified by the 'extreme urgency' of responding to the coronavirus, at least 115 Government contracts worth over £1 billion have been directly awarded without tender to private companies.[53] The largest of these include Edenred, the French catering company awarded a contract worth £234 million by the Department for Education to feed children eligible for school meals; the US–owned Brake Brothers and the

---

51. See David Renton, 'Thousands of renters could be evicted in June. Will the government protect them?', *The Guardian* (8 May, 2020).

52. See Kate Ng, 'Government denies reports it has pulled funding from emergency coronavirus homeless sheltering programme', *The Independent* (15 May, 2020).

53. See Cabinet Office, 'Procurement Policy Note 01/20: Responding to COVID-19' (18 March, 2020); and Rob Evans, Juliette Garside, Joseph Smith and Pamela Duncan, 'Firms given £1bn of state contracts without tender in Covid-19 crisis', *The Guardian* (15 May, 2020).

South African-run BFS Group, which have been directly awarded contracts worth a combined £208m by the Department for Environment, Food and Rural Affairs to deliver food boxes to vulnerable people; and Randox Laboratories, a UK-owned healthcare firm directly awarded a contract worth £133 million by the Department of Health and Social Care to produce testing kits for SARs-CoV-2.[54] Other contacts include £60 million directly awarded by the Department for Education to Computacenter to supply computers; a combined £57 million awarded by Health and Social Care Jobs in Northern Ireland to Bloc Blinds to supply face shields; £23 million directly awarded by the Department of Health and Social Care to Oxford Nanopore; and £20 million directly awarded by HSCNI to Techniclean, again for the supply of face masks.

And as the private sector is being awarded contracts paid for with public money, so a public sector starved of funding is having its services outsourced to private companies. That this should be perpetrated against the NHS while it is being elevated to heroic status by Government propaganda should not surprise anyone who has watched the creeping privatisation of health services in the UK over the past 40 years.

On 2 December, 10 days before the country voted the Conservative Government into office in the 2019 General Election, Siva Anandaciva, Chief Analyst at the King's Fund think-tank, a member of the Office of Health Economics Policy Committee and Chair of the National Payment Strategy Advisory Group for NHS England and NHS Improvement, wrote that the NHS 'heads into winter with A&E performance at its worst level since current records began, 4.6 million people on hospital waiting lists and with 100,000 vacant staff'.[55] This, he explained, was not only because of years of sustained disinvestment in the NHS, but more immediately because the extra Government funding typically released late in the year in anticipation of winter influenzas and respiratory diseases had been withheld as a result of the Election and subsequent cancellation of the Autumn Budget. Add to that the Government changes to NHS pensions and the effects of Brexit, and Anandaciva told *The Guardian*:

---

54. See Rupert Neate, Juliette Garside, Felicity Lawrence and Rob Evans, 'Healthcare firm advised by Owen Paterson won £133m coronavirus testing contract unopposed', *The Guardian* (11 May, 2020).

55. Siva Anandaciva, 'Five reasons why this NHS winter may be different', *The King's Fund* (2 December, 2019).

In recent years the NHS has defied the odds and somehow managed to cope despite warnings about the impact of winter pressures. This time it is heading into what is likely to be the worst winter since modern records began in the eye of a perfect storm.[56]

We've already looked at some of the cumulative effects of underfunding in the NHS on excess deaths both unexplained and attributed to COVID-19; but the entrepreneurs in Government know a business opportunity when they see one. Having denied any connection between the failures to adequately fund public health services and the perfect storm predicted last winter, the Government has taken advantage of what it has insisted is an NHS 'overwhelmed' by COVID-19 deaths, and which could only be 'saved' by the lockdown, to outsource health services to private contractors.[57]

Despite the new policy requiring any contracts awarded under emergency regulations to be published by the contracting authority 'within 30 days of awarding the contract', the financial values of some of the key contracts in the Government's response to the coronavirus 'crisis' have yet to be disclosed. Specifically, contracts to operate drive-through coronavirus testing centres have been awarded to the accountancy and management consultancy firm Deloitte, which is managing payrolls, rotas and other logistics at national level, and has appointed the outsourcing firms G4S, Mitie, Serco, Sodexo, plus the pharmacy retailer Boots, to run the centres. Together with tech companies Palantir and Faculty, all these private companies have been running test centres and creating a COVID-19 data store since March, yet the relevant Government departments have refused to disclose the value of the contracts.[58] While in April, Serco was directly awarded a contract by the Department for Work and Pensions potentially worth £90 million to provide emergency contact centre services for vulnerable

---

56. See Denis Campbell, 'NHS winter crisis: extra beds created by 52% of UK hospitals', *The Guardian* (2 December, 2019).

57. See Juliette Garside and Rupert Neate, 'UK government "using pandemic to transfer NHS duties to private sector"', *The Guardian* (4 May, 2020).

58. See Tabby Kinder, 'Consultants in line of fire over projects to tackle coronavirus', *Financial Times* (4 May, 2020).

people who are self-isolating.[59] Deloitte is also co-ordinating the UK Lighthouse Labs Network, a coalition of public bodies and private companies formed to conduct testing for SARS-CoV-2, and which have been subcontracted to GlaxoSmithKline, AstraZeneca, Amazon and Boots.[60] Dozens of private companies have been awarded contracts to build, run and support the largely empty Nightingale Hospitals, including consultancy firm KPMG, Mott MacDonald, Archus and Interserve, with private security being supplied by G4S. Deloitte is also overseeing the production of protective equipment and other stock, with Clipper Logistics one of the supply chains awarded contracts to deliver protective equipment to NHS trusts, care homes and other healthcare workers.

Perhaps the clearest indicator of this further step forward in privatising health services under the cloak of the lockdown is that the Department of Health and Social Care has instructed NHS trusts that, from 4 May, 16 items of equipment, including PPE, ventilators, computerised tomography scanners, mobile X-ray machines and ultrasounds, must no longer be purchased directly by local NHS managers. Instead, under its new Government contract, Deloitte will centrally oversee all procurement, effectively outsourcing the health and safety of the UK population to private contractors.

Many of these companies, both those whose contracts have been published and those that haven't, have a history of incompetence, malpractice, fraud, price-fixing, prosecution, financial mismanagement, misconduct, bribery, illegality, breaches of security, confidentiality and contract, abuse of human rights, dubious ethical practices and conflicts of interest that, were the tendering process properly scrutinised by the Institute for Government, should preclude them from even bidding for Government contracts, let alone being awarded them without competition, oversight or disclosure.[61] I've written about these before, but they bear repeating and remembering.

---

59. See Peter Geoghegan and Russell Scott, 'Revealed: Serco under fire over fresh £90m COVID-19 contract', *Open Democracy* (28 May, 2020).

60. See Shaun Lintern, 'Inside the coronavirus mega-labs', *The Independent* (29 June, 2020).

61. See Nick Davies, Oliver Chan, Aron Cheung, Gavin Freeguard and Emma Norris, 'Summary — Government Procurement: The scale and nature of contracting in the UK', *Institute for Government* (December 2018).

- Edenred, the French-owned catering company with just 145 employees and revenues of £11.8 million given the responsibility of distributing food vouchers to 1.3 million children eligible for school meals, has been accused of woeful preparation that has left thousands of UK children going hungry.[62]
- BFS Group; the UK-based foodservice wholesaler and distributor and wholly-owned subsidiary of the South-African holding company Bidcorp, suffered losses of £14.8m in the year to June 2018 largely due to its logistics division, which reported operating losses of £37.7 million.[63]
- Randox, a UK company in the in vitro diagnostics industry, in February 2017 faced charges against two employees arrested on suspicion of perverting the course of justice amid allegations of data tampering within its testing services used by police in England and Wales, and currently pays Owen Paterson, the Conservative MP for North Shropshire and former Secretary of State for Environment, Food and Rural Affairs, and who has a history of lobbying Government Ministers on behalf of companies he advises, a £100,000 per year consultancy salary.[64]
- Deloitte, despite being the largest professional services network in the world, in 2016 failed to protect itself against a cyberattack that breached the confidentiality of its clients and 244,000 staff, allowing the attackers to access usernames, passwords, IP addresses and health information.[65]
- G4S, the UK's largest security services company, has been accused of using detained immigrants as cheap labour in prisons, extreme misconduct in child custodial institutions in the UK and the US, and of collaborating in police telephone data manipulation.[66]

---

62. See Rob Davies, 'Government awarded school meal voucher contract without tender', *The Guardian* (7 May, 2020).

63. See Bidfood owner BFS Group suffers £14.8m loss driven by logistics weakness', *The Grocer* (12 April, 2019).

64. See 'Randox forensics inquiry: Drug-drivers to challenge convictions', *BBC News* (22 November, 2017).

65. See Nick Hopkins, 'Deloitte hit by cyber-attack revealing clients' secret emails', *The Guardian* (25 September, 2017).

66. See Kevin Rawlinson, 'Private firms "are using detained immigrants as cheap labour"', *The Guardian* (22 August, 2014); Eric Allison and Simon Hattenstone, 'Managers at G4S-run Medway youth jail paid bonuses despite failings', *The Guardian* (21 October, 2016); and Alan Travis,

- Mitie, the UK strategic outsourcing company that has businesses in immigration detention and deportation, prisons and custodial health services, in 2016 was found by the prison inspectorate to have facilities that were 'dirty', 'rundown' and 'insanitary'.[67]

- Serco, the UK provider of public services in prisons, border security, military defence and information technology, in 2013 was found by the prison inspectorate to be locking 60 per cent of prisoners in their cells up to 23 hours per day in HMP Thameside, was accused of covering up sexual abuse in the Yarl's Wood Immigration centre, and in 2019 was fined £22.9 million by the Serious Fraud Office for charging the Government for electronically tagging people who were dead, in jail, or outside the UK.[68]

- Sodexo, the French food services and facilities management company and one of the world's largest multinational corporations, whose subsidiary, Sodexo Justice Services, was criticised by the UK Ministry of Justice in February 2019 for failing to prevent repeated and systemic breaches of the human rights of inmates at HMP Peterborough, including illegal strip-searches of prisoners and leaving a woman to give birth alone in her cell without any kind of medical support.[69]

- Boots, the UK pharmacy retailer, in February 2018 was criticised for charging elevated prices for low-value products supplied to the NHS.[70]

- Palantir, the US software company that provides tracking and surveillance infrastructure to the US military and local police departments, in 2018 admitted one of its employees helped Cambridge Analytica obtain the Facebook data of 50 million US voters, and last year was criticised for its

---

'G4S police control room staff suspended over claims of bogus 999 calls', *The Guardian* (23 May, 2016).

67. See Gill Plimmer, 'Mitie criticised for 'insanitary' immigration centre', *Financial Times* (29 February, 2016).

68. See Mark Townsend, 'Detainees at Yarl's Wood immigration centre "facing sexual abuse"', *The Guardian* (14 September, 2013); and Kat Hall, 'Serious Fraud Office fines Serco £22.9m over electronic tagging scandal', *The Register* (3 July, 2019).

69. See 'HMP Peterborough inmates were illegally strip-searched', *BBC News* (22 February, 2019); and Hannah Devlin and Diane Taylor, 'Baby dies in UK prison after inmate "gives birth alone in cell"', *The Guardian* (4 October, 2019).

70. See Paul Morgan-Bentley, 'Boots faces inquiry over cancer drug price hike', *The Times* (25 May, 2018).

support for US Immigration Customs and Enforcement's brutal deportation regime.[71]

- Faculty; the British artificial intelligence start-up employed by Dominic Cummings, the Prime Minister's Special Advisor, to work with him on the Vote Leave campaign, and in which Theodore Agnew, the Cabinet Office Minister in charge of the Office for Artificial Intelligence and Government Digital Service, has £90,000 of shares.[72]

- GlaxoSmithKline, in 2012 was fined $3 billion, until then the largest settlement in history, after admitting bribing US doctors and encouraging the prescription of unsuitable anti-depressants to children, and, amid numerous other controversies and fines, in 2016 was fined over £37 million by the Competition and Markets Authority for paying bribes to keep generic varieties of paroxetine out of the UK market.[73]

- AstraZeneca, the British-Swedish multinational pharmaceutical and biopharmaceutical company, in 2010 agreed to pay £505 million to settle a UK tax dispute related to transfer mispricing.[74]

- Amazon, the US multinational conglomerate technology company, despite numerous controversies and accusations, including of supplying law enforcement with facial recognition surveillance technology, the appalling working conditions in its warehouses, sacking workers who tried to unionise, opposing market competition, selling counterfeit products and avoiding federal income taxes, in July 2019 was awarded a contract by the Department of Health and Social Care that gives it free access to information about healthcare published by the NHS.[75]

---

71. See David Pegg and Carole Cadwalladr, 'US data firm admits employee approached Cambridge Analytica', The Guardian (28 March, 2018); and Julie Bort, 'Palantir's tech was used by ICE in the controversial arrests of 680 people at a Mississippi chicken farm according to an immigrants' rights group', Business Insider (October 2019).

72. See Rob Evans and David Pegg, 'Vote Leave AI firm wins seven government contracts in 18 months', The Guardian (4 May, 2020).

73. See Julie Bradshaw, 'Watchdog fines GSK £37m for paying to keep generic drugs out of UK market', The Telegraph (12 February, 2016).

74. See Richard Wachman, 'AstraZeneca agrees to pay £505m to settle UK tax dispute', The Guardian (23 February, 2010).

75. See Amy Walker, 'NHS gives Amazon free use of health data under Alexa advice deal', The Guardian (8 December, 2019).

- KPMG, the multinational professions service network, in 2004 admitted criminal wrongdoing in creating fraudulent tax shelters to help wealthy clients avoid $2.5 billion in taxes between 1996 and 2002, and subsequently agreed to pay $456 million in penalties to avoid indictment.[76]
- Mott MacDonald, the UK multidisciplinary consultancy, in 2017 was suspended from bidding for Government contracts in Hong Kong when it was found to have disclosed confidential population and employment data to outsiders.[77]
- Interserve, the multinational group of support services and construction companies, in 2009 was fined £11.6 million for engaging in illegal anti-competitive bid-rigging activities, and in 2019 went into administration.[78]
- Clipper Logistics, the UK haulage firm whose founder and Executive Chairman, Steven N. Parkin, over the past five years has donated £725,000 to the Conservative Party.[79]

This is a cross section of just some of the private companies to whom the Government is handing over not just the national response to the coronavirus 'crisis' but, increasingly, the running of the UK's public sector, with a third of Government spending, £284 billion per year as of 2018, going on these and other external private contractors even before the current coronavirus sell off got underway.[80]

---

76. See Carrie Johnson, 'Charge Against KPMG Dropped', *Washington Post* (4 January, 2007).

77. See Cannix Yau, 'Hong Kong government temporarily suspends two consultancy firms from making bids for projects', *South China Morning Post* (27 March, 2017).

78. See Adam Jones, 'Builders fined £130m for rigging bids', *Financial Times* (22 September, 2009).

79. See Nafeez Ahmed, 'Conservative Party Donor Cashes in on UK Government-Made PPE Shortages Amidst COVID-19 Crisis', *Byline Times* (2 April, 2020).

80. See Anoosh Chakelian , 'Interserve, and the other companies running Britain that you've never heard of; Or: why are construction firms involved in your welfare?', *The New Statesman* (11 March, 2019); and Nick Davies, Oliver Chan, Aron Cheung, Gavin Freeguard and Emma Norris, 'Summary – Government procurement: the scale and nature of contracting in the UK', *Institute for Government* (12 December, 2018).

11. The Security Ratchet

And, finally, there are the social and infrastructure changes required to implement the surveillance and control of the population should anyone in the UK take it into their heads to try to organise opposition to this wholesale privatisation of the country's assets and public services. Although it didn't include it among its 9 metrics for calculating the Government imposed Social Distancing measures, *Our World in Data* did produce a map of what countries have Government policies for contact tracing all potentially infected citizens.[81]

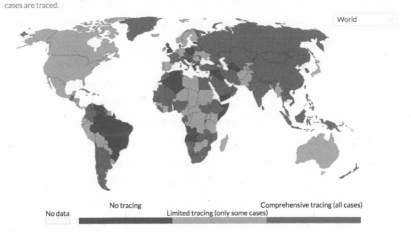

Which countries do COVID-19 contact tracing?, Jun 1, 2020
'Limited' contact tracing means some, but not all, cases are traced. 'Comprehensive' tracing means all cases are traced.

Source: Hale, Webster, Petherick, Phillips, and Kira (2020). Oxford COVID-19 Government Response Tracker – Last Updated 1st June.

Source: Oxford COVID-19 Government Response Tracker, University of Oxford

This does not include voluntarily downloaded mobile phone apps of the kind currently being promoted by the Department for Health and Social Care in the UK, but which are not yet mandatory. Ironically, therefore, we appear on this map as an island of civil liberties in a world that, over the past five months, has seen governments impose levels of intrusion into their population's personal data and

81. See Edouard Mathieu, Hannah Ritchie, Lucas Rodés-Guirao, Cameron Appel, Daniel Gavrilov, Charlie Giattino, Joe Hasell, Bobbie Macdonald, Saloni Dattani, Diana Beltekian, Esteban Ortiz-Ospina and Max Roser, 'Policy Responses to the Coronavirus Pandemic: COVID-19: Testing and Contact Tracing', *Our World in Data*.

movements that are unprecedented and most probably irreversible, and which, far from being reined in as the deaths attributed to COVID-19 fall, have steadily increased.

I've already written about the threat the Government's Test and Trace programme, the personal data from which Public Health England last week announced it will now be retaining for 20 years, presents to what's left of our freedoms in this country, so I won't repeat my warnings here. But I want to add something about its functioning and purpose.

At present, the Test and Trace programme is merely instructing members of the public who think they have COVID-19 to self-isolate for 7 days, with members of their household having to quarantine themselves for 14 days.[82] Asking the British public to diagnose themselves with symptoms indistinguishable, at least to the layman, from a common cold or the flu or any number of other illnesses is almost as ridiculous as empowering a police constable who has 'reasonable grounds' for suspecting that a member of the public has coronavirus to compel them — if necessary using 'reasonable force' — to get tested and self-isolate. But the purpose of this act of self-diagnosis, which is ostensibly at the heart of the Government's attempts to 'contain' a virus that has been in the country for at least 5 months, will become clearer when the new 'coronavirus app' has been released.

As the Department of Health and Social Care has clarified, the NHS COVID-19 smartphone app, which at present the Government says won't be mandatory to upload, will issue two stages of alert to fellow users, a yellow and a red.[83] If a user of the app diagnoses themselves as showing symptoms of COVID-19, such as a cough or a high temperature, and declares their 'status', the software will issue a yellow alert to every other user of the app that has come into proximity with them over an as-yet-undisclosed period of time, notifying them that they are now 'potentially infected persons'. After this, under Schedule 21 of the Coronavirus Act 2020, the person who self-diagnosed will be compelled to take a test for SARS-CoV-2, and if it comes back positive — which doesn't mean they have COVID-19 — everyone previously notified will then be issued a red alert and also be compelled to self-isolate for 14 days. However, while this will potentially

---

82. See UK Health Security Agency, 'NHS Test and Trace: what to do if you are contacted' 27 May, 2020).

83. See Matt Hancock, 'Health and Social Care Secretary's statement on coronavirus (COVID-19): 1 May 2020' (1 May, 2020).

lead to exponentially increasing numbers of the British public — over 83 per cent of whom live in close proximity to each other in urban areas — being under house arrest, causing further damage to the economy, the real purpose of the COVID-19 app isn't to halt the spread of a virus with an infection fatality rate between 0.1 and 0.2 per cent and far lower among the 80 per cent of the population that is under 65 and without pre-existing illnesses, but to keep a terrorised public under control.[84]

Anyone who has let out a cough in a supermarket during the lockdown will know the levels of paranoia about health currently pertaining in the British public. As the numbers of deaths attributed to COVID-19 continue to fall, and the level of infection with SARS-CoV-2 either shrinks or is shown by further testing to be far higher — and therefore less virulent — than the Government claimed, all it will take for a UK population tracked by this app to be put on yellow alert, and therefore confined to their homes as a 'potentially infectious person', is for a tiny percentage of that population to self-diagnose themselves with symptoms of COVID-19. A *BBC News* report about a ticket collector 'killed by COVID-19' should be sufficient for the purpose.[85] From there, via the issuing of yellow alerts, the app will digitally spread their merely suspected self-diagnoses, exponentially increasing the numbers of people subject to compulsory quarantine under coronavirus legislation.

This is the biopolitics of the 'New Normal' being prepared for us, whose functioning will be overseen by the Joint Biosecurity Centre the Government is currently establishing with its private partners, and which, significantly, is to be headed by the Director General of the Office for Security and Counter-Terrorism.[86] In effect a public-private partnership for the UK Biosecurity State, this is the ratchet that will protect and 'lock in' all the financial and power gains made by the private sector under the Government-imposed 'lockdown'.

---

84. See John P.A. Ioannidis, 'The infection fatality rate of COVID-19 inferred from seroprevalence data', *MedRxiv* (13 May, 2020).

85. See 'Coronavirus: Victoria ticket worker dies after being spat at', *BBC News* (12 May, 2020).

86. See Alex Thomas, 'Joint Biosecurity Centre', *Institute for Government* (12 May, 2020); and Beckie Smith, 'Counter-terrorism director general to lead coronavirus risk response unit', *Civil Service World* (12 May, 2020).

12. Manufacturing Compliance

I can't end an article about the lockdown without saying something about the false comfort taken by liberals from the belief that a Government composed of such fools and incompetents couldn't possibly have managed to manipulate and capitalise on the coronavirus 'crisis' with such speed and cunning. From the Reich Cabinet of Adolf Hitler and the Republican Administration of George W. Bush to the Leader of the Free World currently cowering in the bunker beneath the White House, history has demonstrated again and again that stupidity and ignorance are no hindrance to cunning. The widely-made claim that the UK Government doesn't know what it is doing rests on the false premise about what it is trying to do. We shouldn't mistake the incompetence and venality of Dominic Cummings, Dominic Raab, Rishi Sunak, Priti Patel, Michael Gove, Matt Hancock, Gavin Williamson, Robert Jenrick and all the other crooks with which Boris Johnson has surrounded himself for an inability to push through their plans for our final transition to a Britain of fully privatised public services and even greater economic and social inequality in a population ruled by emergency powers, managed by the surveillance state and governed under a permanent State of Emergency.

In my previous article on 'The State of Emergency as a Paradigm of Government' I analysed in detail the legislation, measures and programmes already made by this Government in the 3 months from 10 March to 10 May. But as further evidence of its intentions, the Government has belatedly published the albeit redacted minutes and supporting documents produced by SAGE, the Scientific Advisory Group for Emergencies responsible for briefing the Cabinet Office.[87] Chaired by Patrick Vallance — who until March 2018 was the President of Research and Development at GlaxoSmithKline, the pharmaceutical company awarded an untendered contract of undisclosed value by the Government he advises — SAGE members also included Professor Neil Ferguson, until he resigned for breaking the lockdown measures his discredited research justified. In addition to its official members, on the day the lockdown was announced the SAGE meeting was attended by Marc Warner, a data scientist and the Chief Executive Officer of Faculty, another of the companies awarded an untendered and undisclosed contract by the Government; and by Dominic Cummings, the

---

87. See UK Government, 'Scientific Advisory Group for Emergencies'.

Prime Minister's Chief Advisor, with whom Warner worked closely on the Leave campaign.[88] Indeed, despite requirements that SAGE is politically neutral, SAGE members have reported both men attending meetings as far back as February.

A full analysis of the content of these documents is, once again, outside the scope of this article; but they provide a fascinating insight into the Government's management of the coronavirus 'crisis'. On 22 March, the day before the lockdown of the UK was announced, the Scientific Pandemic Influenza Group on Behavioural Science (SPI-B), one of two main sub-groups of SAGE, prepared a paper titled 'Options for increasing adherence to social distancing measures'. Discussed at the following day's meeting, prior to the Prime Minister's announcement of the lockdown that evening, this paper contained the following recommendations:

> A substantial number of people still do not feel sufficiently personally threatened; it could be that they are reassured by the low death rate in their demographic group. The perceived level of personal threat needs to be increased among those who are complacent, using hard-hitting emotional messaging.
>
> Communication strategies should provide social approval for desired behaviours and promote social approval within the community.
>
> Experience with UK enforcement suggests that, with adequate preparation, rapid change can be achieved. Some other countries have introduced mandatory self-isolation on a wide scale without evidence of major public unrest, and a large majority of the UK's population appear to be supportive of more coercive measures. For example, 64% of adults in Great Britain said they would support putting London under a 'lock down'.[89]

During the SAGE meeting the following day, at which, in addition to Cummings and Warner, Neil Ferguson was also present, as well as Ian Diamond, the Chief Executive of the Office for National Statistics, the minutes record the following under the subtitle 'Excess deaths planning':

---

88. See Severin Carrell, David Pegg, Felicity Lawrence, Paul Lewis, Rob Evans, David Conn, Harry Davies and Kate Proctor, 'Revealed: Cummings is on secret scientific advisory group for Covid-19', *The Guardian* (24 April, 2020).

89. See Scientific Pandemic Influenza Group on Behavioural Science, 'Options for increasing adherence to social distancing measures' (22 March 2020).

The science suggests that a proportion of the estimated fatalities from Covid-19 would be among those expected to die within a year.

NHSX and ONS data need to be combined by modelling groups to give a clear picture of deaths caused directly and indirectly by Covid-19.

Actuarial analysis is required to estimate numbers of deaths caused indirectly by Covid-19, including those caused by social interventions. In due course, analysis of the effects of the interventions on other causes of death should be undertaken.[90]

SAGE then recommended that the NHSX provide the ONS with the data on mortality required to establish excess deaths. But if this data was handed over and the modelling ever carried out, it has not been published, not by SAGE, not by the ONS, and not by the NHS. However, these minutes make it clear that, even before the lockdown had been imposed, the advisors primarily responsible for justifying the Government's decision were aware that it would kill sufficient numbers of people to warrant recording and analysis.

Finally, on 6 May, the same sub-group (SPI-B) produced a paper summarising 'Key behavioural issues relevant to test, trace, track and isolate'. Examining public perceptions of the intrusiveness of the so-called 'NHS Test and Trace' programme being run by the Government and its coterie of private contractors, the AI technology the programme employs and the collection and privacy and use of the personal data it stores, the paper concluded with its recommendations of how to counteract these fears — not by changing the programme in any way, but by managing public perceptions to ensure collaboration and compliance:

First, contact tracing is viewed as more acceptable when framed in terms of an appeal to duty; for example, that contact tracing is 'the right thing to do'. This appeal to duty can also intersect with the perception that when in doubt, it is better to know one way or the other. In the context of a national epidemic, appeals to duty can include responsibilities to family, community and nation. It will be

---

90. See Scientific Advisory Group for Emergencies, 'Addendum to eighteenth SAGE meeting on Covid-19, 23rd March 2020 Held in 10 Victoria St, London, SW1H 0NN' (23 March, 2020).

important as well from an ethical perspective as well to consider the perception of coercion in relation to patients' participation in contact tracing.

Contact tracing is also viewed as more acceptable against a background of high levels of trust in an individualised provider. Personalising that provider as, for example, a health visitor or other public health clinician can also increase confidence and acceptability of contact tracing, even where contact tracing is undertaking (*sic*) using a technological solution. In designing a test and track programme, it may be appropriate to capitalise on trust in the NHS and in local health personnel.[91]

These are not the words of a Government responding on the hoof to a 'crisis' out of their control. On the contrary, behind the practised bumbling of its game-show host Prime Minister, these are measured considerations on how to increase and capitalise on the population's fears in order, first, to implement a lockdown, and then, under its cloak, to induce that population into the voluntary or, if need be, mandatory adoption of the structures, prohibitions and practices of a surveillance state. As I have previously argued, these deserve the description 'totalitarian'. More even than the thousands of unnecessary and unexplained deaths and the enforced destruction of the businesses, public services, jobs and livelihoods of the mass of the UK population, this voluntary embrace of our own chains may turn out to be by far the greatest and most irreversible cost of the lockdown.

— 2 June, 2020

---

91. See Scientific Pandemic Influenza Group on Behavioural Science, 'Key behavioural issues relevant to test, trace, track and isolate' (6 May, 2020).

5. The New Normal: What is the UK Biosecurity State?

Part 1: Programmes and Regulations

The UK, and with it the nation states of Western capitalism, are undergoing a revolution. In comparison to the momentousness of this change, the neoliberal revolution overseen in this country by the Governments of Margaret Thatcher and Tony Blair merely created the political hegemony for the expansion and administration of a global economy. But the world of parliamentary democracies, of civil liberties and human rights, including our rights of assembly, speech, thought, privacy and a fair trial, of the separation of powers between an executive, legislature and judiciary, of media scrutiny of Government, of freedom from censorship, of political activity itself, is now over. What we are entering into is something quite different. Like all revolutions, it's been a long-time brewing, with the legislation necessary to administer it, the technology required to police it, and the manufacture of popular consent to its implementation having been in preparation for at least two decades. But the wheel has now turned, and the world we lived in no longer exists. This is the New Normal.

1. Historical Precedents for Emergency Powers

On 15 June, 2020, opening the Secondary Legislation Scrutiny Committee debate on the motion to approve Amendment No. 2 to the Health Protection (Coronavirus, Restrictions) (England), Lord Bethell, Parliamentary Under-Secretary of State in the Department of Health and Social Care, one of only 814 hereditary peers in the UK and the 5th Baron Bethell, declared:

> The amending regulations we are discussing were made by the Secretary of State on 13 May. These remain an exceptional and necessary package of measures brought forward to protect public health. The regulations we are debating have been amended two further times since, on 31 May and 12 June. This is an unusual

situation, so I will address this early in my speech because I know that it is a cause of concern.

This sequencing has been a necessary consequence of the speed at which the Government have had to respond to the changing impacts of the pandemic on our country. Use of the emergency procedure has rarely been so necessary. These are not usual times. However, I believe that the situation has demonstrated that our flexible unwritten Constitution is a strength in extraordinary times such as these, and that our parliamentary democracy can retain its oversight while bringing about measures necessary to meet these unprecedented circumstances.

I assure noble Lords that this expedited process does not set some kind of inappropriate precedent for the future, when we reach a greater state of normality.[1]

We are — we are constantly being told — living in 'unprecedented times', facing 'unprecedented circumstances' requiring 'unprecedented measures' for which there is no historical precedent and for which — is the unstated implication — the Government cannot be held to account for the consequences of its responses. It didn't know that emptying NHS hospitals of elderly patients already infected by SARS-CoV-2 would start an epidemic in UK care homes. It didn't know that denying medical and emergency care for tens of thousands of patients with cancer, heart disease, diabetes and dementia would kill more people than COVID-19. It didn't know that putting the country into lockdown for three months would send the UK economy spiralling into the worst depression in over 300 years, bankrupt thousands of small businesses and push unemployment up to an estimated 4-5 million people. And it apparently hasn't considered that closing schools for four months because of a disease to which children are statistically immune will have an as-yet-unknown impact on the education and lives of millions of school children. The situation is unprecedented, and the Government is doing the best it can.

'Unprecedented', however, is one of those words that should set alarm-bells ringing in the head of the historical materialist, implying, as it does, that we are in a moment about which history can teach us nothing, but which signals, in

---

1. See UK Parliament, 'Health Protection (Coronavirus, Restrictions) (England) (Amendment) (No. 2) Regulations 2020. Volume 803: debated on Monday 15 June 2020', *Hansard* (15 June, 2020).

practice, that the speaker either hasn't a clue what they're talking about (the journalist) or is deliberately dissembling what they are in fact doing (the politician). But in either case, whether the present is a product of ignorance or deceit, history inevitably has a lot to tell us about supposedly 'unprecedented' moments, and so it is with the coronavirus 'crisis'. Bear with me, then, as we take a brief detour through the history of emergency powers, the better to arm ourselves for confronting their use in the present.

It took less than five years for France to pass from the revolutionary overthrow of the constitutional monarchy of King Louis Philippe I in February 1848; through the subsequent foundation of the French Second Republic in May 1848; the bloody repression of Parisian workers in the June Days uprising; the election by popular vote of Louis-Bonaparte as President of the Republic in December 1848; to the latter's *coup d'état* in December 1851 and subsequent election as Emperor Napoléon III in December 1852 — five years to pass from a king to a republic and back to an emperor — and throughout most of that revolution the citizens of Paris were living under a 'state of siege'.

The best commentary on the constitutional origins and use of emergency powers — as he has been throughout the coronavirus 'crisis' on the juridico-political changes implemented under its cloak — is that by the Italian philosopher, Giorgio Agamben. In *State of Exception*, in which he traces the history of emergency powers back to the French Revolution of 1789, Agamben writes:

> The institution of the state of siege has its origins in the French Constituent Assembly's decree of 8 July, 1791, which distinguished among *état de paix*, in which military authority and civil authority each acts in its own sphere; *état de guerre*, in which civil authority must act in concert with military authority; and *état de siège*, in which 'all the functions entrusted to the civil authority for maintaining order and internal policing pass to the military commander, who exercises them under his exclusive responsibility.'
>
> The subsequent history of the state of siege is the history of its gradual emancipation from the wartime situation to which is was originally bound in order to be used as an extraordinary police measure to cope with internal sedition and disorder, thus changing from a real, or military, state of siege to a fictitious, or political one. In any case, it is important not to forget that the modern state of

exception is a creation of the democratic-revolutionary tradition and not the absolutist one.

The idea of a state of suspension of the Constitution was introduced for the first time in the Constitution of 22 Frimaire Year 8, Article 92 of which reads: 'In the case of armed revolt or disturbance that would threaten the security of the State, the law can, in the places and for the time that it determines, suspend the rule of the Constitution. In such cases, this suspension can be provisionally declared by a decree of the Government if the legislative body is in recess, provided that this body be convened as soon as possible by an article of the same decree.'

The city or region in question was declared *hors la Constitution* [outside the Constitution]. Although the paradigm is, on the one hand (in the state of siege) the extension of the military authority's wartime powers into the civil sphere, and on the other a suspension of the Constitution (or of those constitutional norms that protect individual liberties), in time the two models end up merging into a single juridical phenomenon that we call the *state of exception*.[2]

Following the Restoration of the Bourbon monarchy, Article 14 of the Royal Charter of June 1814 gave the king, as head of state and commander-in-chief of the armed forces, the exclusive power to 'make the regulations and ordinances necessary for the execution of the laws and the security of the state'. The following April, after Napoleon Bonaparte's return from Elba, Section 66 of the Additional Act required that, in the case of civil disturbances, the Government's declaration of a state of siege had to be made by law. This was the constitutional position when, thirty-three years later, on 22 February 1848, in response to striking workers and republican students taking to the streets of Paris, the French Government declared a state of siege. Unfortunately for King Louis Philippe, the National Guard sided with the revolutionaries, protecting them from the French Army. Following the fall of the so-called 'July Monarchy', a decree of the Constituent Assembly on 24 June, 1848, placed Paris back into a state of siege and assigned to General Cavaignac, the newly-appointed Minister of War, the task of restoring order in the city, which he did at the cost of 10,000 killed and wounded. An article establishing

---

2. Giorgio Agamben, *State Of Exception*, Homo Sacer II, 1; translated by Kevin Attell (University of Chicago Press, 2005), p. 5.

the conditions, forms and effects of the state of siege was subsequently incorporated into the new French Constitution of 4 November, 1848. This state of siege, renewed in June 1849 when the socialists and radical republicans made a half-hearted attempt to seize power, lasted until 12 October 1849.

That year, the law of 9 August established that a political state of siege could only be declared by Parliament or the head of state. Louis Bonaparte made considerable use of this law as both President and Emperor, but particularly in the former capacity. Following his military coup in December 1851, resistance in the Departments of France was crushed by, once again, declaring a state of siege; and the following January, Section 12 of his Constitution had the effect of transferring the prerogative of declaring a state of siege from the legislature to the head of state exclusively, with the Senate in the role of mere advisor, thereby turning it against those who had created the idea in the Constituent Assembly. This was the situation on which Karl Marx, that same year, commented at length and with no little irony in *The Eighteenth Brumaire of Louis Bonaparte:*

> The state of siege. A splendid invention, periodically employed in every ensuing crisis in the course of the French Revolution. But barrack and bivouac — which were thus periodically laid on French society's head to compress its brain and render it quiet; sabre and musket — which were periodically allowed to act as judges and administrators, as guardians and censors, to play policeman and do night watchman's duty; moustache and uniform — which were periodically trumpeted forth as the highest wisdom of society and as its rector: were not barrack and bivouac, sabre and musket, moustache and uniform finally bound to hit upon the idea of rather saving society, once and for all, by proclaiming their own regime as the highest, and freeing civil society completely from the trouble of having to govern itself?[3]

Marx's metonyms of barrack, musket and uniform refer, of course, to the French soldiers that, under the direction first of Parliament and then of the head of state, imposed the state of siege on the rebellious French population. But 170 years later, there is little distinction between the police forces that implement

---

3. Karl Marx, 'The Eighteenth Brumaire of Louis Bonaparte', in Karl Marx and Frederick Engels, *Selected Works*, Vol. 1 (Progress Publishers, 1983), p. 412.

government guidance with or without legislation and the armed forces that can be deployed under a State of Emergency that in France was extended five times in the two years between November 2015 and November 2017, the longest in its history. As we have already seen over the last 20 months of violent assaults on the *Gilets jaunes* protests by the neo-liberal Government of President Emmanuel Macron, what has become the standard police armoury of cuffs, baton, CS-gas and taser can very quickly become flash ball, semi-automatic rifle, tear gas and TNT grenade, civil disobedience can quickly be reclassified as terrorist threat, military forces can be deployed on home soil, and keeping the peace used to justify violent assault, targeted mutilation and state-authorised shooting by police officers and gendarmerie very clearly acting *hors de constitution*.[4] Between 22 March and 10 July, 2020, in response to the coronavirus 'crisis', France was once again placed under a State of Emergency.

As for the UK, where we like to think we police by compliance rather than enforcement, like France and the rest of Europe we spent the Great War of 1914-18 under emergency measures that had been prepared in advance by the relevant ministers and then nodded through Parliament almost without debate. The most important of these was the Defence of the Realm Act 1914, which severely limited the rights of UK citizens, including granting military tribunals jurisdiction over civilians, and greatly reduced the activities of Parliament for the duration of the war. No sooner was the war over than, in response to widespread civil disturbance and the perceived threat of revolution, the UK Government made the Emergency Powers Act 1920. In the event of any action or threat of action that might 'deprive the community, or any substantial portion of the community, of the essentials of life', these empowered the king and head of state to declare a 'state of emergency'. These emergency powers first introduced the state of exception proper into UK law, and were subsequently used during the General Strike of 1926 as the basis of the strike-breaking force. The Emergency Powers Act was amended in 1964 and bolstered by the creation in the 1970s of the Cabinet Office Civil Contingencies Unit, which was replaced in 2001 by the Civil Contingencies

---

4. See Anthony Torres, 'Macron to deploy French army against "yellow vest" protests', *World Socialist Website* (21 March, 2019); and Alex Lantier, 'French army receives authorization to shoot "yellow vest" protesters', *World Socialist Website* (23 March, 2019). For photographic documentation of the more than 2,500 injuries inflicted by Macron's police and armed forces, see the website *Le mur jaune*.

Secretariat.[5] In the more than 80 years of its jurisdiction, the Emergency Powers Act was used 12 times to declare a State of Emergency, all of them in response to industrial action, the last time during the coalmining and energy workers' strikes of 1973–74.[6] In 2004 it was repealed and replaced by the Civil Contingencies Act, which remains in force today.

Far from being unprecedented, therefore, the emergency measures justified by the declaration of the coronavirus 'crisis' and enacted by ministers, police and judiciary have been anticipated and provided for in UK legislation every bit as much as they were in the French Constitution that brought Napoleon III to power in the 1850s and legalises Macron waging civil war against the French people today. As I have covered at length in my article on 'The State of Emergency as a Paradigm of Government: Coronavirus Legislation, Implementation and Enforcement', this legislation includes the Coronavirus Act 2020, which is primary legislation, as well as the (at the time of publication) 163 coronavirus-related Statutory Instruments made into law as secondary legislation.[7] No less than 25 of these have been made under the Public Health (Control of Disease) Act 1984, and 13 under emergency procedure set out in Section 45R. This permits a Statutory Instrument to be made without a draft having been laid before and approved by Parliament 'if the instrument contains a declaration that the person making it is of the opinion that, by reason of urgency, it is necessary to make the order without a draft being so laid and approved.'

Four months since Parliament voted itself into extended recess on 25 March, and nearly two months since it returned on 2 June under social distancing rules that limit the House of Commons to 50 MPs with the consequent restriction of Parliament's ability to hold the Government to account, the UK Government continues to circumvent the legislature, with an extraordinary 94 Statutory Instruments made into law without a draft having been presented to Parliament at

---

5. See Cabinet Office, 'Civil Contingencies Secretariat: The Lead Government Department and its role – Guidance and Best Practice' (March 2004).

6. See UK Parliament, 'Emergency Powers Act 1920', *Hansard* (12 June, 1979).

7. See Hansard Society, 'Coronavirus Statutory Instruments Dashboard, 2020-2022' (4 March, 2022).

least 21 days prior to coming into effect, as is required under parliamentary rules.[8] Of the 21 Statutory Instruments requiring parliamentary approval to remain law, 17 were made using the emergency powers conferred on Ministers by the Public Health (Control of Disease) Act 1984. This is what the phrase 'unprecedented circumstances' means in practice: government by legislative dictatorship, in which the legislature is brought in after the fact to rubber-stamp laws already implemented by the executive without scrutiny of the evidence for their justification or proportionality, without an assessment having been made of their impact, and without approval by our democratically elected representatives in Parliament.

2. The Civil Contingencies Act

On Thursday, 25 June, 2020, as temperatures reached 33 degrees centigrade in the UK, and crowds descended on the beaches at the seaside town of Bournemouth in Dorset, Vikki Slade, the Liberal-Democrat leader of the Coalition-run Bournemouth, Christchurch and Poole (BCP) council, announced:

> The irresponsible behaviour and actions of so many people is just shocking, and our services are stretched to the absolute hilt trying to keep everyone safe. We have had no choice now but to declare a major incident and initiate an emergency response.[9]

The key phrase in this statement is the one about 'trying to keep everyone safe', in the implementation of which the council is authorised to declare a 'major incident' justifying an 'emergency response'. One might think these are just phrases to describe a range of actions, but they aren't. In using these terms, council-leader Slade is activating very specific and extraordinarily powerful legislation.

---

8. See UK Parliament, 'Government request call of Parliament' (28 May, 2020); and Alice Lilly and Hannah White, 'Parliament's role in the coronavirus crisis: holding the government to account', *Institute for Government* (21 May, 2020).

9. See BCP Council, 'Major incident declared after services overstretched by thousands flocking to Bournemouth beaches' (25 June, 2020).

First of all, a 'major incident' is defined in Emergency Response and Recovery: Non-statutory guidance accompanying the Civil Contingencies Act 2004, which was revised and published in October 2013. This states:

> The term 'major incident' — is commonly used by emergency services personnel to describe events or situations which would constitute an emergency as defined in the CCA regime; this is the threshold of event or situation that will initiate a response under their major incident plans. These terms refer to the same threshold and are essentially interchangeable.[10]

In Section 1 of the Civil Contingencies Act 2004, an 'emergency' is defined as:

a) An event or situation which threatens serious damage to human welfare in a place in the UK;

b) An event or situation which threatens serious damage to the environment of a place in the UK, or

c) War, or terrorism, which threatens serious damage to the security of the UK.[11]

By declaring the beaches at Bournemouth a 'major incident', therefore, Councillor Slade, a former school governor, was placing them on the same level, for the purposes of jurisdiction over the situation, as the site of a terrorist attack. I think it's safe to assume that BCP council didn't believe they were under either a terrorist attack or at war, or that serious damage was being done to the beaches of Bournemouth; so we can only assume that the emergency they declared a 'major incident' was constituted by the threat of serious damage to human welfare. To qualify as such, however, the situation must have involved, caused or threatened to cause a) loss of human life; b) human illness or injury; c) homelessness; d) damage to property; e) disruption of a supply of money, food,

---

10. HM Government, 'Emergency Response and Recovery: Non statutory guidance accompanying the Civil Contingencies Act 2004' (October 2013).

11. UK Public General Acts, Civil Contingencies Act 2004, Part 1, Section 1(1).

water, energy or fuel; f) disruption of a system of communication; g) disruption of facilities for transport, or g) disruption of services relating to health.

Again, the only threat the beaches may conceivably have presented to holiday-goers was b) injury or illness, and perhaps, through the latter, a) loss of life. We'll get to what exactly the threat was that justified such a response; but by declaring a major incident, BCP council initiated action by an 'emergency responder agency'. This describes all Category 1 and 2 Responders as defined in Schedule 1 of the Civil Contingencies Act and associated guidance. These include local authorities, police services, fire and rescue authorities, health bodies, the Maritime and Coastguard Agency, the Environment Agency, utilities, telecommunications, transport providers, the Highways Agency and the Health and Safety Executive.

In the event, Bournemouth, Christchurch and Poole council didn't bring in the army; but they did deploy the Dorset Local Resilience Forum, which jointly made the decision to declare the beaches a major incident. LRFs are multi-agency partnerships made up of representatives from local public services, including the emergency services, local authorities, the NHS and others.[12] These agencies also work with other partners in both the military and voluntary sectors in preparing for emergencies. The aim of LRFs is to plan and prepare for localised incidents and 'catastrophic emergencies' by identifying potential risks and producing emergency plans either to prevent or to mitigate the impact of any incident on their local communities. LRFs are Category 1 Responders, indicating that it was under the Civil Contingencies Act that the emergency response was initiated.

The Civil Contingencies Act, however, has far greater power than declaring a major incident. Part 2 of the Act contains the Government's generic legislation on emergency powers. These are described as a last-resort option for responding to the most serious of emergencies where existing legislative provision is insufficient. Emergency powers are a mechanism for making temporary legislation in order to prevent, control or mitigate an aspect or effect of the emergency. To this end, the Government can make laws granting them new powers without laying the legislation before Parliament for scrutiny or approval. In the Non-statutory guidance to the Act it states:

---

12. See Cabinet Office, 'Local resilience forums: contact details' (20 February, 2013).

Emergency powers ensure the Government can respond quickly in emergency situations where new powers or amendments to existing powers are needed and there is not time to legislate in the usual way in advance of acting. They ensure the Government can act legally and accountably in situations where temporary new legal provision is required without the time for Parliament to provide it beforehand.[13]

Under such legal provision, the Civil Contingencies Act allows Ministers to amend primary legislation, issue curfews, ban travel, require the movement of people to or from specified places, suspend our rights of assembly and 'other specified activities', confiscate property without compensation, create offences for failure to comply with these regulations and, most significantly, deploy the armed forces on homeland UK. We shouldn't forget that in March this year, under the banner of a 'COVID Defence Force', 23,000 British military personnel were placed on standby in anticipation of civil unrest in response to the Government-imposed lockdown of the UK.[14] Crucially, Section 19 allows the Secretary of State to extend the list of events classed as an 'emergency' in the event that the UK faces an unforeseen threat.

As an example of which — as if this were the first time in history that an English beach had been crowded on a summer's day, a council had failed to provide sufficient bins for the amount of rubbish thrown away, hadn't opened the public toilets to the public, or that there weren't enough carparks for visitors — Assistant Chief Constable Sam de Reya, of the Dorset Police, didn't hesitate to declare:

> These are unprecedented times, and we are urging people to stay away from the area of Bournemouth Beach and other Dorset beaches. We continue to work very closely with BCP Council and other partners to ensure the safety of the public. We are also deploying additional resources to provide increased patrols in the vicinity to help tackle any issues of anti-social behaviour and other offences being committed. The declaration of a major incident allows us to bring agencies

---

13. See Cabinet Office, 'Preparation and planning for emergencies: responsibilities of responder agencies and others' (20 February, 2013).

14. See Ministry of Defence, 'Military stands up COVID Defence Force' (19 March, 2020).

together so we can take actions available to us to safeguard the public as much as possible.[15]

I have written to Councillor Slade and asked what threat of injury, illness or loss of human life the apparently unprecedented incident of a crowded beach presented to the holiday-goers on 25 June, 2020; but she has refused to answer.[16] In the absence of any reports of any of the above, I also asked her whether it was the threat of contagion by SARS-CoV-2 presented by the close proximity of sunbathers on the beaches, but again she refused to answer. This assumption of rights over constituents without the obligation to divulge under what laws they are assumed is, in my experience, typical of the lack of transparency and accountability under which councils enact their authority. But what makes the Bournemouth beaches incident so instructive for how the UK biosecurity state might work in the future is that all it took to go from 'trying to keep everyone safe' to having the right to deploy the UK armed forces on the streets of Britain was a busy beach and the real or feigned shock of the leader of a local authority backed by an Assistant Chief Constable.

In response, Matt Hancock, the Secretary of State for Health and Social Care who has been speaking and acting like a minor dictator for some time now, and who does have the authority to make regulations introducing emergency powers, threatened to close England's beaches. He could do much more. Flexing its own muscles, BCP Council issued 993 fixed-penalty notices for illegally-parked cars in a single day, belatedly opened the public toilets and carparks, drafted in a team to pick up rubbish from the beach, and various other measures hardly consistent with a major incident justifying an emergency response.[17] But under regulations made under the Civil Contingencies Act as an emergency response to a designated 'major incident', anyone arrested, assaulted or otherwise injured or even killed by the deployment of emergency responders has, effectively, the rights of a terrorist — which, as we have seen in shooting after shooting by our police

---

15. See BCP Council, 'Major incident declared after services overstretched by thousands flocking to Bournemouth beaches' (25 June, 2020).

16. See the exchange between my subsequently permanently suspended Twitter account and that of Council Leader Vikki Slade, @vikki4mdnp (15-16 July, 2020).

17. See Sarah Cartlidge, 'Bournemouth beach: the latest rules for visitors', Bournemouth Echo (12 July, 2020).

and security forces, means none whatsoever. In the interests of 'ensuring the safety of the public' — that is to say, of enforcing the regulations of the UK biosecurity state — our individual civil liberties and human rights can and will be taken away from us — including, if necessary, our right to life.

As we have seen, the vast number of new laws made by the Government without scrutiny or approval by Parliament during the coronavirus 'crisis' have been largely made by Statutory Instruments making amendments to existing legislation. This, however, is to my knowledge the first time a local authority has had recourse to legislation in the Civil Contingencies Act 2004, which has never previously been used.[18] The Act has its limitations, since under Section 26 any regulations made under its jurisdiction lapse after 30 days — although they can be renewed with the approval of Parliament; and under Section 30 these must be made by Statutory Instrument, meaning they are secondary legislation and therefore considered subordinate to the Human Rights Act 1998. Indeed, it is these limitations that have persuaded the UK Government to respond to the coronavirus 'crisis' using other legislation.[19]

On 18 July, the Government made yet more regulations into law, again under Section 45R of the Public Health (Control of Disease) Act 1984, again without laying a draft before Parliament, again without approval by either House, again without an assessment of their impact having been made, all of which is justified 'by reason of urgency' four months since the Government-imposed lockdown. The Health Protection (Coronavirus, Restrictions) (England) (No. 3) Regulations 2020 empower a local authority, or the Secretary of State to direct a local authority, if they consider that there is a serious and imminent threat to public health and for the purpose of preventing or protecting against the spread of coronavirus, to give directions imposing prohibitions, requirements or restrictions to close or restrict entry to premises, events or public outdoor places.[20] The exception is for land owned by the Crown, which presumably is immune to the spread of a common disease. If one were attentive to how laws are being made

---

18. See Bennett Institute for Public Policy, 'The history or emergency legislation and the COVID-19 crisis', University of Cambridge (28 April, 2020).

19. See Raphael Hogarth, 'Parliament's role in the coronavirus crisis', *Institute for Government* (17 April, 2020).

20. See Statutory Instruments, 'The Health Protection (Coronavirus, Restrictions) (England) (No. 3) Regulations 2020' (18 July, 2020).

under the cloak of the coronavirus 'crisis', one might conclude that the wildly disproportionate, completely unjustified and altogether absurd response of Bournemouth, Christchurch and Poole council and the Dorset Local Resilience Forum to a crowded beach on an English summer's day, which received front-page and headline coverage on every media outlet in the country, was stage managed to justify the Government making regulations that will allow every local authority in England to act in an equally authoritarian, unjustified and disproportionate manner to any deviation from both existing laws and whatever new ones the Government dreams up in the future without the limitations imposed by the Civil Contingencies Act 2004.

3. Legislation for the UK Surveillance State

The legislative preparation for this permanent State of Emergency has been a long time coming, and any selected moment of origin will inevitably have precursors; but over the last 20 years there have been no less than 12 terrorism Acts, amendments and measures brought into UK law, and the attack on the World Trade Centre in September 2001, as for so much else, signalled the beginning of the state's assault on the rights and liberties of its citizens. I have written about this legislation elsewhere, in our report *Inequality Capital*; but my focus here is on the overlapping legislation for the UK surveillance state.[21]

In December 2014, the Investigatory Powers Tribunal, the judicial body that oversees the intelligence services in the United Kingdom, ruled that, under the Regulation of Investigatory Powers Act 2000, the legislative framework in the United Kingdom does not permit mass surveillance, and that while the Government Communications Headquarters (GCHQ) collects and analyses data in bulk, its practices do not constitute 'mass surveillance', and are compliant with Articles 8 (Right to Privacy) and 10 (Freedom of Expression) of the European Convention of Human Rights.[22] This judgement was corroborated in March 2015 by the Intelligence and Security Committee of Parliament. Both organisations were responding to the raft of legislation passed in the wake of the attack on the

---

21. See Simon Elmer, *Inequality Capital: A Power Walk by Architects for Social Housing* (18 April 2019).

22. See UK Public General Acts, 'Regulation of Investigatory Powers Act 2000' (28 July, 2000).

World Trade Centre in New York on 11 September, 2001, as well as subsequent terrorist attacks in the UK, most notably in London on 7 July, 2005. This included the Anti-Terrorism, Crime and Security Act 2001, which granted powers for the Secretary of State to regulate telephone companies and internet providers in order to retain data for the purpose of national security, and which Adam Tomkins, a Professor of Law at the University of Glasgow, called 'the most draconian legislation Parliament has passed in peacetime in over a century'; the Protection of Freedoms Act 2012, which sought to regulate surveillance, including the retention of biometric data; the Justice and Security Act 2013, which extended the powers of the GCHQ, allowed the Government to withhold trial evidence it considered to be sensitive, empowered courts to decide cases without informing the defendant what the case against them is, and was described by 57 special advocates as leaving Britain with 'more draconian rules than any other country in the world, more suited to despotic regimes such Iran and North Korea'; the Data Retention and Investigatory Powers Act 2014, which tried to remove regulation of surveillance, and which was subsequently repealed in December 2016 following a High Court judgement that sections 1 and 2 were unlawful; and the Counter-Terrorism and Security Act 2015, which requires internet service providers to retain data showing which IP address was allocated to a device at a given time.[23]

The following November, however, these judgements, however inaccurate, were rendered redundant when Parliament passed the Investigatory Powers Act 2016.[24] Nicknamed the 'Snoopers' Charter', this requires internet service providers and mobile phone companies to keep records of everyone's browsing histories for 12 months, including on social media, e-mails, voice calls and mobile phone messaging services; and gives the police, security services and a range of government departments unprecedented access to the data, as well as new powers to hack into computers and phones to collect communication data in bulk. Authorities able to access the internet connections records of UK citizens include the Metropolitan Police Service, the City of London Police, the British Transport

23. See UK Public General Acts, 'Anti-Terrorism, Crime and Security Act 2001' (14 December, 2001); Professor Adam Tomkins, 'Legislating against Terror: the Anti-terrorism, Crime and Security Act 2001', *Public Law* (Summer 2002), pp. 205-220; 'Protection of Freedoms Act 2012' (1 May, 2012); 'Justice and Security Act 2013' (25 April, 2013); 'Data Retention and Investigatory Powers Act 2014' (17 July, 2014); 'Counter-Terrorism and Security Act 2015' (12 February, 2015).

24. See UK Public General Acts, 'Investigatory Powers Act 2016' (29 November, 2016).

Police, the police forces of Scotland and Northern Ireland, of the Ministry of Defence, of the Royal Navy, Military and Air Force, the Security Service, the Secret Intelligence Service, GCHQ, the Home Office, the Ministries of Defence and Justice, the National Crime Agency, the Department of Health, and 26 other authorities.

The Investigatory Powers Act was described by Edward Snowden — the former US National Security Agency contractor turned whistle-blower who in 2013 revealed that GCHQ had been routinely collecting, processing and storing vast quantities of global digital communications, including e-mail messages, posts and private messages on social networks, internet histories, and phone calls — as the 'most intrusive and least accountable surveillance regime in the West'.[25] In December 2015, the Chinese Government cited the Draft Communications Data Bill — which was superseded by the Investigatory Powers Act — in defence of its own intrusive anti-terrorism legislation.[26] In April 2018, the UK high court ruled that the Investigatory Powers Act was incompatible with European Union law.[27] In response, the Government made The Data Retention and Acquisition Regulations 2018 into law.[28] These increased the threshold for accessing communications data to the purposes of serious crime and only following approval by the Investigatory Powers Commissioner; but also included a loophole through which rapid approval can be made internally without independent approval.

Significantly, over this period the UK became the country with the highest density of closed-circuit television (CCTV) cameras per capita in Europe, with half a million in London alone, or 1 camera for every 18 people, with the average Londoner caught on camera 300 times a day.[29] Globally, it is estimated there are 1 billion CCTV cameras, and 6 million of them are in the UK. With a population of 67.5 million, that's 1 camera for every 11.25 UK citizens. By comparison, China, with an estimated 200 million CCTV cameras for a population of 1.4 billion, has 1

---

25. See Amnesty International, 'Why we're taking the UK government to court over mass spying' (18 May, 2020).

26. See Alex Hern, 'China introduces its own "snooper's charter", *The Guardian* (29 December, 2015).

27. See Ian Cobain, 'UK has six months to rewrite snooper's charter, high court rules', *The Guardian* (27 April, 2018).

28. See UK Statutory Instruments, 'The Data Retention and Acquisition Regulations 2018' (31 October, 2018).

29. See Caught on Camera, 'How many CCTV cameras in London?'

for every 7 citizens. But, as always, it is the USA that is the forefront of the surveillance of its population of 330 million people, with 50 million cameras, or 1 camera for every 6.5 citizens, an extraordinary level of intrusion.

Legislation for the use of CCTV in the UK includes the Protection of Freedoms Act 2012; the Surveillance Camera Code of Practice 2013, which was issued by the Biometrics and Surveillance Camera Commissioner under Section 30 of the 2012 Act, and clarified that 'the Government is fully supportive of the use of overt surveillance cameras in a public place'; and the Data Protection Act 2018, which legislates our right to see information held about us, including on CCTV recordings.[30] The use of private companies to implement the surveillance state, in a country where all land is privately-owned and the public has mere rights of way over it, provided the model of how to implement the UK biosecurity state; but the coronavirus 'crisis' was the ideal opportunity to extend these intrusions further into our private lives.

Under the Coronavirus Act 2020, which was 'nodded' through Parliament by mutual agreement of all parties on 25 March after just three days of debate between both Houses before becoming law, the following provisions have increased the investigatory powers of the UK Government as follows:[31]

- Section 22. Empowers the Home Secretary to increase the number of Judicial Commissioners, and to vary the appointment process at the request of the Investigatory Powers Commissioner, who oversees and authorises almost all investigatory powers. This allows the Commissioner to directly appoint temporary Judicial Commissioners for a term of up to 6 months, renewable to a maximum period of 12 months.

The Act claims this provision is to cover for a shortage of Judicial Commissioners as an anticipated result of the effects of COVID-19.

- Section 23. Empowers the Home Secretary, by regulations made by Statutory Instrument, to change the time limits relevant to the issue, approval,

---

30. See UK Public General Acts, 'Protection of Freedoms Act 2012' (1 May, 2012); Biometrics and Surveillance Camera Commissioner, 'Surveillance Camera Code of Practice 2013' (13 August, 2021); and 'Data Protection Act 2018' (23 May, 2018).

31. See UK Public General Acts, 'Coronavirus Act 2020' (25 March, 2020), Sections 22-24.

duration, renewal and modification of warrants under the Investigatory Powers Act 2016. At the request of an Investigatory Powers Commissioner defined under this Act, the lifespan of a warrant can be extended from 5 days to up to 12 working days. In addition, such regulations may make consequential, supplementary or transitional provision lasting for a period up to 12 months.

The Act claims this provision is also to cover for an anticipated shortage of Judicial Commissioners as a result of the effects of COVID-19. The Government has not released the figures on how many Judicial Commissioners have fallen ill or died from COVID-19.

- Section 24. Empowers the Home Secretary, again by regulations made by Statutory Instrument, to extend the time limit for the statutory retention of biometric material such as fingerprints and DNA under the Police and Criminal Evidence Act 1984, the Terrorism Act 2000, the Counter-Terrorism Act 2008, and the Terrorism Prevention and Investigation Measures Act 2011, for a period up to 6 months and not longer than 12 months in total.

The Act claims this provision is in order to mitigate the anticipated impact of the coronavirus pandemic, by protecting national security and prevent serious crime during 'a period of potential widespread upheaval.'

As yet another example of how the Government is bypassing parliamentary scrutiny through the use of Statutory Instruments, a mere two days later, on 27 March, The Investigatory Powers (Temporary Judicial Commissioners and Modification of Time Limits) Regulations 2020 were made into law under Sections 22 and 23 of the Coronavirus Act 2020.[32] Mimicking the process by which they themselves were made, these Regulations extend the length of time that a warrant issued under the Investigatory Powers Act 2016 has to be authorised *ex post facto* by a Judicial Commissioner from 3 working days to 9 working days. In addition, where the Investigatory Powers Act 2016 requires that a Judicial Commissioner cannot be appointed by the Prime Minister unless jointly recommended by the

---

32. See UK Statutory Instruments, 'The Investigatory Powers (Temporary Judicial Commissioners and Modification of Time Limits) Regulations 2020' (27 March, 2020).

Lord Chancellor, the Lord Chief Justice of England and Wales, the Lord President of the Court of Session, the Lord Chief Justice of Northern Ireland and the Investigatory Powers Commissioner, one can now be appointed directly by the Commissioner on a temporary basis. Once again, in the Explanatory Memorandum this extension of powers under the Investigatory Powers Act is justified on the grounds of the anticipated effects of COVID-19 and 'to protect national security and prevent serious crime during this period.'

A further 5 days later, on 2 April, The Coronavirus (Retention of Fingerprints and DNA Profiles in the Interests of National Security) Regulations 2020 were made into law under Section 24 of the Coronavirus Act 2020.[33] These Regulations announced the decision of the Home Secretary to exercise the extension of the deadline for retaining biometric data that would otherwise be destroyed within 12 months of the Coronavirus Act coming into effect on 25 March to a further 12 months. In the Explanatory Memorandum it argues that these Regulations have not been laid before Parliament 21 days before coming into effect because:

> Any delay between the laying and coming into force of this instrument would result in the loss of biometrics (fingerprints and DNA profiles) from police databases which may have otherwise been retained on national security grounds by the making of a national security determination.[34]

Additionally, on 21 April, under Part 1 of Schedule 4 of the Investigatory Powers Act 2016, The Investigatory Powers (Communications Data) (Relevant Public Authorities and Designated Senior Officers) Regulations 2020 were made into law.[35] These extended the power to obtain communications data to five additional public bodies, including the Civil Nuclear Constabulary, the Environment Agency, the Insolvency Service, the Pensions Regulator and the UK National Authority for Counter Eavesdropping.

---

33. See UK Statutory Instruments, 'The Coronavirus (Retention of Fingerprints and DNA Profiles in the Interests of National Security) Regulations 2020' (1 April, 2020).

34. See UK Statutory Instruments, 'Explanatory Memorandum to the Coronavirus (Retention of Fingerprints and DNA Profiles in the Interests of National Security) Regulations 2020' (1 April, 2020).

35. See UK Statutory Instruments, 'The Investigatory Powers (Communications Data) (Relevant Public Authorities and Designated Senior Officers) Regulations 2020' (21 April, 2020).

The provision within the Coronavirus Act 2020 for the making of Statutory Instruments in anticipation of a purely fictional situation that was never in any danger of materialising was and is a cynical use of a viral disease to justify extending the powers of what was already the 'most intrusive and least accountable surveillance regime in the West'; and, once again, this has been done without prior scrutiny by our elected representatives in Parliament, who have obediently approved them when finally called on to do so. However, the foundations for the UK biosecurity state are not confined to regulations made under the cloak of the coronavirus 'crisis', but are also, and primarily, being laid through the technology and programmes by which the UK population is being monitored and controlled, and which are changing our status as citizens under UK law.

4. The Presumption of Guilt

On 6 April, in an article titled 'Coronavirus and the Future of Surveillance' published first in *Foreign Affairs* (a forum for discussion of US foreign policy) and then in *Belt & Road News* (an organ of China's global strategy for infrastructure development and investments in nearly 70 countries and international organisations), Nicholas Wright, a medical doctor and neuroscientist who works on emerging technologies and global strategy at University College London and the Georgetown University Medical Center, and is a contributor to the New America think-tank, argued that one of the significant 'legacies' of the coronavirus 'crisis' will be the spread of digital surveillance enabled by artificial intelligence, and that Western liberal democracies must keep pace with East Asia

> Western democracies must rise to meet the need for 'democratic surveillance' to protect their own populations. One of COVID-19's most important long-term impacts will be the reshaping of digital surveillance across the globe, prompted by the public health need to more closely monitor citizens.
>
> Just as the September 11 attacks ushered in new surveillance practices in the United States, the coronavirus pandemic might do the same for many nations around the world. Afflicted countries are all eager to better control their citizens.

Every functioning state now has a public health strategy to tackle COVID-19 that emphasises both monitoring residents and trying to influence their behaviour.

Western liberal democracies must be unafraid in trying to sharpen their powers of surveillance for public health purposes. There is nothing oxymoronic about the idea of 'democratic surveillance'.[36]

To get an idea of where we're heading in the UK, these are just some of the surveillance technology and programmes already being used by the governments of China, Hong Kong, South Korea and Taiwan to track, monitor and control their populations during the coronavirus 'crisis':

- Mass surveillance of mobile phone, rail, and flight data to track down individuals who had travelled to affected regions;
- Deployment of hundreds of thousands of neighbourhood monitors to log the movements and temperatures of individuals;
- Integration of health and other databases so that hospitals, clinics and chemists can access the travel information of their patients;
- Tracking down individuals suspected of being infected through access to their credit card transactions and CCTV footage;
- Enforcement of self-quarantine through location-tracking smartphone apps in compulsory wristbands;
- Requirement of Government-issued identity cards in order to buy SIM cards or tickets on state-run rail companies and airlines;
- Employment of colour-coded smartphone apps that tag people as green, indicating they are free to travel through city checkpoints, or as orange or red, indicating they are subject to degrees of restriction on movement;
- Use of facial recognition algorithms to identify commuters who aren't wearing a mask or who aren't wearing one properly;
- Use of robotic dogs to patrol parks to ensure compliance with social distancing measures and other Government guidance and regulations;
- Making refusal to comply with these measures an offense punishable by a fine or arrest.

---

36. See Nicholas Wright, 'Coronavirus and the Future of Surveillance: Democracies Must Offer an Alternative to Authoritarian Solutions', *Foreign Affairs* (6 April, 2020).

So what equivalent and similar measures has the UK Government introduced under the cloak of the coronavirus 'crisis'? The so-called 'NHS Test and Trace' programme has been one the most expensive and so-far useless initiatives of the Government in response to the coronavirus 'crisis', yet the Government's commitment to its implementation shows no sign of weakening.[37] I say 'so-called', because from the start the NHS tag has been a cynical use of the UK public's trust in this public service to deflect concerns about its implementation. As I discussed in 'Lockdown: Collateral Damage in the War on COVID-19', on 6 May the Scientific Pandemic Influenza Group on Behavioural Science presented a paper to the Scientific Advisory Group for Emergencies titled 'Key behavioural issues relevant to test, trace, track and isolate'. Reviewing the barriers to compliance with this programme, the paper advised that:

> Contact tracing is also viewed as more acceptable against a background of high levels of trust in an individualised provider. Personalising that provider as, for example, a health visitor or other public health clinician can also increase confidence and acceptability of contact tracing, even where contact tracing is undertaking (*sic*) using a technological solution. In designing a test and track programme, it may be appropriate to capitalise on trust in the NHS and in local health personnel.[38]

The Test and Trace programme was initially announced on 12 April, under the subsequently dropped title of 'Track and Trace', by the Secretary of State for Health and Social Care.[39] This programme utilises a mobile application that is uploaded onto a smart phone that allows the downloader to notify a centralised data base of their self-diagnosis of the symptoms of COVID-19, at which time they will be required to self-isolate for 1 week. The 'app' then notifies every other user of the technology that has come into an unspecified proximity to the phone of the

---

37. See UK Health Security Agency, 'NHS Test and Trace: what to do if you are contacted' (27 May, 2020).

38. Scientific Pandemic Influenza Group on Behavioural Science presented a paper to the Scientific Advisory Group for Emergencies titled 'Key behavioural issues relevant to test, trace, track and isolate' (6 May, 2020), p. 6.

39. See Matt Hancock, 'Health and Social Care Secretary's statement on coronavirus (COVID-19): 12 April 2020', Department of Health and Social Care (30 April, 2020).

self-diagnoser over the previous 48 hours that they have come into contact with someone who may be infected with SARs-CoV-2. This is established through Global Positioning System (GPS) location data and Bluetooth signals in their smartphones, the technology for which — the Exposure Notifications API (application programming interface) — has already been downloaded automatically, without informing users in advance, into all Apple and Android smart phones.[40] At this point, the phones of all the people with whom the phone of the person diagnosing themselves as infected has been in contact are issued with a code-yellow warning, and the owner of the phone instructed to self-isolate for two weeks. They are not allowed to leave their home, enter shops, use public transport, go to work, visit parents, pick up children from school, or meet with anyone outside their immediate household. A single self-diagnosis, therefore, by a person with no medical qualifications, of a disease whose symptoms are indistinguishable from influenza, the common cold and numerous other illnesses, will result in the quarantining of perhaps hundreds of immediate and possibly thousands of secondary contacts.

During this period of yellow alert, the person who made this self-diagnosis is contacted by a member of the privately employed tracking team and asked for their name, date of birth and address, the identities of other members of their household, as well as the names and contact details of anyone they have come into contact with in the 48 hours before their 'symptoms' started and where they came into contact with them. This is only a show of consent, however, since the app automatically records the unique ID of the phones with which it has been in close proximity over the previous 48 hours, and notifies them. It also records how long the phones were in communication with each other, how close they were and where. The person diagnosing themselves is then sent a home-test kit and required, under Schedule 21 (Powers relating to potentially infectious persons), paragraph 10, section 2 of the Coronavirus Act 2020, to send a biological sample, such as blood or a nasal swab, to a testing laboratory that confirms or denies the diagnosis. No time-frame has been given for this process, during which everyone contacted by the app and their household must remain in quarantine, but it is estimated to take several days at the least. The self-diagnoser is contacted every

---

40. See Google, 'Exposure Notification API launches to support public health agencies' (20 May, 2020).

few days by the contact tracing team to ensure their compliance with quarantine. A negative result to the test lifts the quarantine, while a positive result issues their phone with a code-red alert, confirming them as being infected with 'coronavirus', and confining all their contacts to their respective households for two weeks from the moment of contact. Furthermore, a message is also sent to the phones of everyone they have been in contact with over the previous four weeks, recommending that they self-isolate.

Revealingly, for the true purpose of this programme, the Government has instructed those the contact tracing team have alerted but who show no symptoms that they '*must not seek a test*, as the scientific evidence shows that the test may not be able to detect whether you have the virus.' In other words, hundreds of people who may have come into contact with someone who thinks they have the symptoms of coronavirus will be legally confined to house arrest on the basis of a test in which the Government has so little faith that they are instructing those same people not to use it in order to establish whether or not they have been infected. We shouldn't forget that, under coronavirus legislation, we can be compelled not only to provide a biological sample for analysis, but also to remain in quarantine for as long as the Secretary of State regards it necessary, and, should we break this quarantine, to be incarcerated in an isolation centre. In effect, everyone in the UK is assumed to be infected and therefore, under coronavirus legislation, under a permanent state of house arrest that will only be lifted following the negative result from a test to which they do not have the right of access. What this means is that, from a presumption of innocence until proven guilty under Article 6 of the Human Rights Act 1998 ('Right to a fair trial'), in the UK biosecurity state there is a presumption of guilt until proven otherwise by the private companies running the COVID-19 test programmes. Without legislation being made to this effect, therefore, the programmes for testing, tracing and isolating UK citizens are fundamentally changing our status under UK law.

In both 'The State of Emergency as a Paradigm of Government' and 'Lockdown: Collateral Damage in the War on COVID-19' I discussed at some length the potential this programme has not only for mistaken diagnoses by the public, but also for abuse of the data by the tech companies running the app for commercial and financial purposes, and manipulation of the population by the governments mandating its use, and I will not repeat my concerns here. But like

170

the crowded beaches of Bournemouth, the mere perception of a threat to the physical health of the individuals using this app is sufficient to suspend the civil liberties of the public it monitors and controls. This equation is the essence of the biosecurity state, in which the citizen no longer has the right to life (familial, social, economic, political), and in which the state has absolute power over the biopolitical body of the subject. Agamben describes this as the transition from the citizen's right to health to the legal obligation of the subject to biosecurity.

The facade of this being an NHS programme was quickly dropped when, on 18 June, the Government announced that the trials on the Isle of Wight initiated on 5 May had failed and that NHSX, the digital arm of the NHS, didn't have the capabilities to develop the app, and that the technology for tracing us was instead being developed by the US tech firms Google and Apple.[41] The testing component of the programme had already been outsourced to other multinational companies, with the Government awarding the contracts to the US multinational conglomerate Amazon, the British-Swedish multinational biopharmaceutical company AstraZeneca, the UK pharmacy retailer Boots, the multinational professional services network Deloitte, the UK artificial intelligence start-up Faculty, the UK pharmaceutical giant GlaxoSmithKline, the UK company Oxford Nanopore, the UK strategic outsourcing company Mitie, the US software company Palantir, the US scientific supplies company ThermoFisher, the UK *in vitro* diagnostics company Randox, the Swiss multinational healthcare company Roche, and the UK public services provider Serco. Behind the facade of a public initiative administered by the National Health Service and overseen by the Government, the Test and Trace programme is a private enterprise of contractors and subcontractors with an appalling record of incompetence, malpractice, fraud, price-fixing, financial mismanagement, conflicts of interest, misconduct, bribery, breaches of contract, breaches of security, breaches of confidentiality, abuse of human rights and questionable ethical practices.

The contracts awarded to some of the companies developing the Test and Trace programme were only released by the UK Government on 5 June in response to the threat of legal action by *Open Democracy*.[42] These contracts

---

41. See Department of Health and Social Care, 'Next phase of NHS coronavirus (COVID-19) app announced' (18 June, 2020); and Google, 'Privacy-Preserving Contact Tracing'.

42. See Mary Fitzgerald and Cori Crider, 'Under pressure, UK government releases NHS COVID data deals with big tech', *Open Democracy* (5 June, 2020).

revealed that Google and Palantir — the latter of which has committed 10 per cent of its workforce to the project — have been paid no more than a nominal £1 for contracts that were awarded directly and without being put out to tender by the Department of Health and Social Care.[43] Evidently, therefore, the private tech companies offering up their considerable resources to this programme are doing so not — as the Government laughingly suggests — to combat the spread of a deadly virus, but to gain access to and use of the biometric data and personal details of the UK population. In response to a legal challenge by the privacy campaigning organisation, Open Rights Group, the Department of Health and Care admitted — two days after its admission that the NHSX app had failed — that the Test and Trace programme had been rolled out without a Data Protection Impact Assessment having been made, and had therefore been deployed unlawfully, with three data breaches involving personal data by private contractors having already occurred.[44]

Even without these technical and legal barriers, however, from the start there was a more insuperable barrier to this mass transferal of private information into the data bases of private companies, and that was the extent to which the Test and Trace programme would be taken up by the UK public. The Secretary of State for Health and Social Care initially avoided answering the question of whether the use of Test and Trace app would be voluntary or mandatory, but on 11 June he admitted the Government hasn't ruled out using an 'enforcement mechanism'. 60,000 people on the Isle of Wight — about half the local population — downloaded the app as part of the Government trial.[45] And in the two weeks after the system went live across the UK on 28 May, 31,000 people were traced, although over 4,800 of them were uncontactable, and many of those that were refused to self-isolate. According to Allyson Pollock, Clinical Professor of Public Health at the University of Newcastle, a member of Independent Sage, a rival group to the Government's Scientific Advisory Group for Emergencies and the author of NHS plc: the Privatisation of Our Health Care (2004), 27,000 call-handlers have been privately employed on a salary of £20,000 per year, and in 12

43. See Oscar Williams, 'Secret data and the future of public health: why the NHS has turned to Palantir', The New Statesman (21 May, 2020).

44. See Open Rights Group, 'Government admits Test and Trace unlawful' (20 July, 2020).

45. See Svar Nanan-Sen, '"It's your DUTY!" Hancock says Brits MUST abide by test, track and trace — threat issued', Express (11 June, 2020).

weeks they've traced fewer than 56,000 contacts, less than 2 per caller, and of those only 1 contact per caller has been reached.[46] The Government has admitted that 60 per cent of the entire population of the UK — over 41 million people — would have to download the app for the Test and Trace programme to fulfil its function. Google and Apple, however, in a collective statement published in April, have already indicated how their technology will overcome this barrier by building the contact tracing function into the underlying platforms after the contact-tracing APIs have been automatically downloaded in the first phase:

> In the second phase, available in the coming months, this capability will be introduced at the operating system level to help ensure broad adoption, which is vital to the success of contact tracing. After the operating system update is installed and the user has opted in, the system will send out and listen for the Bluetooth beacons as in the first phase, but without requiring an app to be installed. If a match is detected the user will be notified, and if the user has not already downloaded an official public health authority app they will be prompted to download an official app and advised on next steps.[47]

Without downloading the Test and Trace app, therefore, the capacity for following and recording the movement, location, contact and proximity to each other of every Apple and Android phone will be built into their operating systems and uploaded automatically. Once again, then, it will be up to the user to opt out of this system of surveillance either by uninstalling the contact tracing application on their phone or by turning off its Bluetooth function. Whether or not they download the health testing app or not is irrelevant. Just 4 per cent of UK households are without a mobile phone, and 77.21 per cent of all mobile phones in the UK are smart phones.[48] In June of this year, Google's share of the mobile operating system market in the UK was 53.24 per cent; Apple's was 46.53 per cent.[49] This is what the US military calls 'full-spectrum dominance', indicating

---

46. See Sophie Inge, 'Independent Sage blasts government Test and Trace system', *Research Professional News* (10 June, 2020).

47. See Google, 'Exposure Notification Frequently Asked Questions' (April 2020), p. 3.

48. See Statista, How many mobile phones in total do you and members of your household use?'

49. See 'Mobile Operating System Market Share United Kingdom' (January-December, 2020).

control over all dimensions of the battlespace. The University of Oxford's Big Data Institute advising the NHSX has said that 80 per cent of smartphone owners need to use the operating system for it to work.[50] This doesn't mean enough to stop the spread of COVID-19 through tracing and isolating those with symptoms; it means a sufficient percentage of the population for it to be economically viable for the Government to make use of the operating system a condition of entry to public spaces or use of public services. Compliance will remain voluntary because non-compliance will be impossible for most of us. This, and not saving us from an imaginary threat to the public's health, is the real purpose of the Test and Trace Programme.

The Government has already spent £10 billion on this programme — more than the £9.4 billion it has allocated to the job retention scheme to keep UK employees on furlough — most of it in contracts awarded to the private companies running the testing component; so it's not going to drop it.[51] For now, though, the tracking component of the programme has been put on the back-burner, with Lord Bethell, who is leading the Department of Health's work on the NHS app, telling the Commons Science and Technology Committee on 17 June that it 'isn't a priority for us at the moment', but that the Government hopes to have it up and running by winter.[52]

Until then, the Government is relying on manual contact tracing to build up a digital data base of the population, its movements and interactions. On 2 July, two weeks after the technical failures in the Isle of Wight trial and the Government's admission of the app's illegality, the Department of Health and Social Care published Guidance on 'Maintaining records of staff, customers and visitors to support NHS Test and Trace'.[53] This instructed the owners, managers and staff of public houses, bars, restaurants, cafés, hotels, museums, cinemas, zoos, hairdressers, barbershops, tailors, town halls, civic centres, community

---

50. See Leo Kelion, 'Coronavirus: NHS contact tracing app to target 80% of smartphone users', *BBC* (16 April, 2020).

51. See Gareth Lacobucci, 'Covid-19: Government is criticised for "scandalous" £10bn spent on test and trace programme', *BMJ* (10 July, 2020); and HM Treasury, 'Policy Paper: A Plan for Jobs 2020' (8 July, 2020).

52. See Matt Honeycombe-Foster, 'Coronavirus: NHS contact tracing app 'not a priority' and may not be ready until winter, minister confirms', *Politics Home* (17 June, 2020).

53. See UK Health Security Agency, 'Maintaining records of staff, customers and visitors to support NHS Test and Trace' (2 July, 2020).

centres, libraries, children's centres and places of worship to refuse entry to, service in, or employment by, their establishments to visitors, customers or staff who refused to supply them with their personal details, including their name and contact number or e-mail, as well as the time of their visit, purchase or shift; to retain this information in their records for 21 days, and to share it with the private companies running the Test and Trace programme when contacted by them. Despite the bullish tone of these instructions, this Guidance is not law. Compliance with these measures, as the text of the Guidance clearly states, is not mandatory but voluntary; and the establishment does not have to impose them as a condition of entry, service or employment. Any information we chose to give does not have to be verified either by us or the establishment collecting it, and at our insistence it can be withheld from the Test and Trace programme.

However, despite its voluntary nature — expressing nothing more than the wishes of a Minister, and without the force of law behind it — this Government guidance has been widely adopted by establishments in England, with many competing to extend the measures to, for example, making the wearing of face coverings a condition of entry into their premises. For those of us politically opposed to such measures, which have no medical proof of their effectiveness, that are wildly disproportionate to the threat to public health, are an intrusion into our privacy, a violation of our civil liberties, and another element in the apparatus of the biosecurity state being imposed under the cloak of the coronavirus 'crisis', this Guidance has effectively banned us from public life. In the next section I will look at the role of the medical profession in supplying the justification for such extraordinary and authoritarian measures of surveillance and control that have so quickly been accepted as part of the 'New Normal'.

Perhaps the most dystopian vision of our future, however, is provided by so-called 'immunity passports', which more tightly bind the tracking element of contact tracing technology to the biosecurity state. On 28 April, the Chief Executive of NHSX, the unit that sets national policy and best practice for the NHS on digital technology, including data sharing and transparency, told the Parliamentary Science and Technology Committee that they were exploring the creation of immunity passports. An extension and expansion of the Test and Trace app, these will signal to anyone authorised to require this information whether a person has immunity to SARS-CoV-2. In order to do so, immunity passports will require an artificial intelligence facial recognition check that matches a Government-approved form of identification linked to biometric data like a fingerprint or photograph. This check will automatically confirm a person's health 'status' via a Quick Response (QR) code whenever they enter any public space using the biosecurity system. Access to such a place, accordingly, will be taken out of the hands of the security, staff, manager or even owner, and placed within the sole jurisdiction of the Artificial Intelligence (AI) technology employed by the company running the programme. And since the user's health status will have to be regularly updated to guarantee immunity, their access to public life will be contingent on a vastly expanded system of health monitoring — rather than service — outsourced to a plethora of private contractors and sub-contractors in a long chain of dwindling transparency and accountability.

Once again, therefore, there will be a presumption of infection and therefore guilt it is the individual's responsibility to disprove through compliance with the various systems of surveillance, testing, monitoring and control. Without the devices necessary to activate those systems, and without the willingness to comply with its directions, the subject of the biosecurity state will be effectively banned from access to a whole range of public spaces and services, including, potentially, public transport, shopping centres, workplaces, job centres, educational institutions, health clinics, hospitals, council premises and airports. Once again, then, making such a passport mandatory will not be necessary, when citizenship in the country in which they are implemented is dependent upon their use.

There are numerous AI companies competing for government contracts for immunity passports around the world and as many terms to describe the products they're selling; but in the UK the front-runners appear to be the digital identity start-up Onfido, which in its proposal to NHSX recommended that its immunity passport be made mandatory, since this would mean 'participation should be possible without further intrusion on a person's civil liberties and freedoms'; the global digital identity company Yoti, which prefers to use the term 'Digital Health Passes' to reflect doubts among medical professionals of the extent to which the presence of antibodies in a previously infected person confers immunity; and the cyber-security company VST Enterprises, which already supplies its product, COVI-PASS, to 15 countries, including Italy, France, Spain, Portugal, Sweden, the

Netherlands, the USA, Canada, Mexico, South Africa, India and the United Arab Emirates.[54] In its cartoon promotional video, VST Enterprises boasts that its VCode technology gives their company the edge in ensuring 'fluid crowd control and movement of people'.[55] The crowds it depicts the pass controlling are workspaces and businesses open to the public such as department stores, supermarkets and public bars; but as the video says, the product's 2.2 quintillion codes offer 'infinite possibilities, once assigned'. It doesn't take much imagination to apply their boast to every movement of every member of the public in every public space.

5. The Religion of Medicine

In his 2013 book, *Microbial Storms: Essay on Health Security Policies in the Transatlantic World*, Patrick Zylberman looked at how new political strategies of governance based on the health security of the population has given rise to the fictive scenarios required to justify them:

> Health security is today both the object of, and the pretext for, a vertiginous descent into fiction. Exaggerated figures, groundless analogies and bioterrorism threat narratives are all noted examples of this. But where do all these worst-case scenarios come from? And what are their implications when applied to our own defence systems against microbial threats?[56]

To answer these questions, Giorgio Agamben, in another article on the coronavirus 'crisis', 'Biosecurity and Politics', published on 11 May, summarised these strategies as follows:

---

54. See Onfido, 'The role of Digital Identity in Immunity Passports', UK Parliament Committees (April 2020); Chris Burt, 'UK immunity passport proposals leverage biometric facial recognition', *Biometric Update* (30 April, 2020); 'Yoti CitizenCard — the UK's ID solution', *Citizencard*; and 'Deal struck to integrate technologies onto digital health passport', *Med-Tech News* (12 May, 2020).

55. See VST Enterprises, 'COVI-PASS™ Digital Health Passport', *YouTube* (26 May, 2020).

56. Patrick Zylberman, *Tempêtes microbiennes. Essai sur la politique de sécurité sanitaire dans le monde transatlantique* (Paris, Gallimard, 2013), p. 24.

1. The construction, on the basis of a potential risk, of a fictitious scenario in which data would be presented in such a way as to encourage behaviours that would make it possible to govern an extreme situation;

2. The adoption of the logic-of-the-worst as a regime of political rationality;

3. The total organisation of the body of citizens in a way that reinforces the fullest adherence to institutions of government, producing a sort of superlative good citizenship in which imposed obligations are presented as proof of altruism, and the citizen no longer has a right to health ('health safety') but is instead forced by law obliged to be healthy ('biosecurity').[57]

Three months later, this reads like a three-point plan for the UK Government's response to the coronavirus 'crisis', which — let us remind ourselves:

1. By changing the classification and registering of COVID-19 and therefore its appearance as the 'underlying cause of death' on the death certificates of people in whose death its causality is not proven but only suspected, has transformed a respiratory disease that statistically threatens only those over 60 years of age with at least one pre-existing illness into an epidemic justifying the lockdown of 68.8 million UK citizens;

2. On the basis of an 'imminent and serious threat' to the health of all UK citizens, has placed the UK into an 'emergency period' whose continuation only the Government has the ability to end, and during which laws can be made without parliamentary scrutiny or approval, effectively placing the UK under a constitutional dictatorship;

3. Has used this legislative freedom to issue Guidance, impose regulations and implement programmes in violation of our human rights and civil liberties, either enforced by our police forces or made a condition of our access to public services and venues, in which compliance is promoted as a civic duty and refusal punished with a fine or the threat of arrest by propaganda campaigns that denounce dissent as a threat to public health.

---

57. Giorgio Agamben, 'Biosecurity and Politics', *Quodlibet* (11 May, 2020); collected in *Where Are We Now? The Epidemic as Politics*; second updated edition; translated by Valeria Dani (Eris, 2021), p. 56. In the original Italian, both 'health safety' and 'biosecurity' are written in English.

In June this year, at the request of the Government, the Academy of Medical Sciences established an Expert Advisory Group to look at, among other things, how systems of surveillance and other non-pharmaceutical interventions could respond to estimates of a worst-case scenario for the winter of 2020-21. Chaired by Stephen Holgate, Clinical Professor of Immunopharmacology at the University of Southampton, on the 14 July this group published their findings in a document titled 'Preparing for a challenging winter 2020-21'.[58] What the report calls its 'reasonable worst-case scenario' comprises a large resurgence of COVID-19 deaths in a second wave of infection starting this autumn; disruption of health and social care systems caused by the need to respond to this resurgence; the backlog of medical care unrelated to COVID-19 that has accumulated with the suspension of medical service under the lockdown; and a possible influenza epidemic. The compounded result of this worst-case scenario is that from September onwards the rate of infection from SARS-CoV-2 will rise to 1.7 (it is currently 0.8-0.9), resulting in an estimated total number of hospital deaths (excluding care homes) between September 2020 and June 2021 of 119,900, 'over double the number occurring during the first wave in spring 2020', with an upward estimate of over a quarter of a million people.[59]

We've heard similarly exaggerated estimates before. In the report published on 16 March, the Imperial College COVID-19 Response team estimated that, unless the Government imposed a lockdown of the UK, around 510,000 people would die from COVID-19.[60] Unsurprisingly, this latest report takes as proven the effectiveness of social distancing measures, confidently asserting that they 'resulted in an 80% reduction in transmission and that 470,000 deaths had been averted in the UK up to 4 May 2020 due to such restrictions.' In this respect, the group is repeating the claim of the Prime Minister, in his address to the nation on 10 May, that the lockdown of the UK saved 'half a million fatalities'.[61] However, the only evidence the report provides for this assertion is an unedited manuscript

58. See Academy of Medical Sciences, 'Preparing for a challenging winter 2020-21' (14 July, 2020).

59. See UK Health Security Agency, 'The R value and growth rate' (15 May, 2020).

60. See Neil Ferguson, et al., 'Report 9. Impact of non-pharmaceutical interventions (NPIs) to reduce COVID19 mortality and healthcare demand', Imperial College London (16 March, 2020).

61. See Boris Johnson, 'Prime Minister's statement on coronavirus (COVID-19): 10 May 2020' (10 May, 2020).

accepted for publication in *Nature* on 8 June under the title 'Estimating the effects of non-pharmaceutical interventions on COVID-19 in Europe'.[62] Not surprisingly, this was co-written by the same Imperial College team whose gross overestimates of the number of deaths from COVID-19 were used by the Government to justify the lockdown of the country, the suspension of Parliament and the raft of legislation made into law in its continuing absence. It's also not surprising that Professor Neil Ferguson, the leader of the Imperial College team for the initial and long since discredited estimates of COVID-19 deaths, was also one of the contributors to this latest assertion of the efficacy of the lockdown. The Government's go-to man for exaggerated predictions of deaths from diseases — he estimated 65,000 deaths from swine flu (457 have died), 150,000 from mad cow disease (178 have died), and 200 million from bird flu (282 have died) — Ferguson, just two days after this manuscript was published in *Nature*, told a committee of MPs that, if the lockdown of the UK had been imposed a week earlier, deaths from COVID-19 would have reduced 'by at least a half'.[63]

I won't repeat here my previous analysis of the lack of evidence for the effectiveness of lockdown for anything other than increasing the number of deaths in the countries in which it was imposed, which in the UK, in particular, has been largely due to the withdrawal of medical diagnosis and treatment for life-threatening illnesses in order to free up hospital beds for an epidemic that never materialised. But I want to say something about the complete irrationality of these assertions, which are religious in their basis and rationalisations. Like the threat of an eternity of suffering in a hell from which only God's love can save us, the estimation of a worst-case scenario by the medical profession is being used by our Government to justify any measures that will avert catastrophe. And just as the Church, unsurprisingly, tells us that only obedience to their laws will appease the wrath of God, so the Government, equally unsurprisingly, insists that only obeying its emergency measures will stop the worst-case scenario from coming to pass. Of course, like the priest, the politician's proof that such measures work is that nothing even approaching the prediction of 510,000 deaths from COVID-

---

62. See Seth Flaxman, *et al.*, 'Estimating the effects of non-pharmaceutical interventions on COVID-19 in Europe', *Nature* (8 June, 2020).

63. See Steerpike, 'Six questions that Neil Ferguson should be asked', *The Spectator* (16 April, 2020); and James Gallagher, 'Coronavirus: "Earlier lockdown would have halved death toll"', *BBC* (10 June, 2020).

19 came to pass, and asks us to imagine how much worse it would have been as we gaze at the images of eternal damnation the Government and media have painted for us on every available surface and screen.

A rational response to such evangelical fearmongering is to look at the countries where nothing like the level of lockdown measures in the UK were imposed, and where the deaths attributed to COVID-19 are nothing like as high, suggesting not only that the lockdown did nothing to stop the virus but that it increased the number of excess deaths in the countries where it was most strongly imposed. This is precisely what I did in my article 'Lockdown: Collateral Damage in the War on COVID-19'; and in response to the growing number of articles making the same argument the Government has now identified the wearing of masks in countries where the governments didn't impose a lockdown, and in particular in Japan, South Korea and Taiwan, as the real barrier to the spread of the virus. In other words, obedience to the rules of the Church of Medicine is the basis to our entry into the Kingdom of Biosecurity, but a little prayer helps too (and wearing a home-made face covering to stop a virus is nothing more than a prayer), which our local priest is happy to perform on our behalf for a small donation. 'The world, alas, is full of suffering and death!', these peddlers of purgatory gravely inform us. 'But imagine how much worse it would be if we weren't praying for you!' Such are the self-fulfilling prophecies of doom and salvation preached by the evangelists of health.

In one of his commentaries on the coronavirus 'crisis', published in *Quodlibet* on 2 May under the title 'Medicine as Religion', Giorgio Agamben explicitly compares this rationalisation to religious practice:

> It is immediately evident that what we are dealing with here is a cultic practice, and not a rational or scientific necessity. The most frequent cause of death in our country is, by far, cardiovascular diseases, and it is well known that these could be reduced if we practiced a healthier form of life and followed particular diets. But it has never crossed the mind of any doctor that this form of life and diet — which they recommend to the patient — should become the object of a legal rule, one that would decree, as a matter of law, what we must eat and how we should live, transforming our entire existence into a health obligation. And yet precisely this has been done and, at least for now, people have accepted — as if it were

common sense — the renunciation of their freedom of movement, of work, friendships, love and social relations, and of their own religious and political beliefs.[64]

Unfortunately, under a sustained propaganda campaign of co-ordinated adulation — including the weekly 'clap for the NHS' ritual, public expressions of gratitude on everything from house windows to billboards, and the elevation of health professionals to 'front-line' heroes in a 'war' on COVID-19 — the medical profession has been encouraged to view itself as the highest and final arbiter of our response to the coronavirus 'crisis': if not as God, exactly, then as the guardians and arbiters of His laws. And they have not been reticent in adopting this new priestly role. In response to me publishing my article 'Manufacturing Consensus' — which examined how the criteria for attributing deaths to COVID-19 in the UK has been determined by changes to disease taxonomy made by the Department of Health and Social Care and instructions on filling out death certificates for COVID-19 published by the World Health Organization — I was recently attacked on Twitter by a cabal of medical practitioners led by a doctor whose name I won't reveal, but who diagnosed me as 'mentally deficient' and advised me to 'get treatment'. Social media, admittedly, increases the stupidity and aggressiveness with which people speak; but I still find it worrying that a medical practitioner of some seniority should say such things in a public forum at a time of such confusion and doubt among the public about the Government's response to the coronavirus 'crisis'. Not too long ago, the same medical attitude prescribed lobotomies for anyone who didn't knuckle down and toe the line, and collaborated in the incarceration of women who refused to obey their husbands. It is perhaps not surprising that an increasingly secular population should seek hope of salvation from an invisible threat when medicine has become the religion of the biosecurity state; but it is more than concerning that professors and practitioners of medicine should feel authorised to make recommendations on draconian social measures based on irresponsible fearmongering by the Government that is quite blatantly in the service of expanding its powers over the population.

---

64. Giorgio Agamben, 'Medicine as Religion', *Quodlibet* (2 May, 2020); translated in *Where Are We Now?*, p. 52.

These recommendations are made by the Academy of Medical Sciences in Part 4 of their report, titled 'Priorities for prevention and mitigation'. With nothing more than the assurance that face coverings '*could* contribute to reducing viral transmission when population compliance is high' and '*could* reduce onward transmission', the report nonetheless confidently asserts that the 'wearing of face coverings in shared indoor environments, are *vital* to preventing SARS-CoV-2 transmission'.[65] Of more concern, however, is that in the absence of any assessment of their impact or consideration of the proportionality or justification for doing so, the authors bullishly insist that to be effective the wearing of face coverings should not be merely encouraged but made mandatory, so that doing so 'becomes a social norm'. At this point we should remind ourselves that this is a report by professors and doctors of epidemiology, virology, and immunology, not of political science, sociology or law. The exception is Professor Dame Theresa Marteau, Director of the Department of Health and Social Care's policy research unit on behaviour and health at Cambridge University, who also sits on the academic advisory panel of the Cabinet Office's Behavioural Insights Team or so-called 'Nudge Unit' that is leading the Government's management of the coronavirus 'crisis'.[66] Perhaps coincidentally, she once confided to the *British Medical Journal* that her first ambition was 'to become a nun, to atone for sins that in my 9-year-old mind would inexorably lead to eternal damnation'.[67]

It's when the report gets to the question of how to ensure compliance with these measures, however, that the collusion of this new priesthood in the UK biopolitical state becomes most explicit. In response to their own question — 'How do we establish and communicate the "new normal"?' — the authors identify public engagement in the latest version of the Test and Trace programme, now retitled 'Test, Trace and Isolate' (TTI).[68] Having identified the reluctance to put friends and family into quarantine as compromising the effectivity of this programme, the report recommends that public information campaigns should be tailored to the educational, economic and racial characteristics of the targeted communities in collaboration with what it calls 'local leaders', among which it

---

65. Academy of Medical Sciences, 'Preparing for a challenging winter 2020-21', pp. 31-32.

66. See Martin Edwards, 'Behavioural Insights: The Second Team Leading the UK Government's Covid-19 Response', UK Column (3 May, 2020).

67. Theresa Marteau, 'Tackling behaviour change', *BMJ* (21 May, 2014).

68. Academy of Medical Sciences, 'Preparing for a challenging winter 2020-21', p. 32.

includes directors or public health, healthcare practitioners, doctors and religious leaders. However, the report insists that 'TTI will only be effective if it is carried out quickly, accurately, is acceptable to the public, and encompasses a high proportion of symptomatic cases.'[69] To this end, 'testing and tracing capacity will need to be significantly expanded to cope with increasing demands over the winter.'[70] Finally, the report advises that there are 'substantial opportunities for TTI to act synergistically with a broader surveillance system'.[71] One is tempted to ask why the authors do not extend the imposition of such measures to reducing dementia, heart disease and cancer — the primary causes of death in the UK, and in far greater numbers than deaths attributed to COVID-19 — by banning unhealthy foods, smoking and alcohol and imposing a healthy diet and exercise by law and developing an app to ensure our compliance. Of course, this is exactly what the Government is now doing with its recently-announced programme to reduce obesity on the grounds that it increases the risk of dying from COVID-19, and we can look forward to new legislation and apps enforcing our compliance.[72]

It's in the chapter on how to 'optimise public health surveillance', however, that the authors of this report firmly nail their colours to the Government's mast. These are some of their highlighted recommendations — in which 'granular' means more detailed, with the more granular the data the closer the examination; and 'real-time' means data that is not kept or stored, but is passed along to the end-user as soon as it is collected. Together, these recommendations describe a more intrusive, more widely implemented, and far more totalitarian system of surveillance:

- To inform these existing surveillance systems, it is important to sustain and improve the quality and completeness of near real-time, granular data collection with more detailed reporting in time, place and person.
- Targeted surveys of populations where COVID-19 incidence is high or unknown will be vital to ensure such groups are carefully monitored for early evidence of a resurgence in cases.

---

69. Academy of Medical Sciences, 'Preparing for a challenging winter 2020-21', p. 36.
70. Academy of Medical Sciences, 'Preparing for a challenging winter 2020-21', p. 37.
71. Academy of Medical Sciences, 'Preparing for a challenging winter 2020-21', p. 36.
72. See Department of Health and Social Care, 'Tackling obesity: empowering adults and children to live healthier lives' (27 July, 2020).

- All collated data need to be made available to local public health and NHS providers in order to rapidly implement outbreak investigation and control. This data must also be made accessible to researchers with the linking of routine surveillance data and research platforms.
- Given the complexity of all the data collection, processing and distribution involved in effective public health management of a winter COVID-19 outbreak, a single central authority overseeing and coordinating efforts would increase the likelihood of success.[73]

---

73. Academy of Medical Sciences, 'Preparing for a challenging winter 2020-21', pp. 46-47. This seems like a good place to name the primary authors of this report, which one day, hopefully, will be presented in evidence at their trials. These are as follows: Professor Stephen Holgate CBE FMedSci, Clinical Professor of Immunopharmacology, University of Southampton; Professor Wendy Barclay FMedSci, Action Medical Research Professor of Virology & Head of Department of Infectious Disease, Faculty of Medicine, Imperial College London; Dr William Bird MBE, Chief Executive Officer, Intelligent Health; Professor Carol Brayne CBE FMedSci, Professor of Public Health Medicine, University of Cambridge; Professor Chris Brightling FMedSci, NIHR Senior Investigator and Clinical Professor in Respiratory Medicine, University of Leicester; Professor James Chalmers, British Lung Foundation Chair of Respiratory Research, University of Dundee; Dr Tristan Clark, Associate Professor, Honorary Consultant in Infectious Diseases, University of Southampton; Professor John Clarkson FREng, Director of Cambridge Engineering Design Centre, University of Cambridge; Professor Dame Jessica Corner FMedSci, Professor of Cancer and Supportive Care; Pro-Vice-Chancellor (Research & Knowledge Exchange), University of Nottingham; Mark Cubbon, Chief Executive, Portsmouth Hospitals NHS Trust; Professor Simon de Lusignan, Professor of Primary Care and Clinical Informatics, University of Oxford; Dr Jake Dunning MBE, Consultant in Infectious Diseases and Head of Emerging Infections and Zoonoses, National Infection Service, Public Health England; Dr Nigel Field, Director, Centre of Molecular Epidemiology and Translational Research, Institute for Global Health, University College London; Professor Azra Ghani FMedSci, Chair in Infectious Disease Epidemiology, Imperial College London; Professor Bryan Grenfell OBE FRS, Kathryn Briger & Sarah Fenton Professor of Ecology and Evolutionary Biology and Public Affairs, Princeton University; Professor Andrew Hayward, Professor of Infectious Disease Epidemiology and Inclusion Health Research, University College London; Dr Matthew Hort, Head of Atmospheric Dispersion and Air Quality, Met Office; Professor Matthew Hotopf CBE FMedSci, Vice Dean of Research, Institute of Psychiatry, Psychology and Neuroscience, King's College London; Professor Dame Anne Johnson DBE FMedSci, Professor of Infectious Disease Epidemiology, University College London; Professor Kamlesh Khunti FMedSci, Professor of Primary Care Diabetes & Vascular Medicine, University of Leicester; Professor Dame Theresa Marteau DBE FMedSci, Director of Behaviour and Health Research Unit, University of Cambridge; Professor Graham Medley, Professor of Infectious Disease Modelling, London School of Hygiene & Tropical Medicine; Dr Pablo Murcia, Senior Lecturer at the Centre for Virus Research, University of Glasgow; Professor Catherine Noakes, Professor of Environmental Engineering for Buildings,

Given the reports' willingness to provide the Government with the medical opinion it needs to implement the next stage of the UK biosecurity state, the authors' recommendation for this central overseeing and co-ordinating authority isn't surprising: the Government's new Joint Biosecurity Centre.[74]

Announced by the Prime Minister on 11 May, the Joint Biosecurity Centre (JBC) is a monitoring system designed to require businesses to collect a wide range of data, including biometric samples, on their employees, customers and visitors. The Centre is responsible for advising Ministers, local authorities and businesses to close schools, workplaces or other establishments. Like the Test and Trace programme, of which it is a part, the Joint Biosecurity Centre is a public-private partnership — which means it will be run by private contractors and have the backing of the Government, including, if necessary, the regulations made to accommodate its intrusion into our privacy or enforce its use as a condition of access to public spaces.

To this end, the Joint Biosecurity Centre, which is based on the Joint Terrorism Analysis Centre, is responsible for setting what the Government calls the COVID-19 Alert level. This parallels and has much the same function as the UK Terror Threat Levels that the Government introduced in 2006, and which have never since dropped below level 3 ('Substantial'), indicating that a terrorist attack is 'a strong possibility'. Unsurprisingly, since the COVID-19 Alert level was introduced nearly three months ago, it too has never dropped below 3, indicating that the coronavirus is in 'general circulation'. The Government, however, is not bound by this setting level. Supposedly determined by scientific analysis of the

---

University of Leeds; Professor Peter Openshaw FMedSci, Professor of Experimental Medicine, Imperial College London; Dr Mary Ramsay, Head of Immunisation, Public Health England; Professor Steven Riley, Professor of Infectious Disease Dynamics, Imperial College London; Mandy Rudczenko, Co-Chair, Patient and Carer Reference Group; Dr Janet Scott, Clinical Lecturer in Infectious Diseases, University of Glasgow; Sudhir Shah, Co-Chair, Patient and Carer Reference Group; Dr Laura Shallcross, Consultant in Public Health Medicine, University College London; Professor Aziz Sheikh OBE FRSE FMedSci, Chair of Primary Care Research and Development, University of Edinburgh; Professor Rosalind Smyth CBE FMedSci, Director, UCL Great Ormond Street Institute of Child Health; Linda Swanson, Director of Nursing Infection Control, The Northern Care Alliance Professor Russell Viner, President, Royal College of Paediatrics and Child Health; Professor Lucy Yardley, Professor of Health Psychology, University of Southampton and University of Bristol.

74. See Alex Thomas, 'Joint Biosecurity Centre', *Institute for Government* (12 May, 2020).

rate of infection in the UK, the number of confirmed cases of SARS-CoV-2, and the number of deaths attributed to COVID-19, the COVID-19 alert level is set by the same Chief Medical and Chief Scientific advisors to the Government (Professor Chris Whitty and Patrick Vallance) that have so far justified the enforcement of social distancing by police officers beyond the requirements of legislation, the lockdown of the UK for three months, the suspension of medical treatment for life-threatening diseases other than COVID-19, the closure of UK schools for 4 months, the mandating of face coverings in public spaces, and the collecting of personal information in public premises as a condition of entry. So we can expect the same level of supine compliance with Ministerial wishes and willingness to justify disproportionate Government policy. More indicative of the purpose and function of the Joint Biosecurity Centre is that it was initially headed by Tom Hurd, the Director General of the Office for Security and Counter-Terrorism, before being handed over this June to Clare Gardiner, a senior spy at the Director of National Resilience and Strategy at the National Cyber Security Centre, which is a branch of GCHQ.[75] It is from the nexus of science, medicine, security and technology represented by these four civil servants, in which the population is kept in a permanent state of war with itself, that the UK biosecurity state is being built. In 'Medicine as Religion' Agamben writes:

> The epidemic, as the etymology of the term suggests (*demos* is in Greek the people as a political body and *polemos epidemios* is in Homer the name for civil war) is first and foremost a political concept that is about to become the new terrain of world politics — or non-politics. It is possible, however, that the epidemic that we are experiencing is the actualisation of a global civil war that, according to the most attentive political analysts, is taking the place of traditional world wars. All nations and all peoples are now perpetually at war with themselves, because the invisible and elusive enemy with which they are fighting is within us.[76]

---

75. See Beckie Smith, 'Counter-terrorism director general to lead coronavirus risk response unit', *Civil Service World* (12 May, 2020); and Helen Warrell and Sarah Neville, 'Senior spy appointed to lead the UK's joint biosecurity centre', *Financial Times* (5 June, 2020).

76. Giorgio Agamben, 'Medicine as Religion', *Quodlibet* (2 May, 2020); translated in *Where Are We Now?*, pp. 53-54.

6. The Utopia of Shame

As part of the production of its report, the Academy of Medical Sciences employed Ipsos MORI, the market-research company, to conduct three online workshops with 36 members of the public. Among the key findings from these consultations was the following observation:

> There was a general perception that 'other people' were not abiding by the rules of social distancing, evidenced for many by the scenes of crowds on Bournemouth beach and also typified for some by the conduct of high-profile individuals they felt should be setting better examples. This fed a general demand among the groups that the social distancing rules be made clearer and that they should be demonstrably enforced, including through fines and arrests.[77]

The 'public' did not have long to wait. On the same day, 14 July, the Secretary for State for Health and Social Care announced to a House of Commons with less than two dozen MPs present that face coverings will become mandatory for customers in shops and supermarkets, with non-compliance punished with a fixed penalty notice up to £100:

> Should an individual without an exemption refuse to wear a face covering, a shop can refuse them entry and can call the police if people refuse to comply. The police have formal enforcement powers and can issue a fine. This is in line with how shops would normally manage their customers and enforcement is of course a last resort, and we fully expect the public to comply with the rules as they have done throughout the pandemic.[78]

In response to this announcement, the Chair of the Metropolitan Police Force told BBC Radio 4:

---

77. Ipsos MORI in Academy of Medical Sciences, 'Preparing for a challenging winter 2020-21', Annex 3, pp. 1-2.

78. Matt Hancock, 'Face coverings to be mandatory in shops and supermarkets from 24 July' (14 July, 2020).

It will be nigh-on impossible for enforcement because you won't have a police officer on every shop door because there isn't enough of us. If a shopkeeper calls the police because someone hasn't got a mask on, they haven't got the power to detain them so that person can just walk away. We'll be driving around and around London looking for people who aren't wearing masks, it's absolutely absurd.[79]

On 22 July, the Commissioner of the Metropolitan Police Force confirmed that her police officers will not respond to calls about shoppers refusing to wear face coverings, and that calling the police should be a 'last resort'. She also told LBC Radio that she hoped shoppers would be 'shamed' into compliance:

My hope is that the vast majority of people will comply, and that people who are not complying will be shamed into complying or shamed to leave the store by the store keepers or by other members of the public.[80]

The following day, on 23 July, The Health Protection (Coronavirus, Wearing of Face Coverings in a Relevant Place) (England) Regulations 2020 were finally published.[81] Once again, these were made by Statutory Instrument under the Public Health (Control of Disease) Act 1984; once again without prior scrutiny by Parliament of the evidence; once again without an impact assessment having been made; and once again with the absence of all of these requirements justified 'by reason of urgency', despite the Regulations being made four months since the Government-imposed lockdown of the UK and as many since the debate on the benefits and dangers of wearing masks in public began.

Under Regulation 1, these Regulations come into force in England and Wales on 24 July, 2020. Under Regulation 3, we cannot enter or remain within a 'relevant place' without wearing a covering over our mouth and nose. Under Regulation 5, a 'relevant person' can deny us entry to, direct us to wear a face covering within, or direct us to leave, a 'relevant place' when not wearing such a covering. Under

---

79. See Rachel Younger, 'Coronavirus: Shops can call police if customers fail to wear face covering, Hancock says', *ITV News* (14 July, 2020).

80. See 'Coronavirus: London police to enforce face masks "as last resort", *BBC News* (22 July, 2020).

81. See UK Statutory Instruments, 'The Health Protection (Coronavirus, Wearing of Face Coverings in a Relevant Place) (England) Regulations 2020' (24 July, 2020).

Paragraph 9, a 'relevant person' is a police constable, community support officer, Transport for London officer or person designated by the Secretary of State for the purpose of these regulations. Under Schedule 1, a 'relevant place' is defined as an enclosed shop, shopping centre (but not a seated bar or cafe within it), bank, post office or transport hub. If we refuse such direction by a relevant person, under Regulation 5 a constable can remove us from such a place using reasonable force. Under Regulation 6, refusing, obstructing or otherwise resisting such powers is an offence that under Regulation 7 is punishable by a fixed penalty notice of £100, which, again, may only be issued by a relevant person. Under Regulation 9, these Regulations must be reviewed by the Secretary of State within 6 months of them coming into force; and under Regulation 10 they will expire in 12 months. None of these powers are granted to an owner, manager or member of staff of a relevant place. Indeed, The Health Protection (Coronavirus, Wearing of Face Coverings in a Relevant Place) (England) Regulations 2020 have nothing to do with the owners, managers or staff of the relevant places they designate. They merely extend the powers of police constables, community support officers, Transport for London officers or other relevant persons over us when in such places.

There are several things to be said about these new regulations. The first is that — like those preceding them — they exclude the shop, bank, post-office, supermarket and shopping-centre staff, public transport employees, community support officers and police constables that are the most constant human presence in these designated 'relevant places' and are therefore — if we are to believe the Secretary of State for Health and Social Care — the primary source for the spread of the 'serious and imminent threat' the places in which they work are supposed to present. Emergency responders, too, are also exempt. In addition to these exempt persons, the following places are also excluded from the list of relevant places: restaurants with table service, hotel dining rooms, members' clubs, bars and public houses; public libraries and reading rooms; premises providing professional, legal and financial services; premises providing medical services; veterinary services; cinemas, theatres, nightclubs, dance, bingo, concert, exhibition and other public halls; conference and exhibition centres; fitness and dance studios, indoor gyms, leisure centres, indoor swimming pools, water parks, bowling alleys, funfairs, theme parks, amusement arcades, indoor soft-play areas, skating rinks or other indoor premises for indoor sports, leisure, adventure or recreation activities; indoor sports arenas or stadia; casinos, hotels and hostels; spas, nail, beauty and hair salons and barbers; tattoo, piercing and massage parlours; storage and distribution centres; funeral directors; photography studios; and auction houses. Quite evidently, therefore, by the sheer number of public places excluded from these regulations, they have other motivations than protecting 'public health'.

The second thing to say is that, although they can be ignored by the owners, managers and staff of the places they designate as relevant to them, these regulations rely for their implementation not on the various UK police forces — which have admitted that they do not have the constables to police them — but on the owners and managers of shops, supermarkets and other 'relevant places'. However, since their staff do not have the legal powers to detain a customer who refuses to wear a face covering on the premises, or even to deny us entry to the premises under the powers conferred by these regulations, staff can only make wearing one a condition of entry on the grounds that the premises are private property. This is what the Secretary of State referred to when he told Parliament that refusing entry would be 'in line with how shops would normally manage their customers'. As long as doing so does not discriminate against someone under the Equality Act 2010 — that is, because of our age, race, religion, gender, sexuality, etc. — staff can already refuse to serve us, and sometimes do so if, for example, we are drunk, or abusive or threatening. The new regulations have added nothing to an owner's rights over their private property.

What is being presented as a public measure, therefore, will in practice cause further reduction of our public rights of way over private land. This will inevitably lead, at least initially, to increased confrontation and civil disturbance in retail outlets and shopping centres. In the same way, therefore, that more and more private land in the UK is being guarded by private security guards, so too more shops — and not just shopping centres, supermarkets and banks — will employ security guards to enforce this condition. Behind the bogus reason of protecting the public from the spread of a disease that presents no more of a threat than seasonal influenza, these regulations are using the private sector to bear the financial burden of increasing the number of security guards in our public life, thereby expanding the UK surveillance state.

In the UK today, security guards, as a matter of course, wear uniforms as close as is legally permissible to police constables, often with chequered hat bands, high-visibility jackets, dark-blue clothing and jack boots. Given the British public's general ignorance of the laws under which we live, a direction from a private security guard is accepted as having the force of law, when in fact it has nothing of the kind. The owners of private property can insist on someone wearing a face covering as a condition of entry into their shop, and announce this condition on a sign displayed outside the premises, and this makes entry without such a covering trespass. This, however, is only a civil offence. If the owner or his or her representatives — that is to say, the manager, staff or security guard — directs us to leave the premises, to refuse to do so would then incur a charge of aggravated trespass, which is a criminal offence under Section 68 of the Criminal Justice and Public Order Act 1994.[82] However, only a police constable has the power to detain or arrest someone for doing so, and any private security guard who tries to do so is acting illegally.

Anyone who has been following the creeping intrusion of Government measures into the public life and social behaviour of the UK will know that it will not stop here. No sooner had the regulations making face coverings on public transport mandatory come into effect than it was announced that the Government was considering imposing the same in shops and supermarkets. The ink on the regulations imposing the latter has not dried and already the Government has announced it is looking at enforcing the wearing of gloves to combat the spread of the virus.[83] No one should be in doubt that the Government's aim is to make the wearing of masks and anything else its advisors can dream up mandatory in all public places.

Unfortunately, for the overwhelming majority of the UK public a sign outside announcing the wearing of a face covering as a condition of entry, the presence of a private security guard on the door, and the vague awareness of Government regulations to this effect, will most likely be enough to ensure widespread compliance. The English don't do rebellion, except when it comes to football. More effective than all these measures, though, will be the self-policing on which

82. See UK Public General Acts, 'Criminal Justice and Public Order Act 1994' (3 November, 1994), Section 68, 'Offence of aggravated trespass'.

83. See Laura Donnelly, Hayley Dixon and Sarah Newey, 'Gloves may be the next step after masks in the battle against coronavirus', *The Telegraph* (24 July, 2020).

the UK biosecurity state has relied for its implementation since the coronavirus 'crisis' was declared. In England, at least, if perhaps less so in Wales, Scotland and Northern Ireland, the public 'shaming' to which the Chief of the Metropolitan Police Force referred in her interview should not be underestimated as a method of public compliance. As Twitter has tested, demonstrated and confirmed, the shaming of deviations from social orthodoxy is one of the most powerful political tools in this most obedient and ashamed of countries. The uncovered face will become the source of shame every bit as effective for our new socio-political order as clothing is to our naked bodies. Social media is awash with the argument that, just as under existing obscenity laws we cannot enter a shop naked, so now we cannot enter a shop without our face covered. In our radically conservative times, obedience to public shaming is presented as a measure of progress. Whatever unsubstantiated or marginal medical reasons there may be behind the prohibition are no longer relevant. The time for arguing with authority is over. A covered face in public is now the New Normal.

Before it becomes so, however, we should remember that there is nothing in the new regulations compelling or empowering staff, managers or owners of a shop, shopping centre, bank or post office to enforce the wearing of a face covering as a condition of entry or service, and remind them of the fact. Like their equivalents in the pubs, bars, restaurants, cafés and other public premises instructed by the Government to collect customers' private details as a condition of entry or service, those who do so have chosen to police the public beyond what is required by law. Most of the pubs I have visited in London since the Government Guidance on contact tracing was issued had a sign outside saying something like: 'In compliance with Government instructions, we can only serve you if you hand over your contact details'. This is legally incorrect, and around half of the staff I informed that it was, and showed the text of the Guidance clearly stating that it was a 'voluntary' programme, served me without taking my details.[84] The other half, however, refused. But whether it's out of ignorance or choice, indifference or obedience, shame or duty, those who police the public beyond the requirements of the law are the willing instruments of the biosecurity state, in which laws in violation of our human rights are made in contravention of parliamentary

---

84. See UK Health Security Agency, 'Maintaining records of staff, customers and visitors to support NHS Test and Trace' (2 July, 2020).

procedure and police commissioners call on the public to shame those individuals who fail to comply with them.

I have already written at length about face coverings in 'The Science and Law of Refusing to Wear Masks: Texts and Arguments in Support of Civil Disobedience', so will not repeat my discussion of the lack of evidence for their purported efficacy.[85] But the argument for blanket masking remains the same as it was for their mandating on transport or in shops: that no matter how small the difference face coverings make, no matter how marginal their benefits, if they can save even 'one life' they should be made mandatory. Even were it true, this is a purely medical argument, and as such its context is limited to the care of the patient's health. Consideration of these regulations, however, go far beyond the limits of protecting public health; and medical practitioners are not the only people we should be consulting on their justification, proportionality, legality or impact.

First, living is dangerous to an individual's health. Some people like to keep their sofas wrapped in the plastic in which it was delivered from the warehouse, to place coasters between their coffee cups and the coffee table, spray every surface in their home with disinfectant, want to ban smoking cigarettes, drinking alcohol, eating unhealthy foods, stop children playing a game of conkers and all contact sports, but these are pathological reactions to the physical realities and risks of life on which the pharmaceutical, cosmetic and health-and-safety industries ruthlessly prey. It's worth recalling that the most famous wearer of masks in public places was the pop singer, Michael Jackson, who like most billionaire celebrities considered his person to be at risk of contamination from the fans who bought his records, concert tickets and merchandise. If you're rich enough to be able to do so, never leaving your house may eliminate the threat of dying in a road accident, for example, or catching a common cold, but it's hardly conducive to a healthy life, either physically or — as Jackson demonstrated — mentally. And as for an individual so for the nation, physical health must be balanced against mental, social, economic and political health. To take just one example, an immunologist can tell us whether or not outsourcing our children's immune system to a vaccine for a respiratory disease to which they are statistically immune will have negative physiological consequences for them in the future; but

---

85. See Simon Elmer, 'The Science and Law of Refusing to Wear Masks: Texts and Arguments in Support of Civil Disobedience', *Architects for Social Housing* (11 June, 2020).

hopefully we can all understand that raising them — as the Government is instructing us to — to treat their fellow human beings as a source of harm and a threat to their well-being quite clearly has the potential to create a psychological and social time-bomb for the future of the UK. So the medical argument that making the wearing of a face covering mandatory in public is justified on the grounds that it may save 'one life' is a flawed argument that isolates the issue from its wider context.

Second, making the wearing of face coverings in public mandatory is grossly disproportionate to the threat of COVID-19 in the UK. According to estimates by the Office of National Statistics, in the week ending 19 July just 1 in 2,000 people in England, excluding those in hospitals, care homes or other institutional settings, had SARS-CoV-2.[86] This equates to an estimated 27,700 people, with around 0.52 new infections for every 10,000 persons. According to the most recent figures, the number of deaths attributed to COVID-19 in the whole of the UK in the week ending 10 July was 388, the lowest number of deaths attributed to COVID-19 in the last 16 weeks, and constituting just 3.9 per cent of all deaths.[87] By comparison, in the same week 789 people — twice as many — died from a respiratory disease other than COVID-19. The total number of deaths registered in the UK in the same week was 9,919, which is 587 fewer than the average over the last five years.[88] Over a quarter of all deaths attributed to COVID-19 were over the age of 90. Three quarter were 75 and over. All but 35 in a population of 67.8 million were over 64 years old. Indeed, last week it was revealed that there were insufficient numbers of people in the UK infected with SARS-C0V-2 to test-trial the vaccine being developed by AstraZeneca — the multinational pharmaceutical company that has signed a deal with the UK Government to produce 100 million doses of the vaccine — in collaboration with Oxford University.[89] No-one appears to have questioned why we should require a vaccine for a virus so few of us have and which is a threat

86. See Office for National Statistics, 'Coronavirus (COVID-19) Infection Survey, UK: 11 November 2022' (11 November, 2020).

87. See Office for National Statistics, 'Deaths registered weekly in England and Wales, provisional: week ending 10 July 2020' (21 July, 2020).

88. See Office for National Statistics, 'Deaths registered weekly in England and Wales, provisional (2020 edition of dataset up to week ending 1 January 2021).

89. See Helen Lock and Pia Gralki, 'UK's COVID-19 Vaccine Trial Successfully Trains Immune System to Respond to Disease', *Global Citizen* (20 July, 2020); and James Gallagher, 'Coronavirus vaccine: UK government signs deals for 90 million doses', *BBC News* (20 July, 2020).

to even fewer; but this, again, is an indication that the 'severe and imminent threat' coronavirus supposedly presents to the population of the UK is a fictional construct of our Government, given scientific legitimacy by the purchased opinion of senior medical advisors, with the collaboration of the National Health Service, and disseminated by the press and media. What this data doesn't support is the mandatory wearing of face coverings punishable by a fine and prosecution.

Third, the proponents of mandatory face coverings occasionally ask what possible harm wearing one could do. I have yet to see any of them wait to hear an answer. The 'debate' on masks, if it can be called that, addresses the pros and cons of wearing one as if the regulations making face coverings mandatory have been made in isolation from the vast number of laws being made by this Government under the cloak of the coronavirus 'crisis'. One would think — and the noisiest promoters of masks appear to be entirely ignorant of the fact — that these regulations are being made under normal parliamentary conditions by a Government fully accountable to the scrutiny and approval of the legislature, rather than as a distraction from the regulations and programmes which, as I have sought to demonstrate in this article, are tearing down and refashioning the social, legal and political structures of the UK state. The first question to be asked in any debate about whether the wearing of masks should be made mandatory is how doing so serves the Government's ongoing implementation of the UK biosecurity state under the cloak of this 'crisis'. This is a question for political scientists and social activists, not medical practitioners. It is a question that, in its total absence from what debate there is in both our Parliament and our media, all of us should and must ask ourselves and each other before we obediently place the sign of our compliance to that implementation over our mouths.

The press, media and parliamentary opposition have all framed the Government's delay in imposing face coverings on the population as a sign of its indecision and incompetence; while the Government, in turn, has explained its sudden change of opinion as the response to new medical opinion and scientific advice. In truth, it is neither. When the deaths attributed to COVID-19 were sufficiently high to hold the public in the grip of a panic the media did everything to increase and spread, the Government had no need of masks. Now, when the excess deaths on which the press relied for that panic has dropped below the average over the last five years, and even the deaths of 90-year-old Britons attributed to COVID-19 has fallen to figures that even the most imaginative bar-charts have trouble terrifying the public with, the Government needs an easily consumed sign of the presence of what it continues to call in its legislative documents 'a serious and imminent threat to public health'. What better sign of the universal consensus to the existence of that threat than a nation masked and muzzled? Under the silencing and shaming of dissent of which the mask is both symbolic compliance (nakedness covered) and physical enforcer (speech silenced), the Government is free to continue and expand the implementation of the UK biosecurity state.

In a passage widely reproduced over the past six months by students and professors of philosophy thrown into a sudden panic of denial and denunciation by words that appear to have leaped off the pages of their academic research and into the political reality of their own lives, Michel Foucault, in his 1975 book *Discipline and Punish: The Birth of the Prison*, described the result of the measures imposed by the state when the plague appeared in a town in France at the end of the Seventeenth Century:

> The plague-stricken town, traversed throughout with hierarchy, surveillance, observation, writing; the town immobilised by the functioning of an extensive power that bears in a distinct way over all individual bodies — this is the utopia of the perfectly governed city. The plague (envisaged as a possibility at least) is the trial in the course of which one may define ideally the exercise of disciplinary power.[90]

Foucault called this utopia the 'political dream of the plague'. Over three centuries later, in the course of a trial that has already found us guilty, that dream is coming true in the dystopia of our present.

— 31 July, 2020

---

90. Michel Foucault, *Discipline and Punish: The Birth of the Prison*; translated from the French by Alan Sheridan (Penguin Books, 1977), p. 198.

6. The New Normal: What is the UK Biosecurity State?

Part 2. Normalising Fear

What is fear? This is the question the Italian philosopher of biopolitics, Giorgio Agamben, asks in his recent commentary, published on 13 July, on the coronavirus 'crisis'.[1] And his answer is that fear is fear of the 'thing' — which is to say, of an entity that, because we have isolated it from and therefore lost its relationship to the world, threatens us. 'The Thing' is the threat from which we run in horror movies, not realising that we are instead running straight into the trap prepared for us by our own fears, that the danger is not that from which we flee, but the hopeless reality to which our fears deliver us. Engulfed by this fear, which surrounds us on all sides, any and every means of protection is adopted, from locking ourselves in our homes to wearing a mask whenever we leave; for the thing that threatens us is that smallest of entities — a virus. But in doing so we only reaffirm our fear, which grows to a constant feeling of helplessness before the thing. In despair, we reach out for the reassurance of those in authority — the policeman who arrives at the last minute to save us from the thing, or the doctor who will tell us how to kill it — but this does not rid us of our feelings of insecurity. On the contrary, the authorities never tire of telling us that the thing cannot be defeated once and for all, that its threat will always be with us — confirming our impotence in the face of the thing, and increasing its hold over us. Soon, we begin to desire this fear, unable to stop peaking between our fingers at what terrifies us, wanting to live in a permanent state of insecurity. Fear, constant and growing, anticipates and dismisses in advance any argument, any reason, any data that might dispel its illusion. Eventually, we only watch those films that terrify us, and close our eyes to anything that might risk restoring us to a world in which the virus would lose its terrifying aspect and be revealed, instead, for what it is, no longer as an abstract thing but in its concrete relationship to reality. Such fear, argues

---

1. See Giorgio Agamben, 'What is Fear?', *Quodlibet* (13 July, 2020); collected in *Where Are We Now? The Epidemic as Politics*; second updated edition; translated by Valeria Dani (Eris, 2021), pp. 88-95.

Agamben, is distinct from the rational calculation of risk consequent upon our being in the world — the possibility of a falling tree, a flooding river, a sudden assault — against which appropriate precautions can be taken without falling into a blind panic. Worse, fear of the coronavirus has become the new foundation for the biopower of those who, by transforming an emergency situation into the 'New Normal', have created the conditions under which they can remove the laws that guarantee our freedoms. And in their place, fear is first implementing and then normalising the political, juridical and ideological structures of the UK biosecurity state.

But then, we already know this. We've been here before. Or have we already forgotten what awaits us?

1. Historical Precedents for the Biosecurity State

Everybody knows Godwin's Law of Nazi Analogies, even if they don't know it by that name. Coined in 1990 by the US attorney and author Mike Godwin, partly as a counter-meme to lazy comparisons to Nazism as a way of denouncing something, partly as an experiment in memetics, the law asserted that: 'As an online discussion grows longer, the probability of a comparison involving Nazis or Hitler approaches one.'[2] With the subsequent spread of the internet and its mutation into social media, on which every interlocutor is denounced as a Nazi as soon as they voice disagreement, this law is undoubtedly even more applicable now than when it was coined 30 years ago. But like a virus, the meme mutated, producing corollaries, perhaps the most famous of which, adopted by Godwin himself and often confused with the original meme, is that: 'When a Hitler comparison is made, the thread is finished and whoever made the comparison loses whatever debate is in progress'.[3] The popularity of these memes, however, and their widespread use not only on the internet but in policy on, for example, the IHRA definitions of anti-Semitism, has had some unintended effects.[4] While Godwin has stated that the purpose of his experiment was rhetorical and

---

2. Mike Godwin, 'Meme, Counter-meme', *Wired* (1 October, 1994).

3. See Tom Chivers, 'Internet rules and laws: the top 10, from Godwin to Poe', *The Telegraph* (23 October, 2009).

4. See Simon Elmer, 'Oy Vey! No Latkes for Labour', *Architects for Social Housing* (5 September, 2018).

pedagogical, and that he wanted people to 'think a bit harder about the Holocaust' before making glib comparisons, one of its effects has been to do the opposite: first, by reducing the role of comparison to equation (A=B rather than A∝B); and second, by removing the Third Reich from its political, juridical and historical contexts, and turning it into an incomparable act of apolitical, criminal and ahistorical 'evil', in the face of which we must stand in horror and silent reverence for its victims, but from which we must not dare to learn, lest in doing so we dare to compare anything to it, and thereby fall foul of Godwin's Law. In this respect, the prohibition on comparing anything, anywhere, at any time, to any aspect of the 12 years of the Third Reich is comparable to the assertion, which I refuted in Part 1 of this article, that the period we are living through — the period I call the 'coronavirus crisis' to include both the virus and our responses to it — is unprecedented in its circumstances. In reality, just as the emergency powers under which the Government is implementing our transition to a biosecurity state have a long history in the laws and politics of the UK and many other countries, so too this emergent biosecurity state has historical precedents, the most important of which, and the one to which I want to begin by comparing it, is the Third Reich.

There are other examples of the biosecurity state I could use — the most obvious being those countries placed under a state of exception by US law — through the military invasion and overthrow of the governments of sovereign states, through the extraordinary rendition of foreign nationals to countries were torture is legal, and through the indefinite incarceration and torture of prisoners of war as 'enemy combatants' outside the reach of both international and US criminal law — but there are several benefits to comparing the UK today to Germany in the 1930s. The first is that, like so many aspects of contemporary politics, the Third Reich pioneered the governance, techniques, propaganda and programmes of the biosecurity state, and it did it in what, at the time, was the most advanced industrial, scientific and cultural nation in the world. The second reason is that everybody knows something about 'Nazi Germany', however inaccurate that knowledge may be, and has some notion of where such measures can lead once the Government of an advanced industrial nation has dictatorial powers over its population. And the third reason is that the twelve years of the Third Reich are very well-documented, so we have a precise record of how the

National Socialist German Workers' Party (NSDAP) came to form the democratically elected Government of Germany, how it made and enforced its laws within the legal framework of the Weimar Constitution, and how it implemented its programmes of biosecurity — and between these and the UK today there are striking similarities.

Godwin's law, by banning any comparison to this historical period, has had the effect of removing it from history; but historical comparisons are made to draw lessons or issue warnings from a previous moment or period, not to reduce one to another or equate the two. However, the enshrinement of the so-called 'Holocaust' in Western historiography as an incomparable and therefore ahistorical event necessitates me having to say what should be unnecessary, which is that I am not for a moment claiming that we are heading for the same catastrophe — which from a historical point of view alone would be meaningless. Fascism and Nazism belong to a historical period defined by a particular formation of the state emerging from a particular crisis of capitalism. This isn't to say that the state formation we're heading for, as Giorgio Agamben warns us, won't exceed the totalitarianisms of the Twentieth Century in its powers of surveillance, monitoring and population control, corresponding to the far more advanced state of the relevant technologies. But without yet having a word for it other than 'the biosecurity state', what I am arguing is that we are already in a completely altered political landscape from the one we lived in last year, that there are parallels and similarities between the legislative processes by which the respective biosecurity states were and have been implemented, and that the political and legal barriers to the increasingly dictatorial measures being imposed upon us are being as quickly removed. At present, the particular catastrophe we're heading for is limited not by the outrage of a terrified, duped and largely compliant population, but by the wishes of our political and financial masters, and in the UK, at least in my lifetime, we've never had a more corrupt Government or a more spineless Parliament. Finally, therefore, my reason for choosing the Third Reich for comparison is that I wish to awaken people to the reality of what we're facing, and Nazism is a crude shorthand for the dangers of the 'New Normal' that is being imposed upon us.

If you think comparisons with health and racial laws under the Third Reich are unjustified, last month the *Daily Mail*, the most widely-read newspaper in the

UK, reported the findings of a study by researchers at the University of California titled 'Working memory capacity predicts individual differences in social-distancing compliance during the COVID-19 pandemic in the United State'.[5] Published on 10 July in no less a forum than the *Proceedings of the National Academy of Sciences of the United States of America*, this study claims that the choice to obey social distancing measures or to wear a face mask is determined by how much information can be stored in an individual's 'working memory', which also, the authors assert, determines our 'mental abilities such as intelligence'. According to this study, those of us with a low memory capacity have trouble making the decision to obey these measures, while those with a higher capacity are more likely to follow Government advice. In a statement reminiscent of the pseudo-science of Nazi eugenicists, the authors of this study, doctors Weizhen Xie, Stephen Campbell, and Weiwei Zhang, state:

> Noncompliance with social distancing during the early stage of the coronavirus disease 2019 (COVID-19) pandemic poses a great challenge to the public health system. These noncompliance behaviours partly reflect people's concerns for the inherent costs of social distancing while discounting its public health benefits. We propose that this oversight may be associated with the limitation in one's mental capacity to simultaneously retain multiple pieces of information in working memory (WM) for rational decision making that leads to social-distancing compliance.[6]

The rationale behind this conclusion is that, since other psychological and sociological factors (among which the doctors include what they call the 'mood, personality, education and income levels' of the 850 respondents) did not affect the equation between non-compliance and lower memory capacity, the latter must, therefore, be the determining factor. Any student of logic could point out the flaw in this reasoning, in which the range of determinant factors has been delimited in advance, and omits the most obvious one, which is the respondent's

---

5. See Stacy Liberatore, 'Real covidiots! People who refuse to wear a mask or comply with social distancing have lower cognitive ability, new study shows', *Daily Mail* (13 July, 2020).

6. Weizhen Xie, Stephen Campbell and Weiwei Zhang, 'Working memory capacity predicts individual differences in social-distancing compliance during the COVID-19 pandemic in the United States', *PNAS* (10 July, 2020).

rational choice not to believe what the doctors, by contrast, take to be an unquestionable truth: that social distancing measures are proportionate and justified, so not following them must be an irrational choice. It's from this *a priori* belief of the doctors, therefore, and not from their study of non-compliance, that they draw their inevitable conclusion that the more intelligent you are the more you believe the Government — which is hardly supported by everything we know about how the governments of the world operate.

A similarly flawed line of reasoning has been used in the UK to argue that, since Britons of black ethnicity make up a disproportionately higher percentage of deaths attributed to COVID-19, they must be at greater risk to the disease. The Office for National Statistics (ONS), in their report on 'Coronavirus (COVID-19) related deaths by ethnic group, England and Wales: 2 March 2020 to 15 May 2020', reported that for all ages the rate of deaths between 2 March and 15 May attributed to COVID-19 for males of black ethnicity was 3.3 times greater than that for white males of the same age, while the rate for black females was 2.4 times greater than for white females.[7] Even after adjusting for what it calls 'geographic location and population density, living arrangements, socio-economic profile and working conditions', the raised risk of death attributed to COVID-19 for people of black ethnic background of all ages together was 2.0 times greater for males and 1.4 times greater for females compared with those of white ethnic background. From this the ONS concluded that black people in the UK 'appear particularly vulnerable to mortality involving COVID-19'. Scientists haven't been slow to propose biological explanations for this disproportionality, attributing it, no less, to a 'vitamin D deficiency because they have darker skin' — which will no doubt require the further tracking, monitoring and testing of 'dark-skinned' Britons in some future health regulations.[8] Indeed, the lockdown of the North was justified by one Conservative MP, Chris Whittaker, as a response to 'black, Asian and minority ethnic' people not obeying social distancing.[9]

---

7. See Office for National Statistics, 'Coronavirus (COVID-19) related deaths by ethnic group, England and Wales: 2 March 2020 to 15 May 2020' (19 June, 2020).

8. See Fiona Mitchell, 'Vitamin-D and COVID-19: do deficient risk a poorer outcome?', *The Lancet* (20 May, 2020).

9. See Adrian Sherling, 'Muslim and BAME communities not taking coronavirus pandemic seriously, Tory MP says', *LBC Radio* (31 July, 2020).

One might ask why such a breakdown of deaths by ethnicity is even being carried out, and the answer is that race is a protected characteristic under the Equality Act 2010, and the Government's response to the coronavirus must, therefore, be analysed for any signs of inequality. The absurdity of these conclusions becomes more explicit when applied to demographic groups defined not by their ethnicity but by their religion, with the Office for National Statistics reporting that — even taking into account geographical, socio-economic and demographic factors, and what they call the 'increased risks associated with ethnicity' — Jewish males are at twice the risk of death attributed to COVID-19 as Christian males, with atheists having the lowest rate of death attributed to COVID-19.[10] To understand what he confidently calls this 'excess risk', Nick Stripe, Head of Life Events at the Office for National Statistics, concludes that 'additional data and analyses are required'. But either the gods — in order of disproportionality — of the Muslims, Jews, Hindus, Sikhs and Christians are enacting some kind of revenge on their believers, or the ONS analytical framework — which is limited by the Equality Act to considering the ethnicity, religion, age, sex, sexual orientation, gender reassignment, marriage, pregnancy and disability of the deceased — is completely inadequate to analyse the way deaths are attributed to COVID-19 in the UK.

What the ONS conclusion ignores is the conditions that make black people in the UK disproportionately poorer economically, therefore in poorer physical health, living in poorer housing conditions, including in overcrowded homes, concentrated in inner cities in closer proximity to other people, with a lower level of access to increasingly privatised and economically inaccessible health care, employed in jobs where they cannot 'work from home', under 'zero-hour' and insecure contract conditions that mean they cannot claim furlough, where demanding private protection equipment means being dismissed by their employer or agency, and with far less support from the Government to pay their rent meaning they are likely to expose themselves to greater risk. In other words, conditions that have nothing to do with the biology of black people, and everything to do with the social and economic class to which they belong, which is not a protected characteristic under the Equality Act. And — as I have analysed

---

10. See Office for National Statistics, 'Coronavirus (COVID-19) related deaths by religious group, England and Wales: 2 March to 15 May 2020' (19 June, 2020).

at length in my article on 'Manufacturing Consensus: The Registering of COVID-19 Deaths in the UK' — the Office for National Statistics is obliged to take the statistics on COVID-19 deaths at face value, without questioning the extraordinarily lax definitions and deliberately manipulated criteria by which deaths in the UK are attributed to the disease.

The real danger of these studies, however, isn't in the flawed reasoning that produces their irrational conclusions, but in their reduction of political agency to biological determinism, whether that's the inherent 'memory capacity' of the studied subjects or the 'darkness' of their skin. This is the essence of biopolitics, and why the most influential philosopher of its constitutional history, juridical framework and political application over the past 25 years, Giorgio Agamben, has repeatedly gone back to the legislative framework of the Third Reich — and in particular to the legal measures ostensibly imposed to protect the German 'people' — to analyse how the biosecurity state is implemented. In his books *Homo Sacer: Sovereign Power and Bare Life* (1995), *Remnants of Auschwitz* (1998), and *State of Exception* (2003), Agamben has been unafraid to draw comparisons between, and learn lessons from, the State of Emergency under which the twelve years of rule by the NSDAP Government was administered and the increasingly widespread use of this suspension of law in contemporary politics, both of which equate protecting the biological life of citizens with the policing of their civic and political agency. In *Homo Sacer*, Agamben writes:

> National Socialist biopolitics — and along with it, a good part of modern politics even outside the Third Reich — cannot be grasped if it is not understood as necessarily implying the disappearance of the difference between the two terms: the *police* now becomes *politics*, and the care of life coincides with the fight against the enemy.[11]

The last time I made this comparison between Germany in the 1930s and the UK in 2020, in the opening of my article 'Manufacturing Consensus', someone responded that doing so was 'beneath contempt'. I presume he was affecting to protect what he took to be the sanctity of the 'Holocaust' from being profaned by

---

11. Giorgio Agamben, *Homo Sacer: Sovereign Power and Bare Life*; translated by Daniel Heller-Roazen (Stanford University Press, 1998), p. 147.

comparison with any other political or historical context. But what he meant in practice was that the legislative mechanics by which the biosecurity state is implemented was beneath his consideration. It's not beneath mine, however. If we must — as we constantly tell ourselves — ensure that the political conditions under which the concentration camps, the death squads and the extermination camps were implemented never return, it is essential that we rescue the systematic killing of millions from the 'evil deeds of monsters', and try to understand how judicial procedures and other deployments of power created a situation in which, as Agamben writes, 'human beings could be so completely deprived of their rights and prerogatives that no act committed against them could appear any longer as a crime'.[12] The Third Reich was not, as is often and inaccurately asserted, a 'criminal regime', but one legally and constitutionally mandated by a Government democratically elected to a parliamentary majority, constitutionally appointed to form a government by the President of the Reich, and able to function for over a decade under a repeatedly extended State of Emergency; and it is up to us to learn — and not to sanctimoniously or stupidly dismiss — what it has to teach us about the implementation of the UK biosecurity state today.

In the 3-part BBC series *Rise of the Nazis*, first televised in September 2019 before anyone in the UK had heard of COVID-19, Richard Evans, the former Professor of History at the University of Cambridge and author of a trilogy of studies on *The Third Reich*, reflects on this lesson:

> Democracies require, first of all, popular support and popular belief in institutions such as a free press, an independent judiciary, democratic elections. The echoes that we find in our own time of the Nazi seizure of power are in a number of different areas. Emergency powers, for example, and emergency decrees, the State of Emergency that allowed them to put their own plans into action without any serious opposition.[13]

---

12. Giorgio Agamben, *Homo Sacer: Sovereign Power and Bare Life*; p. 171.

13. See Julian Jones, *Rise of the Nazis*, episode 3, 'The Night of the Long Knives', *BBC* (16 September, 2019). The three volumes of Evans' study, published by Allen Lane, are titled *The Coming of the Third Reich* (2003), *The Third Reich in Power* (2005), and *The Third Reich at War* (2008).

2. Implementing the Biosecurity State

Speaking in the House of Commons on 7 July, the Secretary of State for Health and Social Care, Matt Hancock — a former computer software salesman and economic advisor to George Osborne, and like the former Chancellor without any background in economics — said he would 'consider giving badges to people who don't have to wear a mask on public transport, such as small children or those with lung diseases'.[14] That same day, presumably on cue, Dr. Venki Ramakrishnan, the President of the Royal Society of Scientists and member of the Government's Scientific Advisory Group for Emergencies, announced that face coverings should be considered as 'part of the new normal', that wearing them is the 'right thing to do', and that not wearing them in public should be regarded as 'anti-social'.[15] Encouraged and validated by statements such as these from individuals occupying positions of authority, the UK public has not been slow to translate them into their actual meaning within the biosecurity state, with this anonymous Twitter post from 2 August representative of thousands of others in a similar vein:

> If you don't wear a mask, you should not be allowed to fly or ride in a public conveyance. If you persist, you should be arrested, fined and jailed. People like you are hurting other people, killing too many.

It is on this concurrence of Government will, medical opinion and public compliance that the biopolitical state is implemented, as we're seeing with the increasingly violent instances of police enforcement of regulations not only in the UK but across the world, with the recent assault by a police officer of a young woman in Melbourne, Australia, for not wearing a mask outdoors being an example of how rapidly liberal democracies are catching up with the brutality, unaccountability and impunity from prosecution of the police forces in the USA and France.

---

14. See Sam Blanchard, 'Officials WILL look again at whether Britons should wear face coverings or masks in public, Matt Hancock reveals as top scientists argue they should be "part of the new normal"', *The Daily Mail* (7 July, 2020).

15. See Dr. Venki Ramakrishnan, 'President of the Royal Society urges everyone to wear a face covering', *The Royal Society* (7 July, 2020).

It's with this growing ideological hegemony of the UK in mind that I want to review one of the forms by which Jews in the Third Reich and occupied territories were publicly identified, monitored, and ultimately banned from public life. This is the Yellow Star, which, like the mandatory wearing of face coverings and contact tracing enforced as a condition of access to public life in the UK, was introduced progressively — first by suggestion, then by imposition, and finally by regulations which — just like the coronavirus-related Statutory Instruments made into law since this 'crisis' was declared — were introduced under provisions in already existing legislation. Clearly, the legislative process by which Jews, communists, anarchists, socialists, trade unionists, pacifists, refugees, the homeless, Roma, homosexuals, prostitutes, the physically or mentally disabled, those with criminal convictions and the 'socially undesirable' were progressively deprived of their citizens' rights under the Third Reich is beyond the scope of this article; but we can follow the schematic history of the implementation and enforcement of the compulsory wearing of the Yellow Star by Jews.

Over the following pages is a brief timeline of the implementation of this instrument of the German biosecurity state, in which the Jew was branded as a threat to the body politic that had to be identified and banned from participation in the public life of the biologically healthy people (*Volk*), set alongside a parallel timeline of the implementation of the mandatory wearing of face coverings and other measures and technologies of the UK biosecurity state. Once again, what I am doing here is comparing the political strategies and ideological programmes deployed by the respective Governments, not to reduce the one to the other but to reveal the similarities between their use of the excuse of defending the biological health of their respective populations to justify the policing of those populations with regulation after regulation passed under emergency powers without legislative scrutiny or approval by their parliaments.

The German Biosecurity State

- **1933.** On 28 February, in response to the burning of the Reichstag, the home of Germany's Parliament, the Reich President, Paul von Hindenburg, invoked Article 48 of the Weimar Constitution. This allowed him, as Head of State, to enact emergency powers without prior consultation with Parliament 'if public security and order are severely disturbed or threatened'. This wasn't the first time it had been invoked. The President had declared a State of Emergency or issued emergency decrees on more than 250 occasions since the Weimer Republic had been declared in 1919, including to imprison and execute thousands of communists. But the Decree of the Reich President for the Protection of People and State, commonly known as the 'Reichstag Fire Decree', suspended almost all the human rights of German citizens, including the rights of public assembly and of free association, the privacy of postal, telegraphic and telephonic communications, the freedom of expression and the freedom of the press, as well as *habeas corpus*, thereby removing the requirement for an arrested person to be brought before a judge or into court, and to secure their release unless lawful grounds are shown for their detention.
- A month later, on 22 March, Dachau concentration camp was opened by Heinrich Himmler, the Commander of the SS, to hold political prisoners, primarily composed of arrested communists. With an initial capacity of 5,000, the camp was independent of judicial control and juridical order.

The UK Biosecurity State

- **2020.** On 10 February the Secretary of State for Health and Social Care, Matt Hancock, exercising emergency powers conferred by Section 45R of The Public Health (Control of Disease) Act 1984, employed a Statutory Instrument that made The Health Protection (Coronavirus) Regulations 2020 into law with immediate effect, without an impact assessment, and without the approval or scrutiny of Parliament. These empowered the state to detain, isolate and take a biological sample from a person on the grounds that they 'may be' infected with coronavirus.
- On 5 March, under the first Amendment to The Health Protection Regulations 2020, COVID-19 and SARS-CoV-2 were added to the list of, respectively, 'Notifiable' Diseases' and 'Causative Agents' that medical practitioners have a statutory duty to record on a death certificate, as they do not, for example, with pneumonia, the primary cause of death from respiratory diseases. This change to disease taxonomy laid the grounds for attributing deaths in the UK to COVID-19 without causation having been established, thereby leading to the gross exaggeration of its threat to public health that is the basis to the implementation of the UK biosecurity state.
- On 16 March, Public Health England, the executive agency of the Department of Health and Social Care, issued its 'Guidance on social distancing for everyone in the UK'. Despite having no legislative backing, this guidance was enforced through criminal sanctions, including fines and arrests, by police forces across the UK.

210

- On 23 March, the Law to Remedy the Distress of People and State, referred to as the 'Enabling Act', gave the German Cabinet under the newly-appointed Chancellor, Adolf Hitler, plenary powers to pass laws by decree, without the approval of Parliament, and to override fundamental aspects of the Weimar Constitution. Given a four-year lifespan unless renewed by the Reichstag, the Act was extended twice, in 1937 and 1941, and Germany was still under its emergency powers at the end of the Second World War. Together with the Reichstag Fire Decree, these two laws made Germany a constitutional dictatorship.
- On 7 April, the Law for the Restoration of the Professional Civil Service dismissed political opponents of National Socialism (communists, social democrats, etc), Jews and designated 'non-Aryans' from their positions, including as teachers, professors, judges and civil servants.
- On 11 April, the First Order on the Implementation of the Civil Service law extended the terms of this ban to doctors, lawyers, consultants and musicians.
- On 10 May, university students in college towns across Germany burned thousands of books denounced as 'un-German', initiating an era of cultural censorship and control.
- **1934.** On 3 July, the Law on the Unification of Health Care took what had been under the jurisprudence of individual states into centralised federal legislation and administration.
- On 19 August, in a referendum, 90 per cent of the German electorate approved the merger of the offices of Chancellor and President, making Hitler both Head of Government and Head of State.

- On 17 March, the NHS was radically reprioritised, resulting in up to 25,000 hospital patients being discharged into care homes without first being tested for SARS-CoV-2, and over 15,000 deaths being officially attributed to COVID-19 by the end of July.
- On 23 March the Prime Minister announced the 'lockdown' of the UK. This restricted the movements of the public to shopping for basic necessities, one form of exercise per day, receiving or delivering medical needs, and travel to essential work. To ensure compliance, all shops selling non-essential goods were closed, as were libraries, playgrounds, outdoor gyms and places of worship, and gatherings of more than two people in public were prohibited.
- On 25 March, the Coronavirus Act 2020 was enacted into law by Parliament. Among numerous new powers, this extended the time limit for the state's retention of the biometric data of UK citizens; removed the requirement of a jury to establish whether COVID-19 was the cause of a death; prohibited attendance at public gatherings or premises; and postponed elections until May 2021.
- On 26 March, the day after Parliament voted itself into extended recess, the Secretary of State for Health and Social Care made The Health Protection (Coronavirus, Restrictions) (England) Regulations 2020 into law. These initiated an 'emergency period' that will only end at a time specified by the Secretary of State, and during which he is empowered to close premises and businesses, restrict movements and prohibit gatherings of the public, with compliance enforceable by criminal sanctions.

- **1935.** With the expansion of Dachau concentration camp, the use of colour-coded triangles distinguished between inmates: red for political prisoners, including communists, anarchists, socialists, social democrats and trade unionists; green for criminals; brown for male Romani; black for 'anti-social' prisoners, which included the work-shy, the homeless, prostitutes, the mentally ill and disabled; purple for religious pacifists; pink for homosexuals; blue for emigrants; and two yellow triangles, forming the Star of David, for Jews.
- On 15 September, the so-called 'Nuremberg Laws' were enacted at a specially convened meeting of the Reichstag. Under the Law for the Protection of German Blood and German Honour, Jews and other non-Aryans were forbidden from marital and sexual relations with 'citizens of German or related blood'. In addition, the Reich Citizenship Law deprived German Jews of their citizenship, and with it their civil and political rights, and instead made them 'subjects of the state'. This was defined as 'a person who enjoys the protection of the German Reich and who in consequence has specific obligations towards it.'
- On 18 October, the Law for the Protection of the Hereditary Health of the German People required all prospective marriage partners to obtain from the public health authorities a certificate of fitness to marry. Such certificates were refused to those suffering from contagious diseases.
- On 14 November, the first supplemental decree to the Nuremberg Laws defined 'Jews' not as members of a religious or cultural community but as a race defined by hereditary.

- On 30 March, the Cabinet Office announced that the Government's Rapid Response Unit was working with social media companies to remove any information about coronavirus that contradicted its own.
- On 7 April, under Section 22 of the Prosecution of Offences Act 1985, the Coronavirus crisis protocol for the effective handling of custody time limit cases in the Magistrates' and the Crown Court extended the time a defendant can be kept in custody before trial from 56 days to 182 days.
- On 12 April, the Secretary of State for Health and Social Care announced the Government's development of a new centralised contact-tracing app for mobile phones.
- On 21 April, the returned House of Commons, without a vote being held, approved a motion facilitating 'hybrid proceedings'. Under the prohibitions on social distancing imposed by the Prime Minister, these allowed a maximum of 50 MPs to be present in the Chamber at any one time, with 120 MPs able to participate remotely online, and proceedings reduced from 8 to 2 hours. MPs wishing to participate in these hybrid proceedings had to notify the House Service in advance, and all questions were published in advance.
- On 28 April, Matthew Gould, the Chief Executive of NHSX, which sets national policy and best practice for the NHS on data sharing and transparency, told the Parliamentary Science and Technology Committee that the NHSX was exploring the creation of Immunity Passports that will monitor the health status of UK citizens that will determine their access to or ban from entering public spaces.

- **1938.** On 11 July, the Ministry of the Interior banned Jews from attending health spas.
- On 23 July, Jews were ordered to apply for Identity Cards to be shown to police and officials on demand.
- On 12 September, Jews were banned from attending cinemas, concerts and the opera.
- On 9-10 November, in the *Kristallnacht* pogrom, 7,500 Jewish-owned shops and businesses and hundreds of schools, hospitals and synagogues were attacked, and 30,000 Jews were arrested and sent to concentration camps throughout Germany, Austria and the Sudetenland. Following this, the Director of the Secret State Police (Gestapo) that had organised the pogrom recommended that all Jews, and not only those in concentration camps, should wear identifying badges.
- On 12 November, the Decree for the Exclusion of Jews from German Economic Life banned Jews from owning businesses, selling goods or services or having a trade.
- On 15 November, The Ministry of Education banned Jewish children from attending public schools.
- On 28 November, the Ministry of the Interior restricted freedom of movement and travel for Jews.
- **1939.** In September, following the invasion of Poland, Jewish Poles were ordered to wear an identifying mark. There were no consistent requirements as to its colour and shape, which in practice varied from a white armband to a yellow Star of David badge.
- On 23 November, all Jews in occupied Poland above the age of 11 were ordered to wear white armbands bearing a blue Star of David when in public.

- On 11 May, the Prime Minister announced that a Joint Biosecurity Centre would set the new COVID-19 Alert level as part of 'an extended infrastructure to address biosecurity threats to the UK.'
- On 1 June, under the third amendment to The Health Protection (Coronavirus, Restrictions) (England) (Amendment) (No. 3) Regulations 2020, public protests were banned in the UK.
- On 3 June, The Health Protection (Coronavirus, International Travel) (England) Regulations 2020 required anyone arriving in England from designated countries to remain under house arrest ('quarantined') for 14 days from the date of their arrival.
- On 15 June, The Health Protection (Coronavirus, Wearing of Face Coverings on Public Transport) (England) Regulations 2020 made face coverings mandatory on public transport. The Government published design templates demonstrating how to manufacture such masks at home.
- On 29 June, 412,000 people in the City of Leicester were placed under lockdown restrictions on movement, association and closures of premises.
- On 2 July, the Department of Health and Social Care published guidance instructing the owners, managers and staff of public houses, bars, restaurants, cafés, hotels, museums, cinemas, hairdressers, town halls, civic centres, libraries and places of worship to refuse entry to, service in, or employment by, their establishments to visitors, customers or staff who refuse to supply their personal details, including their name and contact number or e-mail, as well as the time of their visit, purchase or shift; and to share this information with the NHS Test and Trace programme.

- **1941.** On 4 June, Jews in the Independent State of Croatia were ordered to wear 'Jewish insignia'.
- On 8 July, Jews in German-occupied Poland, Lithuania, Latvia and Estonia, as well as Soviet Jews in German-occupied areas, were all obliged to wear white armbands or yellow stars.
- On 8 August, Jews in Romania were ordered to wear the Yellow Star.
- On 13 August, the Yellow Star was made the only standardised identifying mark in the German-occupied East, with other badges forbidden.
- On 1 September, Police Regulations on the Labelling of Jews, made on the basis of the Police Regulations of the Reich Ministers of 14 November 1938, and the Regulations on Legislative Law in the Protectorate of Bohemia and Moravia of 7 June 1939, and issued and signed by the President of the International Criminal Police Commission and Director of the Reich Main Security Office, prohibited Jews in the Third Reich and the Protectorate of Bohemia and Moravia who had reached the age of 6 from 'showing themselves in public without a Jewish star.' Directions were given for its manufacture and design, specifying that the badge had to be 'a palm-sized, black-drawn six-pointed star made of yellow fabric with the black inscription *"Jude"*.' It was additionally forbidden for Jews 'to leave the area of their community without having a written permit from the local police'. The punishment for intentionally or negligently contravening these Regulations was to be 'fined up to 150 Reichsmarks or imprisoned for up to six weeks.'

- On 18 July, The Health Protection (Coronavirus, Restrictions) (England) (No. 3) Regulations 2020 empowered local authorities to give directions imposing prohibitions, requirements or restrictions to close or restrict entry to premises, events or public outdoor places.
- On 23 July, The Health Protection (Coronavirus, Wearing of Face Coverings in a Relevant Place) (England) Regulations 2020 made face coverings mandatory in shops, shopping centres, banks, post offices and transport hubs.
- On 27 July, the National Police Chiefs Council announced that in the two months between 26 March, when The Health Protection Regulations had come into force, and 25 May, 17,039 fixed-penalty notices had been issued in England and Wales.
- On 31 July, The Health Protection (Coronavirus, Restrictions) (Blackburn with Darwen and Bradford) Regulations 2020 placed 528,000 people under lockdown restrictions on movement, association and closures of premises.
- On the same day, the Government announced an 'independent panel' to examine reform of judicial review, the means by which citizens can challenge whether a Government decision is within the law as enacted by Parliament, and that the panel would be chaired by Lord Edward Faulks, a Conservative Peer and former Minister.
- On 4 August, The Health Protection (Coronavirus, Restrictions on Gatherings) (North of England) Regulations 2020 placed 6.6 million people under lockdown restrictions on movement, association and closures.

- On 5 September, the German occupation authorities in Luxembourg introduced the Nuremberg Laws, followed by several other anti-Jewish regulations, including an order for all Jews to wear a Yellow Star bearing the word *'Jude'*.
- On 9 September, Jews in Slovakia were ordered to wear the Yellow Star.
- **1942.** Romania started to force Jews who had been denied Romanian citizenship in newly annexed territories to wear the yellow star.
- On 13 March, the Gestapo ordered Jewish Germans and Jews with citizenship of annexed states to mark their apartments or houses on the front door with a white star.
- On 24 April, Jews throughout Greater Germany were prohibited from using public transport.
- On 29 April, Jews in the Netherlands were ordered to wear the Yellow Star.
- On 3 June, Jews in Belgium were ordered to wear the Yellow Star.
- On 7 June, Jews in occupied France were ordered to wear the Yellow Star.
- In August, under German pressure, Bulgaria ordered its Jewish citizens to wear small yellow buttons, but contravention was not prosecuted.
- **1944.** On 7 April, following the occupation of Hungary, Jewish Hungarians and Jews with revoked citizenships in Hungarian-annexed areas were ordered to wear the Yellow Star.

- *Between the Nuremberg Laws in September 1935 and the outbreak of World War Two in September 1939, more than 120 biosecurity laws, decrees and regulations were enacted under the Third Reich, imposing more than 400 legal restrictions.*

- On 8 August, The Health Protection (Coronavirus, Wearing of Face Coverings in a Relevant Place) (England) (Amendment) Regulations 2020 extended the mandatory wearing of face coverings to places of worship, community centres, crematoria and chapels, hotels and hostels, concert and exhibition halls, cinemas, museums, galleries, indoor tourist sites, bingo halls and public libraries.
- On the same day, The Health Protection (Coronavirus, Restrictions on Gatherings) (North of England) (Amendment) Regulations 2020 extended the lockdown of the North to a further 141,000 people.
- On 18 August, the Health Secretary announced the launch of the UK Health Security Agency.
- On 25 August, the Government issued Guidance that children in secondary schools in England must wear face coverings in communal areas.
- On 27 August, The Health Protection (Coronavirus) (Restrictions on Holding of Gatherings and Amendment) (England) Regulations 2020 raised the fine for organising unlawful gatherings of more than 30 people to £10,000.
- On the same day, The Health Protection (Wearing of Face Coverings in a Relevant Place and on Public Transport) (England) (Amendment) Regulations 2020 raised the fine for not wearing a face covering where mandated to a maximum of £6,400.

- *Between 28 January and 28 August 2020, 196 Statutory Instruments justified by the coronavirus have been laid before Parliament, 188 of which were signed into law by UK Ministers of State before being laid before Parliament for scrutiny or approval.*

I'm not the only person to draw comparisons between the enforced wearing of the Yellow Star by Jews under the Third Reich and occupied territories and the mandatory wearing of face coverings in more and more places in the emerging UK biosecurity state; and, once again, those who have done so have been attacked and censored on social media, with at least one account that I know of suspended until the offending comparison was removed. There appeared to be no awareness on the part of the censors of the comparison they were thereby inviting between their own actions and those who censored anything that contradicted the ideology of National Socialism.[16] Once again, the Yellow Star was being removed from history as an object of veneration to which nothing must be compared, and which can therefore teach us nothing in that lesson we're supposed to have learned from that history. One of the more often repeated responses to this comparison was that 'the Jews didn't wear the Yellow Star in order to protect those around them', with the implication being that those who wear a face covering today are. I won't rehearse the reasons why this implication is at best contentious and at worst deliberately misleading, which I have discussed at length in 'The Science and Law of Refusing to Wear Masks'; but this response is equally as wrong about the function of the Yellow Star.

Giorgio Agamben has discussed the inadequacy of 'racism' as a framework through which to understand the Third Reich, and the timeline above should have conveyed how instrumental the imposition of the wearing of the Yellow Star was with the juridical framework of the biosecurity state, the most rigorous formulation of which, Agamben argues, was these words of Adolf Hitler: 'The new State knows no other task than the fulfilment of the conditions necessary for the preservation of the people'.[17]

Within this state, in which care of the 'life of the nation' was coextensive with the policing of the 'body of the people', the Yellow Star was imposed on Jews to protect those around them from infection by this internal enemy. Thanks to the

---

16. In January 2021, in response to the publication of this article, I was accused of 'anti-semitism' by the Architectural Registration Board, the regulator of architectural practices in the UK, which initiated a 6-month investigation that, were we to be found guilty, carried a threat ranging from a £2,500 fine to the removal of the right of our company, Architects for Social Housing, to practice architecture in the UK. See Simon Elmer and Francis Hoar, 'In our Defence: Freedom of Speech in the UK Biosecurity State', *Architects for Social Housing* (16 June, 2021).

17. Quoted in Giorgio Agamben, *Homo Sacer: Sovereign Power and Bare Life*; p. 147.

seemingly endless documentaries about 'The Nazis', it's widely known that Jews were characterised in National Socialist propaganda as carriers of disease, as themselves vermin, who therefore had to be 'exterminated'; but the titles of the legislation by which they were reduced to the legal status where this could be carried out should alert us to the biopolitical aims of the Third Reich that are not reducible to accusations of racism: the 'Decree for the Protection of People and State'; the 'Law to Remedy the Distress of People and State'; the 'Law on the Unification of Health Care'; the 'Law for the Protection of German Blood'; the 'Law for the Protection of the Hereditary Health of the German People'; the 'Decree on the Exclusion of Jews from German Economic Life'; the 'Police Regulations on the Labelling of Jews'. Together, these constitute an epidemiological discourse no less legitimate under law for being entirely manufactured by National Socialist eugenicists: of protection from disease and remedy when infected, and of identifying the infected and isolating (and eventually exterminating) the diseased.

As a function of this discourse, the Yellow Star was the constant and multiplying visual sign of the presence and threat of what is described on every coronavirus-justified Statutory Instrument made into law today as an 'imminent and serious threat to public health'. This alone has justified the making of hundreds of regulations without them having to pass the prior scrutiny and approval of Parliament. Instead, just as Hitler did with the Nuremberg Laws, radically reduced sittings of Parliament are brought in after they have been signed into law to approve their powers by parliamentarians too terrified of being accused of not 'doing their bit' to combat this threat to challenge their lack of justification, their lack of proportionality, their lack of an impact assessment, and the ongoing bypassing of legislative procedure of which they are another instance. Like the Yellow Star, the face coverings being imposed upon us by regulations signed into law by the Health Secretary and being made mandatory in more and more places across the UK are the constant and multiplying sign of the presence of a disease whose threat to public health has been manufactured and grossly exaggerated by changes to disease taxonomy, practices of certification and methods of reporting that allow the Government to continue to implement the juridical apparatus and surveillance programmes of the UK biosecurity state I looked at in Part 1 of this article. Not only are comparisons between the Yellow Star and face masks justified, therefore, but they should alert us to the function the regulations imposing both had then, and are having now, in the respective biosecurity states they helped and are helping to implement.

In 1936, Karl Löwenstein, by then an Associate Professor of Political Science at Yale University, but formerly a lecturer on Constitutional and International Law at the University of Munich before being forced to emigrate by the election of the NSDAP Government, published an article in volume 45 of the *Yale Law Journal* titled 'Law in the Third Reich'. Interestingly, his review covered legal developments in German up to 1 January 1936, yet even with the vast number, range and scope of new legislation made into law by then, Löwenstein, who is now regarded as one of the prominent figures of Constitutional law in the Twentieth Century, still had no idea of what was to come. This makes his comforting conclusion, which I quote here at length, uncomfortable reading, and all the more of a warning to those of us waiting for a return to 'normal' after the coronavirus 'crisis':

> History reveals that revolutionary movements show the greatest co-efficient in celerity and weight in the enthusiasm of the start. Encountering the obstacles of tradition and habits, the movement slackens. Perhaps no other part of social life is less accessible to violent and sudden change than civil or common law, which formalises the daily habits of the people. On the other hand, the political form of the community may comparatively easily be overthrown. It would be tantamount to a refutation of historical experience, as well as of German mores, if National Socialism ultimately succeeded in reversing German law and jurisprudence. By tradition and disposition, German legal habits are based on rationality, formalism, and technicality.
>
> It may be that National Socialist legal values will be at least temporarily accepted, perhaps in view of the amazing pliability of human nature under continued mental pressure. Undeniably the regime is masterly in utilising psychological techniques. But the prediction seems permissible that such a rationally created system of values will scarcely find a permanent foothold in the nation. The racial myth and its implications are not of organical growth; they are artificially invented and politically superimposed. Certainly, a new set of legal values might originate from the creative forces of the national conscience, but an artifice such as the crude romanticism of the racial philosophy cannot turn back

the hands of the clock. There is so far no indication that the new legal values will conquer German jurisprudence.

With due reserve, therefore, we may say that National Socialist legal concepts are only an incident in German legal history. Perhaps a necessary and justified incident, since excessive formalism and technicality needs at times a tonic in the form of a dynamic and even 'unjust' law. In due course, Germany's legal structure is likely to return to a more congenial substance and shape, incorporating — as is usual in revolutions — such elements of the National Socialist experiment which correspond to the national disposition. In spite of or because of its rationalism, National Socialist legal philosophy is nothing more than an unspirited relapse into romanticism, not the first one and probably not the last one in a nation whose unbalanced nature vacillates between the extremes.[18]

3. The English Civil War

In his book *Stasis: Civil War as a Political Paradigm*, which is composed of lectures delivered in the USA in the immediate aftermath of the demolition of three buildings in the World Trade Centre complex in New York on 11 September, 2001, Giorgio Agamben wrote:

The form that civil war has acquired today in world history is terrorism. If the Foucauldian diagnosis of modern history as biopolitics is correct, and if the genealogy that traces it back to an oikonomical-theological paradigm is equally correct, then global terrorism is the form that civil war acquires when life as such becomes the stake of politics. . . . Terrorism is the 'global civil war' that time and again invests this or that zone of planetary space. It is no coincidence that the 'terror' should coincide with the moment in which life as such — the nation (which it to say, birth) — became the principle of sovereignty. The sole form in which life as such can be politicised is its unconditioned exposure to death — that is, bare life.[19]

---

18. Karl Löwenstein, 'Law in the Third Reich', *Yale Law Journal*, vol. 45 (1936), pp. 814-815.

19. Giorgio Agamben, *Stasis: Civil War as a Political Paradigm*, Homo Sacer II, 2; translated by Nicholas Heron (Stanford University Press, 2015), p. 24.

Agamben's focus in this lecture is on what happens when the political state (*polis*) is reduced to the structure of a household (*oikos*), and the former is depoliticised as the economic management of national and global markets, as represented by, for example, the European Union or United Nations. We needn't go into his complex discussion of the etymology of these terms, but the political context for his lecture is what Agamben sees as the ongoing reduction of the political agency, civic duties and human rights of citizens — the political life (*bios*) that constitutes the state — to the bare life (*zoē*) of their natural existence in the home. Historically manifested in, for example, feudal wars between aristocratic families competing for sovereign rule over subjects that have no political agency, from this tendency towards the depoliticisation of the state emerges the civil war (*stasis*) that Agamben argues becomes the paradigm of Western biopolitics.

Today, when neoliberal hegemony has reduced our politics to the management of citizens' biological life — to a biopolitics — the form this civil war has taken is terrorism, in which the distinction between a state of war and a state of peace, between a foreign war and a civil war, is no longer possible to make. This is the legal state of exception in which prisoners of war are removed from the protection of both international and criminal law to be interred indefinitely in Guantánamo Bay, or Julian Assange is imprisoned in Belmarsh Prison awaiting extradition on a charge of espionage under the laws of a country of which he is neither a citizen nor a resident. But in a passage from 'Medicine as Religion' that I already quoted in Part 1 of this article, Agamben updated the terms of this civil war to the global epidemic which, he says 'is preparing to become the new terrain of world politics — or non-politics':

> It is possible, however, that the epidemic that we are experiencing is the actualisation of a global civil war that, according to the most attentive political analysts, has taken the place of traditional world wars. All nations and all peoples are now in an enduring war with themselves, because the invisible and elusive enemy with which they are struggling is within us.[20]

---

20. Giorgio Agamben, 'Medicine as Religion', *Quodlibet* (2 May, 2020); translated in *Where Are We Now?*, p. 54.

On the evening of 6 June, 2020, in response to a Black Lives Matter demonstration outside the Houses of Parliament against the police-killing of George Floyd in Minneapolis, USA, almost the whole of London was placed under a curfew for 24 hours. The notable exceptions were the wealthy boroughs of Westminster and Kensington and Chelsea, and the more affluent and racially White South-west London. However, in the same way that the UK Government hasn't formally declared a State of Emergency in response to the coronavirus, but has instead made legislation and regulations under emergency powers in existing legislation, so too the Metropolitan Police Force didn't issue a curfew but instead placed large swathes of London under a Section 60 order. Legislated by the Criminal Justice and Public Order Act 1994, Section 60 is another provision for the suspension of the law — in this case, 'in anticipation of or after violence' — during which a police constable may 'stop any person or vehicle and make any search he thinks fit whether or not he has any grounds for suspecting that the person or vehicle is carrying weapons or articles of that kind'.[21] It also authorises a constable to direct a person to remove any item of clothing they suspect may be used for concealing their identity — such as a face covering — and to seize that item. With no recourse to the law to oppose, protest or issue a complaint about the exercise of such powers, a Section 60 order effectively places us in a state in which our civil liberties under UK law are suspended.

To Black citizens accustomed to being stopped and searched for being Black, this will make little difference. If you're Black in London and out at night you will be stopped and searched by officers of the Metropolitan Police Force if they see you. The real purpose of the city-wide Section 60 was, first, to stop the protests against the police killing of George Floyd; and second, to demonstrate to White people to what lengths the UK State can and will go in order to impose its control over the population. In the UK, 68.8 million people were placed under lockdown for 3 months because of a virus that is overwhelmingly a threat to people over 65 years of age and, statistically, almost exclusively kills people with pre-existing life-threatening illnesses. On the same lack of justification and proportionality, most of London was under a curfew because of a handful of shootings and stabbings resulting in two deaths in a city of 9.3 million people.

---

21. See UK Public General Acts, 'Criminal Justice and Public Order Act 1994' (3 November, 1994), Section 60, 'Powers to stop and search in anticipation of, or after violence'.

This is like shutting down every road in England because of a fatal accident on the M1, except we have far more fatalities from car accidents in this country than from stabbings (1,870 in 2019 compared to 242).

The abuse of powers set by this precedent wasn't long in arriving. Three weeks later, on 27 June, the Metropolitan Police Force reported that it had received information from an unidentified source about a 'possible' unlicensed music event in Brixton. This was sufficient grounds for it to place the whole of the Coldharbour and Vassal wards in South London under a Section 35 dispersal order for 48 hours. Under the Antisocial Behaviour, Police and Crime Act 2014, the issuing of a Section 35 dispersal order effectively removes a designated area from UK legal jurisdiction and places it under the powers of a police state.[22] The order gives the police the power to direct anyone to leave a designated area based on their 'suspicion' that we are engaged in 'anti-social behaviour'. They can set a time by which we must leave the area, and can even tell us the route we must take. If we have been issued with a 'direction to leave' but fail to comply, we will face arrest. It also empowers police to seize any item of property in our possession. To issue such sweeping powers, they must have reasonable grounds for suspecting that doing so will remove or reduce the 'likelihood' of members of the public being 'harassed, alarmed or distressed' or of 'crime or disorder' occurring.

It is unclear whether the organisers of the Black Lives Matter protests were aware, but on 31 May the Health Secretary had signed into law The Health Protection (Coronavirus, Restrictions) (England) (Amendment) (No. 3) Regulations 2020.[23] Under Regulation 7, 'no person may participate in a gathering which takes place in a public or private place outdoors, and consists of more than six persons', with a gathering defined as 'when two or more people are present together in the same place in order to engage in any form of social interaction with each other, or to undertake any other activity with each other'. The justification for these regulations, once again, was to stop the spread of a virus that by then had been in this country for 5 months. However, this Statutory Instrument was subject to a

---

22. See UK Public General Acts, 'Antisocial Behaviour, Police and Crime Act 2014' (13 March, 2014), Section 35, 'Directions excluding a person from an area'.

23. See UK Statutory Instruments, 'The Health Protection (Coronavirus, Restrictions) (England) (Amendment) (No. 3) Regulations 2020' (31 May, 2020).

'made affirmative' procedure, meaning that it would not remain law unless it was approved by each House of Parliament within 28 days of coming into effect.

On 13 June, the week after the Black Lives Matter protest, a counter protest was held in Westminster by a small group that was quickly identified by the media as 'far-right', and despite its small numbers received widespread coverage in the news and on social media, with 137 arrests being made. Recognising an opportunity when she saw one, Priti Patel, the Secretary of State for the Home Department, the following Monday, 15 June, led a virtual Parliament in what can best be described as a collective and sustained expression of class hatred. Something like the 'Two Minutes Hate' in George Orwell's *Nineteen Eighty-Four*, but lasting for over an hour, protesters were described as 'abhorrent', 'abusive', 'aggressive', 'appalling', 'corrosive', 'criminals', 'disorderly', 'dreadful', 'drunk', 'extremists', 'far-right', 'hateful', 'hooligans', 'ignorant', 'intolerant', 'offensive', 'patently racist', 'prejudiced', 'shameful', 'sickening', 'terrorists', 'thugs', 'ugly', 'vandals', 'vicious', 'vile' and 'violent' — a recital of the A.B.C. of middle-class disgust and revulsion — finally ending with the Home Secretary's assertion that: 'It is right that we continue to reinforce the message that mass gatherings — six or more people — are illegal and people should not be participating in them.'[24]

If anyone was wondering what the point of this expression of class unity was, later that evening a sitting of the House of Commons dutifully resolved that the third amendment to the Regulations be approved. Before they were, however, on 25 June, they were presented for debate and approval by the House of Lords, where they came under criticism as another instance of the Government's repeated use of the emergency procedure to bring regulations into force prior to them being debated in the House. These objections were led by Paul Scriven, a Liberal Democrat peer, who observed:

> My Lords, we play a game of illusion — a pretence that these regulations that put restrictions on citizens and keep parts of the economy closed are enacted with the agreement of Parliament. No. These regulations stem from emergency executive powers. Like lapdogs, we are discussing regulations that we cannot

---

24. See UK Parliament: House of Commons, 'Public Order', *Hansard* (15 June, 2020); and George Orwell, *Nineteen Eighty-Four* (1949), with an introduction by Julian Symonds (Everyman's Library, 1992), pp. 11-19.

influence, revise or halt. Ministers sit in an office and decide the law, knowing that they are immune from normal parliamentary procedures and cannot be held to account.[25]

These reservations didn't stop both Houses approving the new powers, and two days before they were due to expire The Health Protection (Coronavirus, Restrictions) (England) (Amendment) (No. 3) Regulations 2020 were enacted in law, effectively banning protest and demonstrations in England. To clarify, these and other coronavirus regulations and amendments have since been superseded by and consolidated in The Health Protection (Coronavirus, Restrictions) (No. 2) (England) Regulations 2020, which were made on 3 July, and which, under Regulation 5, reduced the restrictions to gatherings of more than 30 people during the ongoing 'emergency period'; but the restrictions may as quickly be reinstated.[26]

Three weeks before, on the morning after the first Black Lives Matter demonstrations in Central London, I cycled into Westminster and passed the Houses of Parliament. There were more police than usual, but not enough to scare the tourists away. But around my way, Waterloo and Lambeth embankment, every back street was lined with police van after police van, scores of them, many belonging to the infamous Territorial Support Group or 'riot police'. The Met is one of the largest and best funded police forces in the world, with over 43,000 personnel as of June 2020 — half the strength of the regular British Army — and an annual budget of £3.8 billion.[27] It'd take about 10-15 minutes to get thousands of police anywhere in Central London. And where I live in Lambeth Cross, every weekend over the lockdown, and every day and night in the weeks when the Black Lives Matter protests moved to the US Embassy, at least one police helicopter, and often more, was hovering over us.

---

25. See UK Parliament: House of Lords, 'Health Protection (Coronavirus, Restrictions) (England) (Amendment) (No. 3) Regulations 2020', *Hansard* (25 June, 2020).

26. See 'The Health Protection (Coronavirus, Restrictions) (No. 2) (England) Regulations 2020' (3 July, 2020). And, in fact, on 14 September, The Health Protection (Coronavirus, Restrictions) (No. 2) (England) (Amendment) (No. 4) Regulations 2020 returned the prohibition to more than 6 persons 'during the emergency period'.

27. See Metropolitan Police, 'Structure' (as of 31 October, 2022).

These are part of the National Police Air Service, which provides all police forces in England and Wales with air support. Their aircraft, the Eurocopter EC135 and EC145, are both fitted with two cameras: a day camera equipped with a powerful zoom lens that can see straight into our living rooms, and a thermal-imaging camera that can detect our body heat at night. Military variants of the EC145 are used in the Royal Air Force, as well as in the armies of the US, Germany and many other countries. In addition, it's been reported that the Metropolitan Police Service branch of the NPAS has been secretly using US-made Cessna F04 aircraft for a number of years, and these are fitted with surveillance equipment capable of intercepting mobile telephone calls and listening in on private conversations. In addition to these manned aircraft, the Met also uses Unmanned Aerial Vehicles or microdrones, which can be fitted with video cameras, thermal imaging devices, radiation detectors, mobile-phone jammers and air sampling devices. Hovering at a height of around 60 metres, they are said to be virtually invisible from the ground.

The Met has refused to disclose how much it costs to keep their helicopters in the air, which is estimated to be in the region of thousands of pounds per hour; but on its website the NPAS justify the use of helicopters as follows:

> In public order situations they provide — literally — an overview enabling commanders to make the most effective deployments and respond quickly to emerging problems.[28]

What these emerging problems include was demonstrated on 18 August this year when the Greater Manchester Police released footage from one of their airborne thermal imaging cameras showing an armed police raid the previous Saturday on a house party at which it claimed approximately 200 people were present, most, to judge by the footage, in the back garden.[29] At the request of the police, the initial 48-hour closure notice placed on the residential property was subsequently extended by Manchester and Salford Magistrates Court to 3 months, prohibiting access to the premises by anyone except the property owner

---

28. National Police Air Service, 'Frequently asked questions'.

29. See GM Police, 'Closure Order Following Gathering in Gorton', *YouTube* (18 August, 2020).

and tenants. The Greater Manchester Police then took the opportunity to invite anyone 'with information about illegal large gatherings' to inform them.[30]

What the Greater Manchester Police didn't report, however, is that The Health Protection (Coronavirus, Restrictions on Gatherings) (North of England) Regulations 2020 under whose powers their raid was made, and which has placed 6.6 million people in the restricted areas under lockdown, have not even been debated by Parliament, and are only due for approval by 28 September, an astonishing 8 weeks after coming into force.[31] This is an example of Government by decree, without legislative oversight, enforced by our police forces using the technologies of the biosecurity state. And yet, in response to this dystopian demonstration of a police state in action, Councillor Nigel Murphy, Deputy Leader of Manchester City Council, had only this to say:

> This was a particularly flagrant breach of Covid-19 restrictions, which are in place to protect everyone in our communities and must be respected. We welcome this tough action, which serves as a reminder that public health must be our first priority and that selfish breaches of the rules will not be tolerated.[32]

On 28 August, The Health Protection (Coronavirus, Wearing of Face Coverings in a Relevant Place and on Public Transport) (England) (Amendment) Regulations 2020 doubled the £100 fine for not wearing face coverings where it is mandated to £200 for repeat offences, rising to a maximum of £3,200 for each repeat offence thereafter.[33] This compares unfavourably to the fine of up to 150 Reichsmarks (about £660 today) for not wearing the Yellow Star in the Third Reich imposed from 1 September 1941. On the same day, The Health Protection (Coronavirus) (Restrictions on Holding of Gatherings and Amendment) (England) Regulations 2020 increased the fine for organising an unlicensed music event, or

---

30. Greater Manchester Police, 'Tell us about a possible breach of coronavirus (Covid-19) measures'.

31. See UK Statutory Instruments, 'The Health Protection (Coronavirus, Restrictions on Gatherings) (North of England) Regulations 2020' (4 August, 2020).

32. Quoted by GM Police in 'Closure Order Following Gathering in Gorton', *YouTube* (18 August, 2020).

33. See UK Statutory Instruments, 'The Health Protection (Coronavirus, Wearing of Face Coverings in a Relevant Place and on Public Transport) (England) (Amendment) Regulations 2020' (28 August, 2020).

an unlawful gathering of 30 or more people, to £10,000, with organisers facing criminal prosecution, and participants subject to fines of £100, doubling on each offence up to a maximum of £3,200.[34] In justifying these measures, the Home Secretary reported that in London the Metropolitan Police Force had raided more than 1,000 unlicensed events since the end of June.[35] The real purpose of these Regulations was made clear on the weekend I published this article, when Piers Corbyn, at the 'Unite for Freedom' protest against coronavirus-justified regulations attended by 35,000 people in Trafalgar Square, was arrested by the Metropolitan Police Force for the third time, and, having been identified by them as the organiser of the demonstration, fined £10,000.[36]

Presumably, these new, extraordinarily punitive regulations, with fines far beyond the financial means of most UK citizens, will be enforced with the help of the National Police Air Service and its advanced technologies of surveillance. If you live in Central London, you almost get used to the sound of helicopter engines, their buzzing the background to every thought. It's become a permanent state to know someone is watching and recording you from the skies, ready to send in armed police at the first sign of disobedience to the latest regulations. Across the UK, there are 145,000 police officers enforcing the huge number of coronavirus-justified laws. Effectively, we're under occupation by our own police and security forces, in a civil war we don't even know has been declared. Under this occupation, we have been progressively stripped of our rights as citizens, and our bare life (*zoē*) — repoliticised, as Agamben wrote, through its exposure to death, first by the threat of terrorism that has ruled our political lives (*bios*) for the past two decades and now by the threat of coronavirus — is being subjected to the programmes and technologies of the biosecurity state. The NSDAP Government's definition of the 'subject of the state' no longer as a citizen with rights and freedoms but as 'a person who enjoys the protection of the state and who in consequence has specific obligations towards it' seems increasingly applicable to our new status under UK law.

---

34. See UK Statutory Instruments, 'The Health Protection (Coronavirus) (Restrictions on Holding of Gatherings and Amendment) (England) Regulations 2020' (28 August, 2020).

35. See Priti Patel, 'Tougher fines ahead of Bank Holiday to crack down on illegal gatherings' (24 August, 2020).

36. See Piers Corbyn, 'Defend the Right to Protest: Justice for Piers Corbyn', *Crowd Justice*.

The standard response to this intrusion of the state into our private lives — or, more accurately, of the constitution of bare life as the object of a biopolitics — is that if you have nothing to hide you have nothing to fear, and that the state already knows everything about us anyway through Facebook, Twitter, Instagram, Apple, Samsung, Pandora, Sony, Microsoft, Amazon, Grindr, Tinder, YouTube, Spotify, Netflix, our mobile phone providers, internet service providers, insurance providers, utilities companies, employers, banks, credit cards, lenders and landlords. But those who find comfort in this thought do so because they have nothing to say, nothing to do, nothing to think, that does not comply with — let alone opposes — this occupation; and it's on their abject compliance and willing collaboration with the technologies of biopower that the UK biosecurity state is being built.

4. The Global Safe Space

In the UK today, the biosecurity state is being implemented not, as it was under the Third Reich, on fear of the Jew and the communist — although recent events in the politics of the UK have demonstrated the continuing hegemony of the British establishment when faced with anything even purporting to resemble socialism — or even of the Muslim and the terrorist — who in the 2000s fulfilled a similar political role to that of the Jew and communist in the 1930s — but on similar feelings of disgust (for the diseased body), fear (of the invisible virus) and hatred (of those responsible for spreading it). For some time now, the body under capitalism has been subjected to an industry of care that exists between the pharmaceutical and the cosmetic, partaking of the discourses of medicine and hygiene, in which all bodily secretions — whether sweat, skin, hair, odour, saliva, mucous, pus, breath, blood, urine or excrement — are considered a form of waste that should be contained at source, concealed at the point of emission, cleansed from the surface of our skin and perfumed around the borders of our bodies. The clearest signifier of wealth in the UK today is not to have to be in proximity to other people, whether that's expressed through the discourse of 'exclusivity' that describes everything from private gyms and trendy restaurants to first-class train compartments and segregated entrances to luxury housing, or through the obsessive cleansing and purification of the spaces we inhabit, beginning with our own bodies.

A noticeable phenomenon of the lockdown of the UK has been the sudden increase in adverts for online yoga classes, as if reducing the spiralling complexities of the world to the limits of our own bodies, which are then spiritualised through ancient and exotic practices, will defend us against the new and very material threats we face. When a population that spends thousands of pounds a year toning our bodies in gyms and yoga classes, smoothing our skin with a catalogue of powders and creams, styling our hair with exorbitantly-priced haircuts and shampoos, concealing our odour and breath with perfumes and mouth sprays, straightening and polishing our teeth with private dentistry, flushing out even our insides with colonic irrigations, spending our last pennies on holidays whose primary purpose is to get a tan — and generally turning our natural bodies (*zoē*) into a signifier of our social class (*bios*) — are suddenly told we're subject to the same viral infection as the rest of the world, then social distancing as a civic virtue, face masks worn as a demonstration of good citizenship, directional arrows on the floors of supermarkets as a method of crowd control, acrylic dividers between tables and bars in pubs in accordance with Government guidance, and all the other new markers of social space, act to reassert our own fading sense of exceptionalism. It is from this disgust, fear and hatred — to which a brief visit to social media will amply testify — and not the altruistic sense of common decency and duty to others appealed to in Government propaganda, that our eagerness comes for the various test-and-trace programmes circling above our future like so many vultures competing for access to the COVID-19 carcass. Disgust, and hatred too — but fear most of all. And what greater fear than the fear of each other, the fear of ourselves?

After the stick comes the carrot. Having been terrified into compliance by the Government-imposed lockdown of the UK and Public Health England's deliberately exaggerated daily reports of COVID-19 deaths out of any statistical or medical context, the 'New Normal' is being implemented on the basis of our love for Big Brother. In behavioural study after behavioural study presented to the Scientific Advisory Group for Emergencies (SAGE) on how to manufacture public engagement and compliance with the raft of new measures and programmes being imposed upon us, the language of national duty, of 'we are all in this together', of social cohesion, community care and mutual support has been consistently recommended as the best means to get the UK population out of our homes and back into work under the radically reduced rights and freedoms and new obligations and impositions under which we now live in the UK biosecurity state. And what is being prepared for us in our velvet-lined prison is the realisation, on a national scale, of our younger generation's demand for what has come to be called a 'safe space'.

In 'Public Disorder and Public Health: Contemporary Threats and Risks', the paper presented to SAGE on 2 July by the Policing and Security sub-Group of the Scientific Pandemic Influenza Group on Behavioural Science (SPI-B), the authors, considering the previous month's protests by both Black Lives Matter (BLM) and what they call the 'extreme-right-wing (XRW)', as well as to recent gatherings at unlicensed music and televised football events, advised that, faced with an erosion of police legitimacy:

> The Government needs to reconstruct a shared sense of responsibility for public health which accentuates its positive virtues, rather than taking a punitive approach.[37]

And on 29 July, the SPI-B, in its 'Consensus Statement on Local Interventions', which responds to SAGE asking about 'specific measures to take to achieve public buy-in and compliance' with localised lockdown measures, recommended a change in terminology from a punitive to a remedial discourse, from the threat of prison to the care of the clinic:

> Terminology should emphasise care, not punishment. Given the punitive connotations of the term 'lockdown', which can be seen to emphasise blame, terms should be adopted that emphasise care, concern and support for the affected communities. Procedural justice and community development evidence stresses that local emergency measures should be framed not as something that is done to people, but with and for them.[38]

---

37. Scientific Pandemic Influenza Group on Behavioural Science, 'Public Disorder and Public Health: Contemporary Threats and Risks' (2 July, 2020), p. 8.

38. Scientific Pandemic Influenza Group on Behavioural Science, 'Consensus Statement on Local Interventions' (27 July, 2020), p. 4.

These recommendations would bear fruit on 18 August when Matt Hancock, the Secretary of State for Health and Social Care, announced the launch of the National Institute for Health Protection to administer this 'New Normal'. A replacement for the dissolved Public Health England, the executive agency of his own Ministry, and merged with both the privately outsourced Test and Trace programme and the Joint Biosecurity Centre, the new institute's 'single and relentless mission', the Health Secretary declared, will be 'protecting people from external threats to this country's health.' In case we were wondering what this new 'terror' was that threatened us, he went on to clarify that it included 'biological weapons, pandemics, and of course infectious diseases of all kinds.' In an echo of Hitler's prioritising of the 'preservation of the people' as the first task of the State, Hancock concluded:

> The first responsibility of any Government is the protection of its citizens. And threats to public health are among the most important of all. Threats like this coronavirus pandemic can emerge anywhere and at any time. So we must be ready. Ready to beat this virus, and protect all of us, all of the time, over the years to come.[39]

In the UK today, the certainties and stupidities of Stalinist cultural orthodoxies have returned in the equal certainty and stupidity with which the politically correct denounce this or that person, work, statement or social media post as 'racist', 'sexist', 'transphobic', 'anti-Semitic', etc. For the dictates of Socialist Realism then we now have the orthodoxies of so-called 'woke' culture; for the Soviet Congress of Writers denouncing apostasy we have Goldsmiths College graduates trolling people on Twitter for political incorrectness; for the Moscow Show Trials of former Bolsheviks we have the indictments, confessions and forced retractions of public figures on social media. In June, it was the sacking of Labour Party MP and candidate for party leader Rebecca Long-Bailey for pointing out what was subsequently established as fact — that the US police practice of kneeling on the necks of citizens — the same tactic that killed George Floyd — was taught to them by Israeli security forces. Before that it was the author, J. K. Rowling, who has been denounced by the former child actors of the

---

39. Matt Hancock, 'The future of public health' (18 August, 2020).

films of her books for asserting that a 'woman' is defined by biology and is not merely a linguistic or cultural construct of patriarchy. Where university students under National Socialism burned books that contradicted their ideology, the 'woke' youth of today are deleting the *Harry Potter* books and other texts of the ideologically non-compliant from their online reading lists.

And just as Stalinism was an inversion of communism that created a totalitarian state out of a philosophy and practice of emancipation from capitalism, so too political correctness — which its acolytes claim to be a practice of liberation from discursive and institutional 'systems' that perpetuate inequalities in our society — has instead become the means by which thought, speech and action is policed online for heresy, corrected with enforced business programmes such as 'diversity training', expiated in corporate-funded spectacles like Black Lives Matter, and appeased, apparently, by the representation of Black, Asian and minority-ethnic individuals in positions of authority within capitalism, while leaving the economic relations of that authority unchallenged and unchanged. It would be interesting to hear whether the advocates of identity politics think the ethnicity of Rishi Sunak, the Chancellor of the Exchequer, Priti Patel, the Home Secretary, or Sadiq Khan, the London Mayor, has altered the neoliberalism of their policies or their ruthless implementation of the biosecurity state.

Our youth — for whom I have some residue of sympathy — raised on national decline, terrorist threat, fiscal austerity and social media in the political vacuum of neoliberalism that has subsumed their rebellion into the radical conservatism of identity politics, doubtless think they're leading us into the promised land; but like the Hitler Youth, Stalin's Komsomol and the Red Guards of Chairman Mao, they're the foot soldiers of the new totalitarianism that's being implemented by the governments of the world with their consent, even at their insistence. That the biosecurity state into which we have been led has been imposed in the name of greater equality, freedom and — that most important value of the 'woke' generation — 'safety' should be of surprise only to those who, like these kids, know nothing about history. Perhaps the clearest demonstration of this is the latest slogan to emerge from their ranks, 'silence is violence', which accuses anyone who does not repeat that 'black lives matter' of being guilty, by default, of racist violence against black people. Apart from betraying the understandable idealism of students who believe the economic forces sustaining racism can be

232

overcome in language, this slogan also reveals something about the dangers not of censoring speech — the inaccurate accusation made against totalitarianism — but the far more accurate one of compelling it in others. It was precisely about this that the French semiotician, Roland Barthes, in his inaugural lecture at the Collège de France, long ago warned another generation of would-be radicals:

> Language is legislation, speech is its code. To speak, and, with even greater reason, to utter a discourse is not, as is too often repeated, to communicate; it is to subjugate. Language — the performance of a language system — is neither reactionary nor progressive; it is quite simply fascist; for fascism does not prevent speech, it compels speech.[40]

The dystopia of the legislated biosecurity state — in which everybody is compelled to clap for the NHS; where everybody must be ready, 'all of the time', to beat the virus; and everybody displays unwavering compliance with every new public measure dreamed up for our protection — is the utopia of the 'woke' generation, its dream of turning the entire planet into a safe space coming true. The face mask is as much its symbol as the Red Book was to the students of Chairman Mao, and like it reducing the political complexities of the 'New Normal' to easily-remembered social directives ('Stay at home. Wash hands. Cover face. Make space.'). And now the New Normal is here, everyone from shop owners, publicans, security guards and council leaders to mobile phone providers, gallery curators, school governors and the architects commissioned to design this dystopia are competing to keep us 'safe'.[41]

Just as multiculturalism was the ideological form of neoliberalism during its heyday in the 1990s, when the untaxed flow of capital through global markets via anonymous offshore accounts was presented as the freedom of movement of peoples between outmoded national borders, so the authoritarianism of political correctness, the radical conservatism of identity politics, the cultural terrorism of no-platforming, the fundamentalism of 'woke' culture, and all the other instruments for creating and policing 'safe spaces', are the cultural forms of

---

40. Roland Barthes, 'Lecture in Inauguration of the Chair of Literary Semiology. Collège de France, January 7, 1977'; translated by Richard Howard in *October*, no. 8 (1979), pp. 3-16.

41. See David Brown, Prina Shah, Steve Connor and Becky Rush, 'This is what coronavirus will do to our offices and homes', *BBC News* (6 August, 2020).

biopolitics. Widely promoted, funded and implemented by the corporate financiers and government administrators of the biosecurity state, these cultural forms, which for some time now have policed behaviour and silenced debate in this country, have both prepared the way for and accustomed their adherents to the 'New Normal' we are now facing. All that was wanting was some 'crisis' to justify entrenching their radical conservatism in legislation. That opportunity has now arrived. The borders being closed by the coronavirus 'crisis' are not only between countries but also between bodies. Police-enforced social distancing, mandatory mask wearing, contact tracing as a condition of access to public life, immunity passports to monitor and protect the biosecurity of the state, enforced quarantining of households, lockdown restrictions on movement and association imposed on millions of people, and all the other programmes being implemented under the cloak of the coronavirus 'crisis', are the technical apparatus of this emergent political form.

5. The Use of Conspiracy Theory

One of the measures of the level of hysteria and lies to which the population has been driven by the coronavirus 'crisis' in this country is that those of us who research the criteria for attributing deaths to COVID-19, or the process by which Government regulations are made into law without parliamentary approval, or what Government contracts have been awarded by Ministers to which companies, or the number of citizens that have died from the suspension of health care under lockdown, are accused by those who rely for their opinions on the *BBC* and fear-mongering rags like the *Guardian*, the *Telegraph* and the *Financial Times* of being 'conspiracy theorists'.

As an example of which, I was recently accused of being such for stating that, 6 months into the coronavirus 'pandemic', as of 19 August, a total of 1,390 people who did not have a pre-existing medical condition have died in hospitals in England while testing positive for SARS-CoV-2, of which just 305 have been under the age of 60. This was so incomprehensible to my accuser that, without waiting for me to provide the proof, he deleted himself from the page on which I wrote this information, presumably to protect himself from hearing confirmation of something that would refute everything he believed about the coronavirus 'crisis'. He would rather remain in willful ignorance of the truth, in other words, than confront the level of lies he's been told, and his own collaboration, therefore, in spreading them.

In fact, this is a very easy fact to prove, though not a particularly easy one to find. If you go to NHS record of daily deaths registered in English hospitals, then click on the fifth link down, 'COVID-19 total announced deaths 20 August 2020 — weekly file', it will take you to an excel spread sheet (to which I can't link directly here, hence this long explanation).[42] On there you will see that, in table three, 'COVID-19 deaths by age group and presence of pre-existing condition', and clicking on this will take you to the page from which I have made this screen grab below.

Breakdown by pre existing condition

Age group	Pre existing condition			
	Yes	No	Unkown presence of pre-existing condition	Total
Total	28,095	1,390	0	29,485
0 - 19 yrs	16	4	0	20
20 - 39	179	34	0	213
40 - 59	2,023	267	0	2,290
60 - 79	10,635	575	0	11,210
80+	15,242	510	0	15,752
Unknown age	0	0	0	0

Source: National Health Service — COVID-19 deaths

To summarise these records of the National Health Service, as of 20 August 2020:

- 29,485 people have died in hospitals in England with their deaths attributed to COVID-19.
- Of these, 26,962 have been 60 years and older, making up 91.4 per cent of all 'COVID-19 deaths'.
- 28,095 of the deaths in hospitals in England attributed to COVID-19 died with one or more pre-existing medical condition, making up 95.2 per cent of the total deaths.
- Only 1,390 people who had their deaths attributed to COVID-19 died without a pre-existing medical condition, 4.7 per cent of the total.
- Of those, 1,085 were 60 years or older, 78 per cent of the total number of deaths without pre-existing medical conditions.

---

42. See NHS England, 'COVID-19 Deaths'.

- 305 people, therefore, under the age of 60 and without any pre-existing medical condition, have had their deaths in English hospitals attributed to COVID-19, 1.03 per cent of the total 'COVID-19 deaths'.

It's on the justification of these figures that, as of 28 August, 2020, 188 coronavirus-justified Statutory Instruments have been made into law in the UK before being laid before or approved by Parliament, this being deemed necessary and proportionate by what the relevant Minister in each and every explanatory memorandum describes as 'the serious and imminent threat to public health which is posed by the incidence and spread of severe acute respiratory syndrome coronavirus 2 (SARS-CoV-2).'[43] The figures I've quoted above expose this excuse to be so blatantly unjustified, disproportionate and absurd that I'll try and anticipate some of the questions in response to this data. The coronavirus 'crisis' has passed far beyond anything resembling reality in this country, where we are now ruled by terror and public displays of virtue; but it is important that those of us who still read these statistics keep repeating their evidence of the reality of the 'thing' from which most of the population have long ago fled in horror.

First, the NHS records don't include those who died outside of hospitals, with the Office of National Statistics reporting 31,253 people dying in hospitals in England as of 14 August having their deaths attributed to COVID-19, compared with 18,149 dying at home, in hospices, care homes, other communal establishments and elsewhere, making a total of 49,402 deaths attributed to COVID-19 in England.[44]

However, 14,707 of these non-hospital deaths have been in care homes, largely because the NHS made the decision, on 17 March, to discharge around 25,000 patients, many of them already infected with SARS-CoV-2, into care homes.[45] Although there is no record — at least that that I know of — of what they

---

43. See Hansard Society, 'Coronavirus Statutory Instruments Dashboard, 2020-2022' (4 March, 2022).

44. See Office for National Statistics, 'Deaths registered weekly in England and Wales, provisional (2020 edition of this dataset up to week ending 1 January 2021)'.

45. See Sir Simon Stevens, NHS Chief Executive, and Amanda Pritchard, NHS Chief Operating Officer, 'To Chief executives of all NHS trusts and foundation trusts, CCG Accountable Officers, GP practices and Primary Care Networks Providers of community health services' (17 March, 2020).

died of, I think it's safe to say that these deaths, and the 2,323 who died at home, were of elderly and frail people, almost certainly with pre-existing medical conditions, who died as a result of the Government's decision to impose a 'lockdown' of the UK with scant regard, if any, to the consequences of doing so for changes to emergency, adult social, elective, primary and community care, which the ONS has estimated will result in 56,000 excess deaths over the next five years.[46] Very few of the deceased are likely to have been under the age of 60 without pre-existing medical conditions.

This is reflected in the ONS breakdown of the ages of the 52,026 deaths attributed to COVID-19 in both England and Wales, of which 43,145 have been 70 years of age or over, 83 per cent or the total; 31,546 have been 80 and over, 60 per cent of the total; and 11,217, 21.5 per cent of the total, have been 90 and over — representing over a fifth of all 'COVID-19 deaths'.

If we, as a nation, instead of giving into the hysteria propagated by the Government and media, had examined the data from Italy, which I analysed in 'Language is a Virus: SARs-CoV-2 and the Science of Political Control', and which we were constantly being warned was our immediate future, we would have seen that COVID-19 does not constitute a threat to the vast majority of the population that is under 65 and in good health, but almost exclusively kills the elderly with existing illnesses, with the average age of death attributed to COVID-19 in Italy 80, and almost always with one or more pre-existing medical conditions.[47] Instead of locking down our entire country in anticipation of an epidemic that never arrived, this data should have made us quarantine and protect this demographic, while at the same time continuing medical care to the tens of thousands of others who have died and will continue to die as a result of the lockdown.

Second, the NHS figures don't include those who died outside of England. Again, as of 14 August, 4,216 deaths in Scotland (76 per cent of which were 75 and over), 2,543 in Wales and 863 in Northern Ireland have been attributed to COVID-19, making a total of 7,622 deaths out of the UK total of 56,503, or 13.5

---

46. See Office for National Statistics, 'Direct and Indirect Impacts of COVID-19 on Excess Deaths and Morbidity: Executive Summary for the Department of Health and Social Care, the Government's Actuary Department and Home Office,' (15 July 2020).

47. See Simon Elmer, 'Language is a Virus: SARS-CoV-2 and the Science of Political Control', *Architects for Social Housing* (3 April, 2020).

per cent.[48] I haven't found data from these countries breaking down how many of these people had pre-existing medical conditions, but I'd be surprised if the percentage was significantly different from that in England.

Even calculated by the 1.03 per cent of deaths attributed to COVID-19 in hospitals in England that were under 60 and without pre-existing medical conditions, which is likely to be an exaggerated percentage of the total deaths so attributed, that only makes an additional 75 people. In the whole of the UK, therefore, 6 months into a supposed epidemic, less than 400 people under 60 without pre-existing health conditions have had their deaths attributed to COVID-19 out of a population of 67.8 million. By any rational measure or risk not based on hysteria and fear, this does not constitute an epidemic justifying the lockdown of the UK.

Even the senior scientific and medical advisors to the Government who have participated in this deception of the public, Patrick Vallance and Chris Whitty, admitted in a press conference as far back as April, when fear of coronavirus was at its peak, that COVID-19 being mentioned on a death certificate as the underlying cause of death doesn't mean the deceased tested positive for SARS-CoV-2.[49] Having researched in some detail the extraordinarily lax and deliberately manipulated criteria for attributing deaths to COVID-19, I have since always used the description 'attributed to COVID-19', rather than dying 'of' or 'with' COVID-19. To be included in the official figures of COVID-19 deaths in the UK does not require a positive test for SARS-CoV-2 (which in any case does not mean the patient had COVID-19), or even a medical diagnoses of COVID-19 by the examining pathologist, but merely the 'suspicion' of the doctor, or in the case of deaths in care homes of the care home provider, or even, according to the Coronavirus Act 2020, of a medically unqualified undertaker, that COVID-19 was the cause of death.

As I explained in detail in 'Manufacturing Consensus: The Registering of COVID-19 Deaths in the UK', on 5 March, COVID-19 was recategorised as a 'Notifiable Disease' and SARS-CoV-2 as a 'Causative Agent' by The Health Protection (Notification) (Amendment) Regulations 2020. Following which, on 20

---

48. See National Records of Scotland, 'Deaths involving coronavirus (COVID-19) in Scotland'.

49. See Dominic Raab, 'United Kingdom Coronavirus Briefing Transcript April 16' (16 April, 2020).

April, the World Health Organization issued 'International guidelines for certification and classification (coding) of COVID-19 as cause of death' stating that COVID-19 must always be listed on death certificates as the 'underlying cause of death' — as the WHO instructs doctors 'whether this can be considered medically correct or not' — while any other medical conditions the patient may have, such as dementia, heart disease, diabetes or cancer, will only be listed as a contributory cause.[50] Even the figure of 1,390 deaths without pre-existing conditions attributed to COVID-19 in English hospitals is undoubtedly an exaggeration, therefore. Numerous NHS doctors have come forward in articles not published in the mainstream press to expose the exaggeration of COVID-19 deaths, but unless you seek them out you will most likely not have heard of them due to the censorship to which anything questioning the Government narrative is being subjected.

Just as damaging to the justification these figures constitute for Government regulations and programmes, on 16 July a paper by Yoon K. Loke, Professor of Medicine and Pharmacology at Norwich Medical School, and Carl Heneghan, Professor of Evidence-Based Medicine and Director of the Centre for Evidence-Based Medicine (CEBM) at the University of Oxford, titled 'Why no-one can ever recover from COVID-19 in England — a statistical anomaly', showed that Public Health England had been regularly looking for people who had ever tested positive for SARS-CoV-2 and, in the event of their death from any cause, listing them in their daily figures as a 'COVID-19 death', no matter how long ago the test was, and whether or not they had been successfully treated and discharged from hospital. 'By this PHE definition', they point out, 'no one with COVID in England is allowed to ever recover from their illness', when in fact, at the time of publication of their paper, more than 125,000 patients had been admitted to NHS hospitals for COVID-19, and 80,000 who had recovered remained in the community.[51] Given the advanced age of most patients discharged, who have then died of other illnesses, this has led to an over-exaggeration of deaths attributed to COVID-19.

---

50. See World Health Organization, 'International Guidelines for Certification and Classification (Coding) of COVID-19 as Cause of Death' (20 April, 2020).

51. Yoon K. Loke and Carl Heneghan, 'Why no-one can ever recover from COVID-19 in England — a statistical anomaly', The Centre for Evidence-Based Medicine (CEBM), University of Oxford (16 July, 2020).

In response to this embarrassing evidence of what at best is incompetence and at worst deliberate manipulation, the Health Secretary, Matt Hancock, ordered a review of how the Public Health England figures have been calculated. The new criterium resulting from this review is that a death can now only be attributed to COVID-19 if the deceased has died within 28 days of a positive test for SARS-CoV-2. While this is still grossly inadequate in establishing the actual cause of death for all the reasons I have mentioned, it has resulted in the reduction of the number of official 'COVID-19 deaths' in the UK from the ONS figures of 56,503 I broke down above, to the Government's current estimation of 41,449 — a reduction of over 15,000 deaths, 12,600 of them in England.[52]

Even more of a barrier to the claims of a 'serious and imminent' threat to public health whose 'urgency' requires the passing of regulations that won't be approved until up to 8 weeks after they come into effect, is the rapid and sustained decline in deaths that, even on the mere suspicion of doctors, care home providers and undertakers, have been attributed to COVID-19. Having now dissolved Public Health England, the Government's new 'COVID-19 dashboard' shows that, under the new criterium, between 1 July and 24 August, 6 deaths in Scotland, 8 in Northern Ireland, 77 in Wales, and 851 in England have been attributed to COVID-19, a total of 942 across the UK. In August this decline has accelerated, with just 196 deaths in England attributed to COVID-19. The COVID-19 dashboard doesn't bother to break these deaths down by the age of the deceased, but according to the Office of National Statistics, in the first two weeks of August only 30 people under the age of 65 had their deaths attributed to COVID-19 in the whole of the UK; 55 such deaths were between 65 and 74 years of age; 89 between 75 and 84; and 134 were 85 years and older: a total of 308 deaths attributed to COVID-19.

To put these figures into context, in the same two weeks, 1,643 people died in England and Wales where the underlying cause of death was a respiratory disease (ICD-10 J00-J99) other than COVID-19 (ICD-10 U07.1 and U07.2), including influenza, pneumonia, bronchitis, emphysema, asthma and other chronic obstructive pulmonary diseases included under this taxonomy. 18,187 people have died of all ages from all causes in these two weeks, meaning deaths attributed to COVID-19 have constituted less than 1.7 per cent of all deaths in

---

52. See UK Government, 'Coronavirus (COVID-19) in the UK'.

England and Wales. Yet in August alone, over 7 million people have been placed under lockdown restrictions on their movements and associations, together with the closure of their businesses and other public premises; the mandatory wearing of face coverings has been extended to more public places, including most recently to secondary schools; and the fines for non-compliance have been raised to punitive levels far beyond the financial means of most of the British public.

. As can be seen by those who take the time to look and read, there is neither justification for, nor proportionality to, such measures to be found in these figures. As the deaths of even elderly and sick people fade to what is, statistically speaking, the end of a respiratory disease that posed no threat to the vast majority of the UK population, the Government is now terrorising us with threats of what it calls, with reference to its carefully crafted charts, a 'second wave' in cases. This is very much the focus of the new COVID-19 dashboard, which reports that, as of 25 August, 327,798 people have tested positive in the UK, with 1,184 reported that day. This has risen from a low of 352 'cases' on 6 July, with a high of 1,441 on 14 August. However, there are several serious flaws in the desired narrative these figures are being used to construct.

Cases in United Kingdom ▾

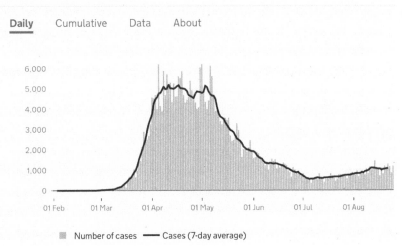

Daily   Cumulative   Data   About

Source: GOV.UK Coronavirus (COVID-19) in the UK

First, 'cases' indicate infection with the novel coronavirus (SARS-CoV-2), not the development of the symptoms of the disease (COVID-19), which is a basic distinction of infectiology, with around 80 per cent of persons contracting the virus either remaining asymptomatic or developing only very mild symptoms, similar to a common cold. As I reviewed in Section 3 of 'The Science and Law of Refusing to Wear Masks', and as studies continue to show, asymptomatic transmission of coronavirus is extremely low, with an infection rate of under 1 per cent. Of the remaining 20 per cent who develop severe symptoms, a smaller percentage again have to be admitted to hospital, with the infection fatality rate currently estimated to be 0.3 per cent. To call all these 'cases', therefore, as the Government's COVID-19 dashboard does, is a grossly and deliberately inaccurate representation of both the number of people with COVID-19, the degree of their illness, and the threat of infection those who currently have the virus represent to others.

Second, the figures say nothing about how many people have recovered from infection by SARS-CoV-2, or how many people are currently infected. As the paper from the CEBM at Oxford criticised, the impression still given by the Government's dashboard is that no-one ever recovers from COVID-19. But from a peak of 3,563 patients with COVID-19 in UK hospitals on 1 April, on 25 August there were just 779, which is a better measure of the current level of threat to public health of COVID-19. Again, to put this in context, between April and June this year there were 118,451 hospital beds available in England, 92,596 of which were for general and acute care, of which 58,146 were occupied.[53] Even at the height of the so-called 'epidemic', in other words, only 62.8 per cent of hospital beds for general and acute care were filled; while on 9 August, according to NHS records, the 655 patients with COVID-19 in English hospitals occupied just 0.7 per cent of such beds.[54]

Third, the recent rise in daily increases in so-called 'cases' are a product of the parallel increase in testing.[55] Quite logically, the more tests are conducted, the more instances of infection are revealed. From 1 August the average daily tests have never fallen below a 7-day average of 170,000, while in July they fell as low as 130,500. Significantly, this sudden rise in testing is also a product of the

---

53. See NHS England, 'Bed Availability and Occupancy Data – Overnight'.
54. See NHS England, 'COVID-19 Hospital Activity'.
55. See UK Government, 'Coronavirus (COVID-19) in the UK (Testing in England)'.

privatisation of the testing process by the awarding of Government contracts. To take 14 August as a typical example, 54,444 tests were conducted by the National Health Service and Public Health England, compared to 104,989 by commercial partners. It's through this commercial incentive that the rise in so-called 'cases' justifying the restrictions on our freedoms has been produced, and which is preparing the UK public for the promised 'second wave' this winter. To represent the increase in positive tests consequent upon the long-delayed increase in testing as a second wave of infections justifying a second lockdown of the UK is, quite simply, a deliberate lie to the UK public that no medical practitioner should be party to.

Testing in United Kingdom ▼

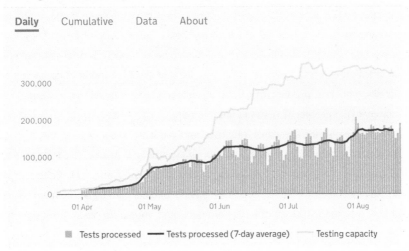

Source: GOV.UK Coronavirus (COVID-19) in the UK

As an example of this political manipulation of testing, on 8 August, The Health Protection (Coronavirus, Restrictions on Gatherings) (North of England) (Amendment) Regulations 2020 placed 141,000 people in Preston City Council under lockdown restrictions on their movements and associations, as well as closures of their businesses and public premises, because of a reported increase in 'cases' in the 'Weekly Coronavirus Disease 2019 (COVID-19) Surveillance

Report' for the week ending 7 August.[56] A summary of COVID-19 surveillance systems, this report, co-produced by Public Health England, the Joint Biosecurity Centre and the NHS Test and Trace programme — which is to say, what is now the UK Health Security Agency, and an example of its function — showed that Preston, with 36 cases per 100,000 of the population as of 30 July, was one of 20 local authorities targeted for lockdown.[57] As suggested the previous month by the Scientific Pandemic Influenza Group on Behavioural Science, this has now been rebranded as 'intervention'. By the following week the *BBC* was reporting that in the 7 days to 4 August this rate had risen to 42.6 'cases' per 100,000 people.[58] What this meant in reality is that 61 people testing positive for SARS-CoV-2 in a city of 141,000 people was enough for police to enforce the catalogue of prohibitions and obligations with fines and other criminal sanctions. Under this national surveillance system, all of England lives under the same threat, which no rebranding can disguise as the arbitrary decree of a State of Emergency that suspends our rights and freedoms until such time as an equally arbitrarily set rate of infection — which bears no relation to level of illness or threat of contagion or fatality, and is a product of a rate of testing whose increase is motivated by commercial interests — restores them to us.

To dismiss the extensive, recorded and verifiable evidence of all this data as a 'conspiracy theory' is not only to remain in wilful ignorance of the truth; it is to collaborate in the lies that have already killed tens of thousands of UK citizens left to die alone in care homes, denied life-saving medical care by empty hospitals or those too terrorised by the Government and media to visit Accident and Emergency wards; that is estimated will push the UK economy into the worst depression in over 300 years; that has already bankrupted thousands of businesses; and which is predicted to push unemployment in the UK to 4-5 million; all while covertly outsourcing our public services to multinational corporations and implementing programmes of digital surveillance and

---

56. See UK Statutory Instruments, 'The Health Protection (Coronavirus, Restrictions on Gatherings) (North of England) (Amendment) Regulations 2020' (8 August, 2020); and Public Health England, Joint Biosecurity Centre, NHS Test and Trace, 'Weekly Coronavirus Disease 2019 (COVID-19) Surveillance Report: Week 32, 2020' (12 August, 2021).

57. See Public Health England, 'National COVID Surveillance Reports' (23 April, 2020).

58. See 'Coronavirus: Preston young people targeted as lockdown imposed', *BBC News* (8 August, 2020).

biosecurity which, as Agamben says, 'far exceed any form of control exercised under totalitarian regimes such as fascism or Nazism.'[59]

I've gone into considerable detail in recalling these figures and discussing what they mean to show that it is not for those of us who take the time to do so to refute the accusation of 'conspiracy theory' thrown at us by childish, arrogant or frightened people — whether it is to take comfort in dismissing this evidence as such or to try to silence anyone who exposes the lies of the Government and media; rather, it is for them to show how these figures support the actions of the UK Government and, just as importantly, their own obedience to the increasingly dictatorial regulations and programmes it is imposing on the British population. For, once again, it is on their unthinking obedience, and on the blind fear that drives their flight into the arms of the Government and its private contractors, that the UK biosecurity state is being implemented.

If you have any sense of yourself as a UK citizen, with a citizen's rights and some remnants of political agency in the administration of the state under which we live; if you have any thought for the tens of thousands of unnecessary deaths caused by the ongoing lies of our Government and media; or if you are concerned by the cynical use of a virus to expand the regulations, programmes and technologies of the biosecurity state in which our children will grow up and live for the foreseeable future — then the wilful ignorance, childish fear and blind obedience that has defined the UK public's response to the coronavirus 'crisis' must stop now. The question is, how?

6. Collaboration and Resistance

In a recent interview with the Austrian television station ServusTV, published on *YouTube* on 3 May (and subsequently removed for 'violating *YouTube* Community Guidelines'), Dr. Sucharit Bhakdi, Professor Emeritus of Medical Microbiology, who served for 22 years as Chairman of the Institute of Medical Microbiology and Hygiene at the Johannes Gutenberg University in Mainz, one of the most cited research scientists in German history and one of the most outspoken critics of

---

59. Giorgio Agamben, 'New Reflections', *Quodlibet* (22 April, 2020); collected in *Where Are We Now?*, p. 43.

'measures' justified by the threat of COVID-19, when asked how long the coronavirus crisis will last, responded:

> This crisis is caused by the politicians. The crisis does not exist as a real crisis, so the crisis will end when the politicians decide it will end. It has nothing to do with the virus. This crisis has never existed. This nationwide epidemic has never existed. Do you understand? It is a phantom. And if you ask me whether I know when a phantom ends, then all I can say is that a phantom never ends until you yourself end it.

That was nearly four months ago, and since then this 'phantom' — Bhakdi used the German word *'Spuk'*, which has the sense of haunting — has become a terrifying reality for more and more people. The implementation of the UK biosecurity state, whose regulations and programmes I discussed in Part 1 of this article, relies on this spirit of fear and collaboration. In its negative aspect, this extends to the self-policing on which all totalitarian states have relied historically, and whose primary agents are the informers assembled from that society. Under the Third Reich, 80 per cent of investigations by the Gestapo were initiated as a result of denunciations of a neighbour or family member by civilians. By the time the Berlin Wall fell in 1989, there were 189,000 civilian informants working for the Ministry for State Security of the German Democratic Republic. In the UK, little more than a month after The Health Protection (Coronavirus, Restrictions) (England) Regulations 2020 were signed into law, the National Police Chiefs' Council announced on 30 April that it had received reports from public informants of more than 194,300 coronavirus-related incidents in England and Wales — over 5,700 reports per day.[60] And in one weekend alone, according to the Home Office, the Metropolitan Police Force received information on more than 200 events across London made unlawful by coronavirus legislation.[61] These are the neighbourhood curtain-twitchers, public-shamers, online video-posters, social-media trolls and police-informants that have emerged in vast numbers at the invitation of our Government, municipal authorities, councils and police forces.

---

60. See Lizzie Dearden, 'Coronavirus: Police issue almost 9,000 fines for lockdown breaches in England', *The Independent* (30 April, 2020).

61. Priti Patel, 'Tougher fines ahead of Bank Holiday to crack down on illegal gatherings' (23 August, 2020).

Forming this active contingent of collaborators from the general public relies, as it always has done historically, on widespread and unrelenting programmes of propaganda and indoctrination on which even the most self-interested collaborator can fall back when justifying — to others or to themselves — their behaviour. As an example of which, the widely reproduced Government propaganda of a person in a mask claiming they are wearing it 'for you' has been universally adopted and parroted by the compliant; yet this mimicked signalling of biosecurity altruism hasn't stopped the same people from accusing those who don't wear a mask of being murderers and terrorists and demanding they be arrested. As Agamben said, politics has become policing, and the care of the life of the population is indistinguishable from the civil war being waged against the enemy within.

Despite its voluntary nature, Government guidance on everything from social-distancing and self-isolating to contact-tracing and mandatory mask-wearing has been widely adhered to by the always obedient UK public, imposed by private and public establishments in the UK beyond the force of law, and enforced by UK police forces even when they don't have the legal powers to do so. For those of us politically opposed to such measures — which have no medical basis, are wildly disproportionate to the actual level of threat to public health, are a violation of our human rights and civil liberties, and are instruments of the biosecurity state being implemented under the cloak of the coronavirus 'crisis' — this guidance, and the regulations made into law following the public's widespread adherence, is increasingly banning us from public life. This includes the public transport we can't take, the shops and supermarkets we can't enter, the pubs and bars where we can't drink, the restaurants in which we can't eat, the museums and cinemas we can't visit, the concerts we can't attend, the events at which we can't speak, the banks, post-offices and libraries we can't use, the hotels where we can't stay, the countries to which we can't travel, the clinics in which we can't consult a doctor, the hospitals in which we can't visit our loved ones, the schools to which we can't return our children. Soon, this will include the workplaces in which we can't find employment. Whether or not to comply with these measures, therefore, presents a dilemma whose response is not merely an ethical choice limited to our individual conscience or whether doing so fits more or less conveniently into our 'lifestyle', but a social and political choice with consequences for all of us.

We don't have to turn to the gradual exclusion of Jews from public and economic life under the Third Reich for a comparison to this programme. Compliance with these measures, both guidance and regulations, is akin to entering a 'Whites-only' diner in the USA in the 1960s, or drinking in an English pub with a sign outside saying 'No Irish, no blacks, no dogs' in the 1970s, or boarding a racially segregated bus in apartheid South Africa in the 1980s, or entering any of the myriad places in Saudi Arabia to which a woman is banned today, or using roads prohibited to Palestinians in Israel, or teaching in a Turkish school where use of the Kurdish language is banned — or, closer to home, using a socially segregated entrance to a luxury residential development in London — in that doing so affirms a system of exclusion and discrimination to which you, individually, are exempt.

One might respond that the black woman cannot change the colour of her skin, the Irishman his nationality, the Palestinian his lack of citizenship, the Saudi woman her sex, or the Kurdish child their mother tongue, while I can choose to hand over my personal details, wear a mask, upload my biological data, maintain the prescribed distance or stay quarantined at home. But those who refused to comply and continue to protest against such discrimination, both black and white, Arab and Jew, men and women, don't seek access to such establishments; they seek to end a form of state control that binds all citizens — both those with access and those without — to a system of social, cultural, economic and political discrimination and exclusion.

One of the more contradictory aspects of the coronavirus 'crisis' is that a Prime Minister who throughout his career — first as a journalist, then as London Mayor, then as the Foreign Minister — has been repeatedly exposed as a liar, who now sits at the head of a Cabinet selected for its venality and ambition, and who throughout his Leadership has lied repeatedly to the nation, is despite this taken at his word about the biggest lie of the Twenty-first Century. This isn't quite true. Boris Johnson and his Government are constantly accused of lying, but about the severity of the 'crisis', not about its veracity. Since it began, the UK commentariat in mainstream and social media have consistently insisted that more people are dying of COVID-19 than the official figures claim, and have called for the

Government to impose harsher restrictions, impose the lockdown for longer, make masks mandatory across public life, issue more punitive fines and punishments, and give the police forces more powers to take away our freedoms. Yet with a few honourable exceptions — in law Jonathan Sumption QC, in medicine Dr. John Lee, in academia Professor John Oxford, in journalism Peter Hitchens — no politician in this country, no mainstream media outlet, no head of a public institution or other figure of authority in British public or cultural life has dared to question the transparent lies, deliberate manipulations, blatant inventions and movie magic that have conjured the coronavirus 'crisis' into the appearance of reality up there on the big screen of ideology.[62] Indeed, it is this highly unlikely, factually baseless and empirically refuted 'phantom' that is the conspiracy theory we should all be denouncing. And yet, the vast majority of the UK public has chosen to go along with it, and throw their hands up in horrified delight at every new garment added to the Emperor's new clothes. Why?

Why do people collaborate? Collaboration during the Second World War was widespread amongst the populations of occupied Europe. Some collaborated because they thought it would benefit them, either financially or in gaining more power under the new puppet government. By far the most denunciations to the Gestapo came from individuals settling scores with neighbours, but others did it for the financial rewards offered for selling their neighbours out. We've seen this revived today in the widespread denunciation of neighbours to the police for breaking lockdown regulations in the UK, and in the financial inducements for the public to take part in test trials.

Many more collaborated out of fear, and the hope that by doing so they'd be spared. To justify this betrayal of their former compatriots, collaborators had to see their neighbours as threats to their security, so that they, and not the occupying forces, became the source of the threat, and therefore had to be eliminated. This has been repeated in the hysterical denunciation on social media of people without their faces covered, whether they're on a protest, a train or at a party, and the calls for their arrest, imprisonment and even death.

---

62. See Jonathan Sumption, 'Former Supreme Court Justice: "This is what a police state is like"', *The Spectator* (30 March, 2020); Dr. John Lee, 'The dangers of a COVID "elimination" policy', *The Spectator* (22 September, 2020); Professor John Oxford, 'A View from the HVIVO', *Novus Communications* (31 March, 2020); Peter Hitchens, 'Face masks turn us into voiceless submissives — and it's not science forcing us to wear them, it's politics', *Mail on Sunday* (19 July, 2020).

Others collaborated in the hope that by appeasing the demands of the occupiers they would lessen the negative effects of that occupation, and with the belief that, if only they could survive this undoubtedly temporary suspension of their rights and freedoms and continue to look the other way at the graver injustices, someone else would eventually come along and liberate them. This excuse is echoed today in the pleas that if we 'only' wear the masks, if we 'just' obey the regulations, soon everything will return to normal and the harsher restrictions will be lifted.

Still others collaborated out of agreement with the new laws. Anti-Semitism, like hatred and fear of communism, was widespread in Europe, and many nationalists and patriots looked to an occupying army to rid Europe of these 'foreign' elements where their own governments wouldn't, and felt it their duty to collaborate with those who would do so. In the UK today, the division between collaborators and those who resist doesn't fall into party allegiances, but undoubtedly many political scores are being settled, with what passes for the UK Left dismissing anyone who refuses to comply with lockdown measures as 'alt-right', etc.

Many collaborated because they were naïve enough — or wanted badly enough — to believe what they read in the newspapers, heard on the radio, were instructed to by their collaborationist government, heard in the gossip of their neighbours, were told by the propaganda agents of the occupying forces, and genuinely believed that all Jews were communists simultaneously running an international conspiracy of bankers. We had something of the same last year when the British press accused Jeremy Corbyn, then the Leader of the Labour Party, of being both a communist and an agent of Putin — presumably forgetting that Russia was no longer a member of the USSR — and everyone voted accordingly. Indeed, the excuse that 'we were lied to' was perhaps the most common one claimed by collaborators after the War, and there may have been some degree of truth in that given the years of propaganda, indoctrination and censorship. Today, with the sheer volume of evidence and arguments against the Government measures available online if not in the mainstream media, there can be no such excuse.

But the widest cause of collaboration, including the whole of Vichy France, was indifferent compliance with the prevailing authority and its new laws, no matter how contrary to logic, freedom, humanity, dignity or their own beliefs. The French may not have greeted Hitler's triumphal march into Paris with the same glee they greeted De Gaulle's five years later, but in between they rapidly settled down to collaboration, and as the past six months have demonstrated, the UK, had it been invaded by the Third Reich, would undoubtedly have done the same.

But whether, eighty years later, you collaborate with the biosecurity state being imposed by the occupying forces of the UK Government and its corporate financiers out of greed, spite, fear, hope, duty, ignorance, indifference or conformity, you're still collaborating. If you wear a mask in public, observe social distancing, comply with the contact-tracing programme, hand over your personal details to enter public spaces, submit a biological sample for testing, inform on your neighbours to the police for breaching coronavirus regulations, and, six months since the lockdown was imposed, continue to refuse to educate yourself about what is happening in this country, you are a collaborator with the UK biosecurity state. Under the current regime of surveillance and censorship, in which anything contradicting Government policy is deleted from the digital record, history is under lock and key in Belmarsh prison with Julian Assange; but if the history of this moment is ever written in the future, it will judge us as it did the collaborators with the Third Reich in the Second World War. I, however, don't think we should wait that long.

The childish exasperation with which willing implementors of the biosecurity state stamp their feet while telling us to 'just wear a mask!'; the frustration with which those who unquestioningly obey every new Government regulation proclaim they 'don't understand' why anyone wouldn't follow suit; the distracted annoyance with which those who live their lives on social media insist they 'don't have time' to read information that contradicts their views; the eagerness with which the Twitterati condemn dissenters as equivalent to 'terrorists'; the rapidity with which comparisons between refusing to wear masks and drink driving are taken up and repeated across mainstream and social media by figures in authority, including doctors; the point-blank refusal of the loudest apologists for the biosecurity state to even consider the consequences of their actions; the vehemence with which self-appointed informants call on the Government to use the police, armed forces and whatever violence is necessary to impose the 'New Normal' — these are all signs of collaboration with an occupying force, as familiar to the French living under the Vichy regime in 1940 as they are to us in the UK in 2020.

Part of the way collaboration works is through the willingness, when it comes down to making a choice, to trust those in authority. The commentariat that for twenty years has declared that everything our Governments have said was a lie — from the justification for the Iraq War to the charges against Julian Assange, from the necessity of fiscal austerity after the Global Financial Crisis to the causes of the housing 'crisis', from capitalist solutions to global warming to the liberalism of the European Union — has, when they've found the consequences of these decisions on their doorstep, chosen to believe everything the latest Government says about the most far-reaching political revolution of our time.

The internet, which has granted to everyone a speed and ease of access to information that was never available to me even when I was a student in the British Library, has had the effect of relativising all knowledge. Without the analytical skills or even the attention span to make a judgement about the rationality and veracity of the arguments being made in any given article — whether my own or in *The Guardian* — the vast mass of non-readers, sifting through the internet for something to corroborate their beliefs and fears, choose to believe what they read based on the criteria of identity politics. That is to say, they make a judgement about their degree of identification with the author or the forum in which the article is published. A generation raised to believe that outing politically incorrect terms constitutes a politics, and only recently having come into positions of influence and power in the media and culture industry, require nothing more than the use of a prohibited word such as 'hysteria', an 'offensive' comparison to the Third Reich, a deviation from the orthodoxies of 'woke' culture, in order to stop thinking; while the older generation, faced with the hitherto unseen consensus of the entire UK media and press in propagating the lies of the UK Government, has apparently chosen to place its trust in the authority of those who, in every other aspect of its perception of the world, it distrusts.

Very much as happened over the three-and-a-half long years of bickering that preceded Brexit, the coronavirus 'crisis' has fragmented the illusory unity of the 'British People' into a multitude in which political allegiances, whether to party or newspaper, mean nothing. While the British Left is united in calling for the most right-wing Government in living memory to impose stronger measures to protect the British People from an epidemic that presents no threat to it, liberals demand the arrest of anyone not complying with regulations unapproved by Parliament, socialists take up the Health Secretary's claim that wearing face masks is an act of solidarity, and even communists affect to see in Government bailouts the precursor to an entirely imaginary vision of a communitarian future — those opposing these measures range across a similar political spectrum, with conservatives announcing their departure from the Party of Government in protest at the destruction of the economy, right-wing libertarians demanding their civil rights be restored, anarchists denouncing the lockdown as the Great Reset of capitalism promised by the World Economic Forum, and even one or two communists seeing in the response to this 'crisis' the implementation of the biosecurity state. Like the upside-down man of Medieval imagery who wears his boots on his head and carries an ass on his back, this inversion alone signals the revolution we're undergoing.

There is, however, only one truth to this situation. Although knowledge is relative to the historical context of its discursive formation, the truth is not. There are not — as journalists too lazy to do their research like to hide behind — two sides to this national argument, which a balanced assessment must walk between. There are lies, and there are truths. The way Public Health England attributes deaths to COVID-19 and now, in its new guise as the UK Health Security Agency, publishes information about those deaths is a lie. The factual records showing the number of individuals under the age of 60 without pre-existing illnesses that have had their deaths attributed to COVID-19 is a truth. The claim that the threat of COVID-19 justifies outsourcing our public health services to private companies is a lie. That the coronavirus 'crisis' has been deliberately exaggerated in order to accelerate and extend the neo-liberalisation of the UK state is a truth. The claim that face coverings are necessary to protect us from a virus that is no worse than the flu for 99.8 per cent of the population is a lie. The truth is that, now the tens of thousands of excess deaths resulting from the suspension and reduction of medical care for life-threatening illnesses under the lockdown have fallen to levels insufficient to sustain public fear, the Government needs a justification for extending the 'emergency period' under which it can make what laws it wishes without the approval of Parliament, and an obediently masked public is the clearest sign of the consensus that COVID-19 still presents a 'serious and imminent threat'. This truth must be recovered from the lies in which it has been hidden, then learned, understood, and used to dispel the propaganda that has indoctrinated the UK public into compliance with the biosecurity state.

I've consistently described the regulations and programmes implementing this revolution being made 'under the cover of the coronavirus crisis'; but in practical terms it no longer matters whether an individual does or does not believe the Government's lies about the threat of COVID-19. The legislation required to make every future restriction enforceable has already been passed. There is no longer any other resort for civil disobedience to these measures than militant resistance; and the British people, who have passively watched the erasure of our democratic rights and forms of political representation while protesting about Brexit and institutional racism and other activities of mass displacement, are not even close to that, if indeed we ever have been. As the sight of Matt Hancock and other Government Ministers handing over billions of pounds of public money in sweetheart deals to national and multinational corporations confirms, there is no longer any accountability in British public life. Public opprobrium can reach hysterical levels on social media, but the UK Government is effectively beyond criticism by a universally compliant media. The Prime Minister's general refusal to appear in public is an indication that he intends to stay well out of the firing line while allowing his subordinates to ransack the country on behalf of his financial backers and political supporters. And the British public appears content to distract itself with Black Lives Matter protests and other displacement activities that make us feel these old and long-outdated forms of political activity still have some influence on the world.

As I wrote at the very start of this article, the coronavirus 'crisis' is a revolution, and it has been undertaken with the full collaboration of the UK State and its political allies against the British people. We are living under occupation by our own Government, with the collaboration of its corporate clients, the civil service, the financial sector, the media, the police, the security services and the armed forces. Whether the British people, collectively or as individuals, agree with the biosecurity state being imposed upon us no longer matters. This is the New Normal.

— 28 August, 2020

Afterword: Acts of Resistance

I had planned to end with a 'vision of the future' designed to have enough of a foothold in the present to be believable and at the same time sufficiently dystopian to convince readers of the seriousness of our situation; but the future is finally here, and it's too late for pessimism. The actor, Peter Ustinov, once said that the pessimist is the man who wakes up every day to rediscover the world is run by bad people, while the optimist knows exactly how bad the world can be and does everything he can to make it better. As a contribution to which, I offer these acts of resistance. This is the hard bit, where words turn into actions or fade into silence.

1. Face coverings

The Health Protection (Coronavirus, Wearing of Face Coverings in a Relevant Place) (England) (Amendment) Regulations 2020, which came into effect on 8 August, have extended the places where a face covering is mandatory to include public transport, transport hubs, shops, supermarkets, shopping centres, banks, building societies, post offices, transport hubs, places of worship, community and youth centres, crematoria and burial-ground chapels, public areas in hotels and hostels, concert and exhibition halls, cinemas, museums, galleries, indoor zoos, aquariums and other tourist and cultural sites, bingo halls, public libraries and reading rooms, nail, beauty and hair salons and barbers, tattoo and piercing parlours, massage parlours, storage and distribution centres, auction houses, spas, funeral directors, veterinary practices and premises providing professional services.[1] However, if you wish to claim exemption from wearing a face covering, the fixed penalty notice for which is now £100, doubling on a second and subsequent 'offence' to a maximum of £3,200, you only have to state that you 'have exemption'. I've done so to every shopkeeper that has asked me, and in general they have accepted this statement without question.

---

1. See UK Statutory Instruments, 'The Health Protection (Coronavirus, Wearing of Face Coverings in a Relevant Place) (England) (Amendment) Regulations 2020' (8 August, 2020).

To those few who ask what the exemption is for, you should answer that they do not, under the Equality Act 2010, have the right to ask you, as it may involve a disability, and therefore, under Section 26, constitute 'harassment', which is defined, under Paragraph 1, Section B, as 'conduct [which] has the purpose or effect' of either (i) 'violating [your] dignity or' (ii) 'creating an intimidating, hostile, degrading, humiliating or offensive environment'.[2] If someone continues to harass you, you may wish to respond that you claim it under Exemption (ii), Section A, Paragraph 1, Regulation 4 of The Health Protection (Coronavirus, Wearing of Face Coverings in a Relevant Place) (England) Regulations 2020.[3] That will shut 99 per cent of collaborators up. For the 1 per cent who ask what exemption 'ii' is, you may wish to ask them why they are trying to enforce Regulations they have not read and do not understand. Exemption 'ii' is that wearing a mask causes 'severe distress', but if someone doesn't know that you have no legal obligation to inform them of the fact.

2. Social distancing

The former Supreme Court Justice of the Peace, Lord Sumption, QC, has clarified that Government guidance on social distancing, which was issued by the Department of Health and Social Care on 16 March, and which mandated keeping a distance of 2 metres between individuals not from the same household, goes beyond coronavirus laws and regulations, and cannot, legally, be enforced by the police. To clarify, under The Health Protection (Coronavirus, Restrictions) (No. 2) (England) Regulations 2020, the police currently have the power to order a gathering of 30 or more people to disperse — and to use 'reasonable force' to compel us to do so — if we are in a private dwelling, including in private gardens, or in public spaces not owned by a private business or run by a public body as a visitor attraction, and in particular in those outdoor places that meet the definition of a 'rave' in Section 63 of the Criminal Justice and Public Order Act 1994.[4]

---

2. See UK Public General Acts, 'Equality Act (2010)' (8 April, 2010), Section 26(1)(b).

3. See UK Statutory Instruments, 'The Health Protection (Coronavirus, Wearing of Face Coverings in a Relevant Place) (England) Regulations 2020' (24 July, 2020), Regulation 4(1)(a)(ii).

4. See UK Statutory Instruments, 'The Health Protection (Coronavirus, Restrictions) (No. 2) (England) Regulations 2020' (3 July, 2020); and UK Public General Acts, 'Criminal Justice and Public

But unless the outdoor place we are in is under a Section 60 order under the Criminal Justice and Public Order Act 1994, or a Section 35 order under the Antisocial Behaviour, Police and Crime Act 2014, or it has been targeted for 'intervention' by the Secretary of State or a local authority under The Health Protection (Coronavirus, Restrictions) (England) (No. 3) Regulations 2020, the police cannot legally order us to disperse.[5] In short, in the UK biosecurity state there are now so many places and times where and when we can be physically stopped from socialising with each other, fined for doing so, and even arrested and prosecuted for such an 'offence', that you might justly and ethically conclude that it is our duty to do so when and where we can.

3. Contact tracing

Under guidance on 'Maintaining records of staff, customers and visitors to support NHS Test and Trace' issued by the Department of Health and Social Care on 2 July, the owners, managers and staff of public houses, bars, restaurants, cafés, hotels, museums, cinemas, hairdressers, town halls, civic centres, libraries and places of worship have been instructed to refuse entry to, service in, or employment by, their establishments to visitors, customers or staff who refuse to supply their personal details, including their name and contact number or e-mail, as well as the time of their visit, purchase or shift; and to share this information with the Test and Trace programme.[6]

However, once again, Government guidance is not law. As the guidance itself says, compliance with these measures is not mandatory but 'voluntary', and the establishment does not have to impose them as a condition of service. Any information you give does not have to be verified either by you or the establishment, and at your insistence any information given must be withheld from

---

Order Act 1994' (3 November, 1994), Section 63, 'Powers to remove persons attending or preparing for a rave'.

5. See UK Public General Acts, 'Criminal Justice and Public Order Act 1994' (3 November, 1994), Section 60, 'Powers to stop and search in anticipation of, or after violence'; UK Public General Acts, 'Antisocial Behaviour, Police and Crime Act 2014' (13 March, 2014), Section 35, 'Directions excluding a person from an area'; and UK Statutory Instruments, 'The Health Protection (Coronavirus, Restrictions) (England) (No. 3) Regulations 2020' (18 July, 2020).

6. See UK Health Security Agency, 'Maintaining records of staff, customers and visitors to support NHS Test and Trace' (2 July, 2020).

the Government's Test and Trace programme. The staff or managers in the establishments where you are asked for this information may not be aware of this, and you may wish to take the opportunity to inform them of the fact, and that by denying you entry or service they are taking upon themselves the policing of the public beyond the requirements of the law. This may result in them serving you, though it also may not. Any privately-owned establishment can refuse service as long as doing so does not violate your protected characteristics under the Equality Act 2010; and public establishments can impose new conditions of entry and use on the same terms.

Should they do so, you may wish to choose another pub to drink in, eat in another restaurant, take a pack lunch and coffee flask, spend the gallery entry fee on a book, wait until the film is released online, get your hair cut elsewhere, or organise a protest of less than 30 people outside the town hall, library or museum to which you have been denied access, demanding to know why a public institution is enacting Ministerial wishes without the force of law. The situation is more complex for employees, which I will address in the next act of resistance.

4. Employment rights

Regulation 3, Paragraph 2 (b) of The Health Protection (Coronavirus, Wearing of Face Coverings in a Relevant Place) (England) Regulations 2020, which came into effect on 24 July, specified that the requirement to wear a face coverings in designated places does not apply to 'a person responsible for a relevant place or an employee of that person acting in the course of their employment'.[7] Even Government guidance doesn't recommend employees wearing face coverings.[8] Instead, the Department for Business, Energy and Industrial Strategy recommends that employers carry out a risk assessment for their business addressing the risks of COVID-19. Face coverings for employees are not required under coronavirus regulations because employers already have a legal obligation to provide a safe working environment. Employers should therefore assess the

---

7. See UK Statutory Instruments, 'The Health Protection (Coronavirus, Wearing of Face Coverings in a Relevant Place) (England) Regulations 2020' (24 July, 2020), Regulation 2(2)(b).

8. See Department of Health and Social Care, 'Face coverings: when to wear one, exemptions and what makes a good one'.

use of face coverings on a case-by-case basis depending on the workplace environment.

According to Law or Fiction, which was founded by the solicitor Stephen Jackson and describes itself as 'a group of concerned lawyers dedicated to separating the Law from the Fiction, particularly in relation to the current Coronavirus lockdown', this gives employees considerable leverage in resisting their imposition by their employers.[9] Since it is unlikely, they say, that an employer has conducted such a risk assessment, they risk a charge of causing 'severe distress' to any employee they compel to wear a face covering as a condition of employment, and would therefore be in breach of contract. Should they try to do so, the employee should ask to see the risk assessment, and establish whether it reflects the information about the risk of COVID-19 given in this and my other articles, as well as the recorded risks of wearing a face covering, some of which may be found in 'The Science and Law of Refusing to Wear Masks: Texts and Arguments in Support of Civil Disobedience'.[10] An employer simply stating that they are 'following Government guidance' is neither sufficient nor accurate, as the guidance is to pass the decision and responsibility to the business. In the opinion of these lawyers, it is unlikely that a business will risk a claim for unfair dismissal for forcing an employee to wear a face covering, or for their insurance providers to risk them having to pay out compensation for doing so or against personal injury claims that may result from wearing masks. As they conclude:

> Insurers might well turn around and ask the business why they required masks to be worn when no risk assessment justified it and when no law required it. Insurers might well be asking themselves now why they are exposing themselves to such claims.[11]

To help resist their imposition, these lawyers have provided further information about how employees can go about responding in writing to their employers, which you may wish to follow, as well as the offer to recommend

---

9. See Laura Dodsworth, 'Liberty in Lockdown', *The Critic* (September, 2020).

10. See Simon Elmer, 'The Science and Law of Refusing to Wear Masks: Texts and Arguments in Support of Civil Disobedience', *Architects for Social Housing* (11 June, 2020).

11. Law or Fiction, 'Time to blow the whistle on shops' (28 July, 2020).

specialist employment lawyers, which you may wish to take up should it come to this.

5. Smart phones

As I reviewed in detail in Part 1 of 'The New Normal: What is the UK Biosecurity State?', 96 per cent of households in the UK have at least one mobile phone, and over 77 per cent of these are smart phones. Between them, Apple and Android phones monopolise 99.7 per cent of this market, and both operating systems are in the process of building a contact tracking function into their respective operating systems. The consequences of what we have known for some time — that mobile phones are tracking devices — has now become a reality, and is already being used to track our movements, record our contacts with other mobile-phone users, including their location, and the proximity, time and duration of each contact. In doing so, smart phone are helping the Government compel us, for example, to go into self-imposed quarantine for two weeks after we return from a country designated, without any medical justification and purely for political reasons, as a biosecurity threat to the UK. If they are not already, these tracking devices will more than likely be used to track the movements of people detained by the police for attendance at, for example, an illegal gathering, in order to ensure they do not meet again either in the same location or with the same people from different households. According to Google and Apple, the tracking facility requires the user to turn on the Bluetooth function for it to communicate with other mobile phones; but that won't stop the operating system functioning to identify the user's movements, for example, away from their homes when quarantined. Again, the providers have stated that it is possible to uninstall the update through which the tracking device has been downloaded into the operating system of the phone; but how many of us know how to do this, and if we do, wouldn't that require re-installing all the phone's functions using a previous operating system? Anyone who has tried to run their laptop on a superseded operating system will know the technical problems this causes. Finally, as the old system becomes obsolete, we will face a choice between access to all the facilities to which we have become accustomed by use and habit and advertising, and the freedom of not being tracked and monitored by the device that provides those facilities.

You may, therefore, choose to use a mobile phone that does not have an inbuilt global positioning system and Bluetooth function, carry an A-Z, learn to read a map, use a music player that does not have a positioning device installed or is integrated with Google Maps, only carry your laptop with you when you need it, and read a book or newspaper rather than be permanently logged on to social media. The difficulty of making what should be a clear and obvious decision shows how psychologically attached we have become to our 'smart' phones, but the time when their influence over us is no longer merely psychological and has becomes operational is here, and the choice must be made now if we are to resist the UK biosecurity state being implemented through our willing use of its instruments.

6. Biometric testing

Whether uploading your health status into an immunity passport carrying your digital identity or submitting a biological swab sample for testing by a private company, handing over your biometric data to the state and its contractors is laying the foundations for the next stage of the biosecurity state. This is more than contributing to the medically meaningless thresholds beyond which the Joint Biosecurity centre locks down millions of people; it is building up the data base on which artificial intelligence systems will dictate where we can and cannot go, what places we can and cannot enter, whether we can leave our homes, use transport, go to work, visit our friends and family, or see our own children. Collaborating in doing so is not only, as I have shown, without any medical justification, and as meaningless as being tested for the flu, but is contributing to excluding those who don't collaborate from public life and spaces as 'potentially infected persons'.

So far, I have suggested what you may wish to do in resistance, but for participating in the testing programme there can be no excuse. Biometric testing, for as long as it is voluntary, must be refused by anyone who is serious about resisting the UK biosecurity state. If that means being refused departure from the country, for example, and having to take your holiday in the UK, be glad that it does not yet mean being refused entrance to your workplace, or the freedom to walk the streets without an immunity passport.

Beyond these acts, there is the work of communicating them to others, both the how and the why of their enactment, so that they can begin to recover a properly political meaning from the biopolitics to which we are being subjected by the UK biosecurity state. Things are not going to get better. On the contrary, they are only going to get far worse. The regulations will increase, expanding their control over more and more of our lives. The fines for non-compliance will increase, and their enforcement will become more brutal, more unaccountable. More and more of UK society will be brought into their implementation. The surveillance and control of our lives will be more closely tied into the technologies of our day-to-day lives. As is already being promised, the winter ahead will be a giant step forward in the entrenchment of the programmes and technologies of the biosecurity state in the UK. An economy being brought to its knees is already being sold to the global corporations that increasingly run our lives, and every remaining province of public service is being outsourced to private contractors as impervious to scrutiny as they are unaccountable to criticism. Politics, in this world, will be nothing more than a televised game show for the credulous masses.

Karl Löwenstein was right about what he called, back in 1936, 'the pliability of human nature under continued mental pressure' when exerted by a biosecurity state 'utilising psychological techniques'. By the time we emerge blinking into the spring of 2021, the world before the coronavirus 'crisis' will seem like a distant dream. But he was wrong, as subsequent history proved, about 'artificial inventions politically superimposed' inevitably returning to 'a more congenial substance and shape', and we shouldn't make the same mistake. There may come a time in the future when we look back at the present as the last chance we had to stop what is happening, to rise up now, not in hundreds or thousands or even tens of thousands, but in millions, to stop what is being done before it cannot be undone. If we don't, the totalitarianisms of the Twentieth Century offer only a glimpse of the degree and breadth of control exerted by the UK biosecurity state under which we will live for the foreseeable future. Never in recent history has there been a threat to our freedom that more justifies, more demands, our civil disobedience and militant resistance to the disaster into which we are being led.

— 10 September, 2020

Bibliography

Academy of Medical Sciences. 'Preparing for a challenging winter 2020-21' (14 July, 2020).

Adam, David. 'UK has enough intensive care units for coronavirus, expert predicts', *New Scientist* (25 March, 2020).

Adi-Tabatabal, Sean. 'Sean Penn: "It's Time To Send Unvaccinated Citizens to Jail"', *News Punch* (20 December, 2022).

Agamben, Giorgio. Giorgio Agamben, *Homo Sacer: Sovereign Power and Bare Life*; translated by Daniel Heller-Roazen (Stanford University Press, 1998).

_____. *State of Exception*, Homo Sacer II, 1; translated by Kevin Attell (University of Chicago Press, 2005).

_____. *Stasis: Civil War as a Political Paradigm*, Homo Sacer II, 2; translated by Nicholas Heron (Stanford University Press, 2015).

_____. *Quodlibet: Una voce, rubrica di Giorgio Agamben* (February 2020-October 2022); selections from which have been translated by Valeria Dani in *Where Are We Now? The Epidemic as Politics*; second updated edition (Eris, 2021).

_____. 'The Invention of an Epidemic', *Il Manifesto* (26 February, 2020); collected in *Where Are We Now?*, pp. 11-13.

_____. 'A Question', *Quodlibet* (13 April, 2020); collected in *Where Are We Now?*, pp. 34-37.

_____. 'New Reflections', *Quodlibet* (22 April, 2020); collected in *Where Are We Now?*, pp. 42-45.

_____. 'Medicine as Religion', *Quodlibet* (2 May, 2020); collected in *Where Are We Now?*, pp. 49-54.

_____. 'Biosecurity and Politics', *Quodlibet* (11 May, 2020); collected in *Where Are We Now?*, pp. 55-58.

_____. 'What is Fear?', *Quodlibet* (13 July, 2020); collected in *Where Are We Now?*, pp. 88-95.

Ahmed, Nafeez. 'Conservative Party Donor Cashes in on UK Government-Made PPE Shortages Amidst COVID-19 Crisis', *Byline Times* (2 April, 2020).

Albrecht, Professor Martin, *et al*. 'Joint Statement' (29 April, 2020).

Allison, Eric, and Simon Hattenstone. 'Managers at G4S-run Medway youth jail paid bonuses despite failings', *The Guardian* (21 October, 2016).

Amnesty International. 'Why we're taking the UK government to court over mass spying' (18 May, 2020).

Anandaciva, Siva. 'Five reasons why this NHS winter may be different', *The King's Fund* (2 December, 2019).

Anon. 'Randox forensics inquiry: Drug-drivers to challenge convictions', *BBC News* (22 November, 2017).

_____. 'HMP Peterborough inmates were illegally strip-searched', *BBC News* (22 February, 2019).

_____. Bidfood owner BFS Group suffers £14.8m loss driven by logistics weakness', *The Grocer* (12 April, 2019).

_____. 'How deadly is the new coronavirus?', *The Economist* (12 March, 2020).

_____. 'Inside YouTube's "numerous policy changes" during the pandemic', *CNN Business* (19 April, 2020).

_____. 'Yoti CitizenCard — the UK's ID solution', *Citizencard*.

_____. 'No quarantine in UK for travellers from France, Macron and Johnson agree', *The Local* (10 May, 2020).

_____. 'Deal struck to integrate technologies onto digital health passport', *Med-Tech News* (12 May, 2020).

_____. 'Coronavirus: Victoria ticket worker dies after being spat at', *BBC News* (12 May, 2020).

_____. 'Coronavirus: London police to enforce face masks "as last resort"', *BBC News* (22 July, 2020).

_____. 'Coronavirus: Preston young people targeted as lockdown imposed', *BBC News* (8 August, 2020).

_____. 'Mobile Operating System Market Share United Kingdom' (January-December, 2020).

_____. 'Russia's 500 Super Rich Wealthier Than Poorest 99.8% – Report', *The Moscow Times* (10 June, 2021).

_____. 'Tracking covid-19 excess deaths across countries', *The Economist* (last published 20 October, 2021).

_____. 'Arrest of UK anti-royal protesters raises free speech concerns', *Al Jazeera* (13 September, 2022).

_____. 'Bank of England ceases bond-buying after spending £19.3bn', *Sky News* (14 October, 2022).

_____. 'New UK Prime Minister Rishi Sunak Pushes Heavily to Introduce CBDC', *Unlock Media* (25 October, 2022).

_____. 'Macron calls for "a single global order" to combat China', news.com.au on *YouTube* (19 November, 2022).

_____. 'New Zealand takes custody of ill baby from anti-vaccine parents', *Manila Standard* (7 December, 2022).

_____. 'Russia enters the top ten economies in the world for GDP at current prices', *Nova News* (31 December, 2022).

Apter, John. 'If you don't heed the government's advice steps could be taken to clamp down on selfishness', *The Telegraph* (24 March, 2020).

Bank of England. 'Monetary Policy Report' (May 2020).

_____. 'UK central bank digital currency' (last updated 1 September, 2022).

_____. 'Quantitative Easing' (last updated 15 December, 2022).

Barthes, Roland. 'Lecture in Inauguration of the Chair of Literary Semiology. Collège de France, January 7, 1977'; translated by Richard Howard in *October*, no. 8 (1979), pp. 3-16.

BCP Council. 'Major incident declared after services overstretched by thousands flocking to Bournemouth beaches' (25 June, 2020).

Beeley, Vanessa. 'Assassinated for telling the truth about Uraine, *The Wall Will Fall* (17 April, 2022).

Benedictus, Leo. 'What we know, and what we don't, about the true coronavirus death toll', *Full Fact* (1 May, 2020).

Bennett Institute for Public Policy. 'The history or emergency legislation and the COVID-19 crisis', University of Cambridge (28 April, 2020).

Benvenuto, Sergio. 'Benvenuto in clausura', *Antinomie* (5 March, 2020).

Berg, Anastasia. 'Giorgio Agamben's Coronavirus Cluelessness', *The Chronicle of Higher Education* (23 March, 2020).

Berkowitz, Roger. 'When Philosophers are blinded by theory', *The Hannah Ardent Center for Politics and Humanities* (18 March, 2020).

Bet, Martina. 'Tory MP urged to apologise and correct record on "dangerous" Covid vaccine claim', *The Independent* (7 December, 2022).

Biometrics and Surveillance Camera Commissioner. 'Surveillance Camera Code of Practice 2013' (13 August, 2021).

Biswas, Soutik. 'India coronavirus: The "mystery" of low Covid-19 death rates', *BBC News* (28 April, 2020).

Blanchard, Sam, and Stephen Matthews. 'Government pledges to publish REAL death totals including non-hospital deaths as Britain suffers 586 more coronavirus deaths after ONS suggest true total may now be 55% higher at more than 33,000', *Mail Online* (28 April, 2020).

Blanchard, Sam. 'Officials WILL look again at whether Britons should wear face coverings or masks in public, Matt Hancock reveals as top scientists argue they should be "part of the new normal"', *The Daily Mail* (7 July, 2020).

Bolton, Paul, and Iona Stewart. 'Domestic Energy. Prices', *House of Commons Library* (25 November, 2022).

Bort, Julie. 'Palantir's tech was used by ICE in the controversial arrests of 680 people at a Mississippi chicken farm according to an immigrants' rights group', *Business Insider* (October 2019).

Bowman, Verity. 'Why do so any NHS Nightingale hospitals remain empty?', *The Telegraph* (29 April, 2020).

Bradshaw, Julie. 'Watchdog fines GSK £37m for paying to keep generic drugs out of UK market', *The Telegraph* (12 February, 2016).

Brecht, Bertolt. 'Five Difficulties in Writing the Truth', *Unsere Zeit*, no. 2-3 (April 1935); collected in *Brecht on Art and Politics*, edited by Tom Kuhn and Steve Giles, translated by Laura Bradley, Steve Giles and Tom Kuhn (Methuen Drama, 2003), pp. 141-157.

Bridgen, Andrew. 'List of supporting references used in vaccine harms debate speech' (16 December, 2022).

British Petroleum. 'Statistical Review of World Energy' (71st edition, 2022).

Brown, David, Prina Shah, Steve Connor and Becky Rush. 'This is what coronavirus will do to our offices and homes', *BBC News* (6 August, 2020).

Brown, Ellen. 'Conservation or Land Grab? The Financialization of Nature', *The Web of Debt Blog* (5 November, 2021).

Burt, Chris. 'UK immunity passport proposals leverage biometric facial recognition', *Biometric Update* (30 April, 2020).

Butchard, Patrick, and Bukky Balogun. 'Research Briefing: What is the proposed WHO Pandemic Preparedness Treaty?', *House of Commons Library* (18 May, 2022).

Cabinet Office. 'Preparation and planning for emergencies: responsibilities of responder agencies and others' (20 February, 2013).

_____. 'Civil Contingencies Secretariat: The Lead Government Department and its role – Guidance and Best Practice' (March 2004).

_____. Cabinet Office, 'Local resilience forums: contact details' (20 February, 2013).

_____. 'Procurement Policy Note 01/20: Responding to COVID-19' (18 March, 2020);

_____. 'Staying at home and away from others (social distancing)' (1 May, 2020).

Calvert, Jonathan, George Arbuthnott and Jonathan Leake. 'Coronavirus: 38 days when Britain sleepwalked into disaster', *The Times* (18 April, 2020).

Campbell, Denis. 'NHS winter crisis: extra beds created by 52% of UK hospitals', *The Guardian* (2 December, 2019).

Carrell, Severin, David Pegg, Felicity Lawrence, Paul Lewis, Rob Evans, David Conn, Harry Davies and Kate Proctor. 'Revealed: Cummings is on secret scientific advisory group for Covid-19', *The Guardian* (24 April, 2020).

Cartlidge, Sarah. 'Bournemouth beach: the latest rules for visitors', Bournemouth Echo (12 July, 2020).

Caught on Camera. 'How many CCTV cameras in London?'

Chakelian, Anoosh. 'Interserve, and the other companies running Britain that you've never heard of; Or: why are construction firms involved in your welfare?', *The New Statesman* (11 March, 2019).

Chalmers, Vanessa. 'Winter death toll highest since 1975: Failure of flu jab to combat severe outbreak resulted in more than 50,000 extra people dying in England and Wales last year', *Daily Mail* (30 November, 2018).

Chandler, Simon. 'U.K. Government Is Using Coronavirus As Excuse To Ramp Up Surveillance', *Forbes* (2 April, 2020).

Chartered Institute of Personnel and Development. 'COVID-19 vaccination: guide for employers' (7 March, 2022).

Child Poverty Action Group. 'Fuel poverty estimates for April 2023 following the Autumn statement' (23 November, 2022).

Chivers, Tom. 'Internet rules and laws: the top 10, from Godwin to Poe', *The Telegraph* (23 October, 2009).

Christaens, Tim. 'Must Society be Defended from Agamben?', *Critical Legal Thinking* (26 March, 2020).

Climate Emergency Fund. 'Protest movements are the fastest, most cost-effective way of creating transformative change'.

Cobain, Ian. 'UK has six months to rewrite snooper's charter, high court rules', *The Guardian* (27 April, 2018).

College of Policing. 'COVID-19 restrictions', 2022.

Conway, Ed. 'Cost of Living: Bank of England shares responsibility for crisis, former governor says', *Sky News* (20 May, 2022).

Cooban, Anna. 'Billionaires added $5 trillion to their fortunes during the pandemic', *CNN Business* (16 January, 2022).

Collins, Paul. 'IPCC climate report 2022 summary: The key findings', *Climate Consulting by Selectra*, 2022.

Compton, Kristin. 'Big Pharma and Medical Device Manufacturers', *Drug Watch* (last modified 8 September, 2022).

Corbyn, Piers. 'Defend the Right to Protest: Justice for Piers Corbyn', *Crowd Justice*.

Craig, Emily. 'Return of the Masks: Health chiefs urge people to wear face coverings and say anyone feeling ill should "stay at home" in echo of pandemic era — as medics claim the NHS is under more pressure than at the height of Covid', *Daily Mail* (3 January, 2023).

Crown Prosecution Service. 'Coronavirus coughs' at key workers will be charged as assault, CPS warns' (26 March, 2020).

D'Arcais, Paolo Flores. 'Filosofia e virus: le farneticazioni di Giorgio Agamben', *MicroMega* (16 March, 2020).

Davies, Nick, Oliver Chan, Aron Cheung, Gavin Freeguard and Emma Norris. 'Summary — Government Procurement: The scale and nature of contracting in the UK', *Institute for Government* (December 2018).

Davies, Rob. 'Government awarded school meal voucher contract without tender', *The Guardian* (7 May, 2020).

Davis, Iain. 'SDG7: The Impossible Energy Transformation', *Unlimited Hangout* (6 January, 2023).

Davis, Iain, and Whitney Webb. 'Sustainable Debt Slavery', *Unlimited Hangout* (13 September, 2022).

Dawkins, Richard. 'The Root of All Evil?', *Channel 4* (2006).

Dearden, Lizzie. 'Coronavirus: Police issue almost 9,000 fines for lockdown breaches in England', *The Independent* (30 April, 2020).

Department for Business, Energy and Industrial Strategy. 'Business population estimates for the UK and regions 2022: statistical release' (6 October, 2022).

Department for Digital, Culture, Media and Sport. 'Government cracks down on spread of false coronavirus information online' (30 March, 2020).

_____. 'Policy Paper: UK digital identity and attributes trust framework — alpha version 2' (last updated 14 June, 2022).

Department of Health and Social Care. 'Coronavirus (CQVID-19) listed as a notifiable disease' (5 March, 2020).

_____. 'Coronavirus (COVID-19): Scaling up our testing programmes' (4 April, 2020).

_____. 'Next phase of NHS coronavirus (COVID-19) app announced' (18 June, 2020).

_____. 'Tackling obesity: empowering adults and children to live healthier lives' (27 July, 2020).

_____. 'Face coverings: when to wear one, exemptions and what makes a good one'.

Department for Work and Pensions. 'Universal Credit: 29 April 2013 to 9 April 2020' (19 May, 2020).

D'Eramo, Marco. 'The Philosopher's Epidemic', *New Left Review* (March/April 2020).

Devlin, Hannah, and Diane Taylor. 'Baby dies in UK prison after inmate "gives birth alone in cell"', *The Guardian* (4 October, 2019).

Devlin, Hannah. 'Extra 10,000 dementia deaths in England and Wales in April, *The Guardian* (5 June, 2020).

Diver, Tony. 'Jeremy Hunt faces Tory rebellion over £7bn government spending on "woke" projects', *The Telegraph* (10 December, 2022).

Dodsworth, Laura. 'Liberty in Lockdown', *The Critic* (September, 2020).

Donnelly, Laura, Hayley Dixon and Sarah Newey. 'Gloves may be the next step after masks in the battle against coronavirus', *The Telegraph* (24 July, 2020).

Dunford, Daniel, Becky Dale, Nassos Stylianou, Ed Lowther, Maryam Ahmed and Irene de la Torre Arenas. 'Coronavirus: The world in lockdown in maps and charts', *BBC* (7 April, 2020).

Edwards, Martin. 'Behavioural Insights: The Second Team Leading the UK Government's Covid-19 Response', UK Column (3 May, 2020).

Elmer, Simon. 'Stand Up To Labour: The Denials of Momentum', *Architects for Social Housing* (10 October, 2016).

_____. 'Oy Vey! No Latkes for Labour', *Architects for Social Housing* (5 September, 2018).

_____. *Inequality Capital: A Power Walk by Architects for Social Housing* (18 April 2019).

_____. 'The Persecution, Incarceration, Torture and Extra-territorial Extradition of Julian Assange: Template for a letter to your Member of Parliament', *Architects for Social Housing* (18 June, 2019).

_____. 'COVID-19 and Capitalism', *Architects for Social Housing* (18 March, 2020).

_____. 'Sociology of a Disease: Age, Class and Mortality in the Coronavirus Pandemic', *Architects for Social Housing* (24 March, 2020).

_____. 'Language is a Virus: SARS-CoV-2 and the Science of Political Control', *Architects for Social Housing* (3 April, 2020).

_____. 'Coronazombies! Infection and Denial in the United Kingdom', *Architects for Social Housing* (9 April, 2020).

_____. 'The Science and Law of Refusing to Wear Masks: Texts and Arguments in Support of Civil Disobedience', *Architects for Social Housing* (11 June, 2020).

_____. 'Five Stories Under Lockdown', *Architects for Social Housing* (1 December, 2020).

_____. 'March for Freedom: London, 29 May, 2021', *Architects for Social Housing* (30 May, 2021).

_____. *The Road to Fascism: For a Critique of the Global Biosecurity State* (Architects for Social Housing, 2022).

_____. 'How the "Pandemic" Has Paved the Way for the New Fascism of the Global Biosecurity State', *The Daily Sceptic* (15 October, 2022).

_____. 'Interview with Simon Elmer', *The Delingpod* (25 October, 2022).

_____. 'Why Did the Left Fail So Utterly to Resist the Global Biosecurity State?' *The Daily Sceptic* (11 November, 2022).

_____. 'Lockdown Wasn't Imposed to Protect the World from a New Virus but Because the Real Economy Had to Be Shut Down', *The Exposé* (19 November, 2022).

_____. 'Biosecurity State: Another Right-wing Conspiracy Theory or How the Left Was Won Over', *The Exposé* (24 November, 2022).

_____. 'Welcome to Planet Oligarch', *The Conservative Woman* (26 November, 2022).

_____. 'Understanding the road to fascism', *The Light* (19 December, 2022).

_____. 'Crisis: Housing, Covid-19 and the Emergence of a New Fascism', *UK Column* (20 December, 2022).

_____. 'Arise, AstraZeneca!', *Off-Guardian* (23 December, 2022).

_____. 'The Victims of AstraZeneca', *Off-Guardian* (23 December, 2022).

_____. 'Covid "Vaccines": Why is the MHRA Lying About Adverse Effects?', *Off-Guardian* (30 December, 2022).

_____. 'What are we up against? How did we get here? What can we do about it?' Presentation to the *Think Twice* Symposium (20 January, 2023).

_____. 'The Road to Fascism: An interview with Simon Elmer', *Thinking Coalition* (5 February, 2023).

Elmer, Simon, and Geraldine Dening. *For a Socialist Architecture: Under Capitalism* (Architects for Social Housing, 2021).

Elmer, Simon, and Francis Hoar. 'In our Defence: Freedom of Speech in the UK Biosecurity State', *Architects for Social Housing* (16 June, 2021).

Evans, Rob, and David Pegg. 'Vote Leave AI firm wins seven government contracts in 18 months', *The Guardian* (4 May, 2020).

Evans, Rob, Juliette Garside, Joseph Smith and Pamela Duncan. 'Firms given £1bn of state contracts without tender in Covid-19 crisis', *The Guardian* (15 May, 2020).

European Court of Human Rights. 'Guide on Article 8 of the European Convention on Human Rights' (August 2019, last updated 2022).

_____. 'Guide on Article 15 of the European Convention on Human Rights: Derogation in time of emergency' (updated on 31 August 2022).

Evans, Milly. 'COVID-19: Can I get tested for coronavirus?', *Patient* (6 April, 2020).

Evans, Richard. *The Coming of the Third Reich* (Allen Lane, 2003).

_____. *The Third Reich in Power* (Allen Lane, 2005).

_____. *The Third Reich at War* (Allen Lane, 2008).

Facts and Details. 'Russian Privatization and Oligarchs' (last updated May 2016).

Feeney, Matthew. 'A Censor's Charter? The case against the Online Safety Bill', *Centre for Policy Studies* (September 2022).

Ferguson, Neil, et al. 'Report 9: Impact of non-pharmaceutical interventions (NPIs) to reduce COVID-19 mortality and healthcare demand', Imperial College COVID-19 Response Team (16 March, 2020).

Fitzgerald, Mary, and Cori Crider. 'Under pressure, UK government releases NHS COVID data deals with big tech', *Open Democracy* (5 June, 2020).

Flaxman, Seth, Swapnil Mishra Axel Gandy, H. Juliette T. Unwin, Thomas A. Melian, Helen Coupland, Charles Whittaker, Harrison Zhu, Tresnia Berah, Jeffrey W. Eaton, Mélodie Monod, Imperial College COVID-19 Response Team, Azra C. Ghani, Christi A. Donnelly, Steven Riley, Michaela A. C. Vollmer, Neil M. Ferguson, Lucy C. Okell and Samir Bhatt. 'Estimating the effects of non-pharmaceutical interventions on COVID-19 in Europe', *Nature* (8 June, 2020).

Foucault, Michel. *Discipline and Punish: The Birth of the Prison*; translated from the French by Alan Sheridan (Penguin Books, 1977).

_____. 'Right of Death and Power over Life', part five of *The Will to Knowledge*, volume 1 of *The History of Sexua*lity, translated by Robert Hurley (Penguin Books, 1998), 133-159.

Gallagher, James. 'Coronavirus: "Earlier lockdown would have halved death toll"', *BBC* (10 June, 2020).

_____. 'Coronavirus vaccine: UK government signs deals for 90 million doses', *BBC News* (20 July, 2020).

Gardiner, Laura, and Hannah Slaughter. 'The effects of the coronavirus crisis on workers', *The Resolution Foundation* (16 May, 2020).

Garside, Juliette, and Rupert Neate. 'UK government "using pandemic to transfer NHS duties to private sector"', *The Guardian* (4 May, 2020).

Gates, Bill. 'Transcript: Bill Gates speaks to the FT about the global fight against coronavirus', *Financial Times* (9 April, 2020).

Geoghegan, Peter, and Russell Scott. 'Revealed: Serco under fire over fresh £90m COVID-19 contract', *Open Democracy* (28 May, 2020).

Getty, Aileen. 'I fund climate activism — and I applaud the Van Gogh protest', *The Guardian* (22 October, 2022).

Gibson Dunn Lawyers. 'BlackRock, Vanguard, State Street Update Corporate Governance and ESG Policies and Priorities for 2022' (25 January, 2022).

Giesecke, Johan. 'The Invisible Pandemic', *The Lancet* (5 May, 2020).

Giles, Chris. 'UK coronavirus deaths more than double official figure, according to FT study', *Financial Times* (22 April, 2020).

_____. 'BoE warns UK set to enter worst recession for 300 years', *Financial Times* (7 May, 2020).

Giles, Chris, and Gill Plimmer. 'Coronavirus deaths more than twice hospital toll, data indicate', *Financial Times* (28 April, 2020).

Glass, Karligash, Anthony Glass, Sam Williams and Alasdair Crookes. 'An Improved Measure of Deaths Due to COVID-19 in England and Wales', *Social Science Research Network* (posted 2 July, 2020).

Global Climate Intelligence Group. 'World Climate Declaration: There is no climate emergency' (1 October, 2022).

Godwin, Mike. 'Meme, Counter-meme', *Wired* (1 October, 1994).

Goldman, Marshal I. 'Putin and the Oligarchs', *Council on Foreign Relations* (November-December, 2004).

Google. 'Exposure Notification Frequently Asked Questions' (April 2020),

_____. 'Exposure Notification API launches to support public health agencies' (20 May, 2020).

_____. 'Privacy-Preserving Contact Tracing'.

Greater Manchester Police. 'Tell us about a possible breach of coronavirus (Covid-19) measures'.

_____. 'Closure Order Following Gathering in Gorton', *YouTube* (18 August, 2020).

Greene, Alan. 'State of emergency: how different countries are invoking extra powers to stop the coronavirus', *The Conversation* (30 March, 2020).

Griffin, Shaun. 'Covid-19: "Huge rise" in deaths at home is not fully explained by virus, say experts', *British Medical Journal* (27 May, 2020).

Hagan, Shelly. 'Nearly One in Two Americans Takes Prescription Drugs: Survey', Bloomberg UK (8 May, 2019).

Hall, Kat. 'Serious Fraud Office fines Serco £22.9m over electronic tagging scandal', *The Register* (3 July, 2019).

Hancock, Matt. 'Health and Social Care Secretary's statement on coronavirus (COVID-19): 2 April 2020' (published 30 April, 2020).

_____. 'Health and Social Care Secretary's statement on coronavirus (COVID-19): 3 April 2020' (published 30 April, 2020).

_____. 'Health and Social Care Secretary's statement on coronavirus (COVID-19): 5 April 2020' (published 30 April, 2020).

_____. 'Health and Social Care Secretary's statement on coronavirus (COVID-19): 10 April 2020' (published 30 April, 2020).

_____. 'Health and Social Care Secretary's statement on coronavirus (COVID-19): 12 April 2020' (published 30 April, 2020).

_____. 'Health and Social Care Secretary's statement on coronavirus (COVID-19): 23 April 2020' (published 30 April, 2020).

_____. 'Health and Social Care Secretary's statement on coronavirus (COVID-19): 1 May 2020' (1 May, 2020).

_____. 'Face coverings to be mandatory in shops and supermarkets from 24 July' (14 July, 2020).

_____. 'The future of public health' (18 August, 2020).

Hansard Society. 'Coronavirus Statutory Instruments Dashboard, 2020-2022' (4 March, 2022).

Harriss, Lydia, and Philippa Kearney. 'Research Briefing: Smart Cities', *UK Parliament* (22 September, 2021).

Henley, Jon. 'Swedish PM warned over "Russian roulette-style" Covid-19 strategy', *The Guardian* (23 March, 2020).

Hern, Alex. 'China introduces its own "snooper's charter"', *The Guardian* (29 December, 2015).

Hersh, Seymour. 'How America took out the Nord Stream Pipeline', *Peoples Dispatch* (10 February, 2023).

Hickel, Jason. 'The World's Sustainable Development Goals Aren't Sustainable', *Foreign Policy* (30 September, 2020).

Hitchens, Peter. 'Face masks turn us into voiceless submissives — and it's not science forcing us to wear them, it's politics', *Mail on Sunday* (19 July, 2020).

Hobson, Francis, and Aaron Kulakiewicz. 'Research Briefing: Potential merits of a universal basic income', *House of Commons Library* (13 June, 2022).

Hogarth, Raphael. 'Parliament's role in the coronavirus crisis', *Institute for Government* (17 April, 2020).

Home Office. 'Guidance: Automated Facial Recognition: ethical and legal use' (25 October, 2021).

_____. 'Public Order Bill: factsheet' (28 October, 2022).

Honeycombe-Foster, Matt. 'Coronavirus: NHS contact tracing app 'not a priority' and may not be ready until winter, minister confirms', *Politics Home* (17 June, 2020).

Hopkins, Nick. 'Deloitte hit by cyber-attack revealing clients' secret emails', *The Guardian* (25 September, 2017).

HM Government. 'Emergency Response and Recovery: Non-statutory guidance accompanying the Civil Contingencies Act 2004' (October 2013).

_____. 'Take care with what you share using the SHARE checklist'.

_____. 'Our plan to rebuild: The UK Government's COVID-19 recovery strategy' (May 2020).

_____. 'Open letters between HM Treasury and Bank of England, December 2022 (15 December, 2022).

HM Treasury. 'Policy Paper: A Plan for Jobs 2020' (8 July, 2020).

_____. 'Autumn Statement 2022' (17 November, 2022).

Hooper, Louise. 'Briefing on the Health Protection (Coronavirus, Restrictions) (England) Regulations 2020', Garden Court Chambers (27 March, 2020).

House of Lords Environment and Climate Change Committee, 'In our hands: behaviour change for climate and environmental goals', 1st Report of Session 2022-2023 (12 October, 2022).

Iacobucci, Gareth. 'Covid-19: Government writes off £10bn on unusable, overpriced, or undelivered PPE', *BMJ* (3 February, 2022).

Inge, Sophie. 'Independent Sage blasts government Test and Trace system', *Research Professional News* (10 June, 2020).

Institute for Government. 'Government emergency powers and coronavirus' (updated 22 March, 2021).

Intrinsic Exchange Group, 'Be Invested' (2022).

Ioannidis, John P.A. 'The infection fatality rate of COVID-19 inferred from seroprevalence data', *MedRxiv* (13 May, 2020).

_____. 'Infection fatality rate of COVID-19 in community-dwelling populations with emphasis on the elderly: An overview' (13 July, 2021).

Johnson, Boris. 'Prime Minister's statement on coronavirus (COVID-19): 10 May 2020' (published 10 May, 2020).

Johnson, Carrie. 'Charge Against KPMG Dropped', *Washington Post* (4 January, 2007).

Johnson, Sarah. 'NHS staff forbidden from speaking out publicly about coronavirus', *The Guardian* (9 April, 2020).

Jolly, Jasper, and Jessica Elgot. 'Profits at world's seven biggest oil forms soar to almost £150bn this year', *The Guardian* (27 October, 2022).

Jones, Adam. 'Builders fined £130m for rigging bids', *Financial Times* (22 September, 2009).

Jones, Julian. *Rise of the Nazis*, episode 3, 'The Night of the Long Knives', *BBC* (16 September, 2019).

Joseph Rowntree Foundation. 'Overall UK Poverty Rates' (2022).

Judge, Lindsay. 'Coping with housing costs during the coronavirus crisis', *The Resolution Foundation* (30 May, 2020).

Just Stop Oil. 'Campaign Background' (2023).

Law or Fiction. 'Time to blow the whistle on shops' (28 July, 2020).

Kelion, Leo. 'Coronavirus: UK confirms plan for its own contact tracing app', *BBC* (12 April, 2020).

_____. 'Coronavirus: NHS contact tracing app to target 80% of smartphone users', *BBC* (16 April, 2020).

Kinder, Tabby. 'Consultants in line of fire over projects to tackle coronavirus', *Financial Times* (4 May, 2020).

Kirby, John, Libby Handros and Lee Davis. 'Perspectives on the Pandemic II: A Conversation with Dr. Knut Wittowski', *Ratical* (1-2 April, 2020).

Kotsko, Adam. 'What Happened to Giorgio Agamben?', *Slate* (20 February, 2022),

Lacobucci, Gareth. 'Covid-19: Government is criticised for "scandalous" £10bn spent on test and trace programme', *BMJ* (10 July, 2020).

Lai, Alvina, Amitava Banerjee, Laura Pasea and Spiros Denaxas. 'Estimating excess mortality in people with cancer and multimorbidity in the COVID-19 emergency', *Research Gate* (28 April 2020).

Lancashire Constabulary. 'Report a COVID-19 incident'; Staffordshire Police, 'Tell us about a possible breach of coronavirus (Covid-19) measures'.

Lantier, Alex. 'French army receives authorization to shoot "yellow vest" protesters', *World Socialist Website* (23 March, 2019).

Lawson, Alex, and Rowena Mason. 'UK inflation will hit 18% in early 2023, says leading bank Citi', *The Guardian* (22 August, 2022).

Lee, Dr. John. 'How deadly is the coronavirus? It's still far from clear', *The Spectator* (28 March, 2020).

Lewis, Nic. 'Imperial College UK COVID-19 numbers don't seem to add up', *Climate Etc.* (1 April, 2020).

_____. 'The dangers of a COVID "elimination" policy', *The Spectator* (22 September, 2020).

Liberatore, Stacy. 'Real covidiots! People who refuse to wear a mask or comply with social distancing have lower cognitive ability, new study shows', *Daily Mail* (13 July, 2020).

Lilly, Alice and Hannah White. 'Parliament's role in the coronavirus crisis: holding the government to account', *Institute for Government* (21 May, 2020).

Lintern, Shaun. 'Inside the coronavirus mega-labs', *The Independent* (29 June, 2020).

Lock, Helen, and Pia Gralki, 'UK's COVID-19 Vaccine Trial Successfully Trains Immune System to Respond to Disease', *Global Citizen* (20 July, 2020).

Loke, Yoon K., and Carl Heneghan. 'Why no-one can ever recover from COVID-19 in England — a statistical anomaly', The Centre for Evidence-Based Medicine (CEBM), University of Oxford (16 July, 2020).

Lovett, Samuel. 'Coronavirus: 25,000 patients discharged into care homes without being tested, report finds', *The Independent* (12 June, 2020).

Löwenstein, Karl. 'Law in the Third Reich', *Yale Law Journal*, vol. 45 (1936), pp. 814-815.

Marsh, Sarah. 'Fears that seriously ill people are avoiding A&E as numbers drop', *The Guardian* (27 March, 2020).

Marteau, Theresa. 'Tackling behaviour change', *BMJ* (21 May, 2014).

Marx, Karl. 'The Eighteenth Brumaire of Louis Bonaparte', in Karl Marx and Frederick Engels, *Selected Works*, Vol. 1 (Progress Publishers, 1983), pp. 394-487.

Mathieu, Edouard, Hannah Ritchie, Lucas Rodés-Guirao, Cameron Appel, Daniel Gavrilov, Charlie Giattino, Joe Hasell, Bobbie Macdonald, Saloni Dattani, Diana Beltekian, Esteban Ortiz-Ospina and Max Roser. 'Policy Responses to the Coronavirus Pandemic', *Our World in Data*.

Matthews, Chris. 'Devon and Cornwall police clarify travel to exercise guidance', *Cornwall Live* (2 April, 2020).

McElroy, Erin, Meredith Whittaker and Genevieve Fried. 'COVID-19 Crisis Capitalism Comes to Real Estate', *Boston Review* (7 May, 2020).

Medicines and Healthcare products Regulatory Agency. 'Pfizer/BioNTech COVID-19 vaccine authorised for use in infants and children aged 6 months to 4 years' (6 December, 2022).

Meredith, Sam. 'Sweden's economy actually grew in the first quarter after it opted against a full virus lockdown', *CNBC* (29 May, 2020).

Metropolitan Police. 'Structure' (as of 31 October, 2022).

Mills, Mark P. 'The "New Energy Economy": An Exercise in Magical Thinking', *Manhattan Institute* (26 march, 2019).

Ministry of Defence. 'Ministry stands up COVID Support Force' (19 March, 2020).

Ministry of Housing, Communities and Local Government. 'English Housing Survey: Headline Report, 2018-19' (January 2020).

Mitchell, Fiona. 'Vitamin-D and COVID-19: do deficient risk a poorer outcome?', *The Lancet* (20 May, 2020).

Mitra, Ritwika. 'Over 1.7 million homeless residents across India struggle to fight coronavirus', *The New Indian Express* (23 March, 2020).

Mohan, Geeta. 'Are Ukraine's vast natural resources a real reason behind Russia's invasion?' *Business Today* (25 February, 2022).

Morgan-Bentley, Paul. 'Boots faces inquiry over cancer drug price hike', *The Times* (25 May, 2018).

Morrisson, Chris. '"There is no Climate Emergency": Hundreds More Sign the World Climate Declaration, Including 20 Professors', *The Daily Sceptic* (31 October, 2022).

Nanan-Sen, Svar. '"It's your DUTY!" Hancock says Brits MUST abide by test, track and trace — threat issued', *Express* (11 June, 2020).

Nancy, Jean-Luc. 'Eccezione virale', *Antinomie* (27 February, 2020).

National Health Service. 'National homecare providers' (last reviewed 1 September, 2021).

National Police Air Service. 'Frequently asked questions'.

National Records of Scotland. 'Deaths involving coronavirus (COVID-19) in Scotland'.

Neal, Rupert, Juliette Garside, Felicity Lawrence and Rob Evans. 'Healthcare firm advised by Owen Paterson won £133m coronavirus testing contract unopposed', *The Guardian* (11 May, 2020).

NetPol undercover research group. 'Policing the corona state: a diary of security and surveillance during Britain's state of emergency'

Newey, Sarah. 'Why have so many coronavirus patients died in Italy?', *The Telegraph* (23 March, 2020).

Ng, Kate. 'Coronavirus: NHS urges people to go to hospital for emergencies as A&E visits fall by 50 per cent', *The Independent* (25 April, 2020).

_____. 'Government denies reports it has pulled funding from emergency coronavirus homeless sheltering programme', *The Independent* (15 May, 2020).

NHS England. 'COVID-19 Deaths'.

_____. 'Bed Availability and Occupancy Data – Overnight'.

_____. 'COVID-19 Hospital Activity'.

Norton, Ben. 'Ukraine's Zelensky sends love letter to US corporations, promising "big business" for Wall Street', *Scheerpost* (27 January, 2023).

Nuki, Paul. 'Two new waves of deaths are about to break over the NHS, new analysis warns', *The Telegraph* (25 April, 2020);

Office for National Statistics. 'The 2008 recession ten years on' (30 April, 2018).

_____. 'Different uses of figures on deaths from COVID-19 published by DHSC and ONS' (31 March, 2020).

_____. 'Deaths involving COVID-19, England and Wales: deaths occurring in March 2020' (16 April, 2020).

_____. 'Deaths registered weekly in England and Wales, provisional: week ending 17 April 2020' (28 April, 2020).

_____. 'Publication of statistics on deaths involving COVID-19 in care homes in England: transparency statement' (28 April, 2020).

_____. 'Deaths involving COVID-19 in the care sector, England and Wales: deaths occurring up to 1 May 2020 and registered up to 9 May 2020 (provisional)' (15 May, 2020).

_____. 'Claimant Count : K02000001 UK : People : SA : Thousands' (19 May, 2020).

_____. 'Coronavirus and the social impacts on Great Britain: 22 May 2020' (22 May, 2020).

_____. 'Coronavirus and the latest indicators for the UK economy and society' (28 May, 2020).

_____. 'Coronavirus (COVID-19) related deaths by ethnic group, England and Wales: 2 March 2020 to 15 May 2020' (19 June, 2020).

_____. 'Coronavirus (COVID-19) related deaths by religious group, England and Wales: 2 March to 15 May 2020' (19 June, 2020).

_____. 'Direct and Indirect Impacts of COVID-19 on Excess Deaths and Morbidity: Executive Summary for the Department of Health and Social Care, the Government's Actuary Department and Home Office,' (15 July 2020).

_____. 'Deaths registered weekly in England and Wales, provisional: week ending 10 July 2020' (21 July, 2020).

_____. 'Coronavirus (COVID-19) Infection Survey, UK: 11 November 2022' (11 November, 2020).

_____. 'Deaths registered weekly in England and Wales, provisional (2020 edition of this dataset up to week ending 1 January 2021)'.

_____. 'User Guide to Mortality Statistics' (last revised 1 July, 2022).

_____. Office for National Statistics, 'Commentary — Monthly Insolvency Statistics October 2022' (15 November, 2022).

Oke, Jason and Carl Heneghan. 'Global Covid-19 Case Fatality Rates', The Centre for Evidence-Based Medicine (7 October, 2020);

Onfido. 'The role of Digital Identity in Immunity Passports', UK Parliament Committees (April 2020).

Open Rights Group. 'Government admits Test and Trace unlawful' (20 July, 2020).

Orange, Richard. 'Will Sweden's herd immunity experiment pay off?', Prospect (1 May, 2020).

Oster, Emily. 'Let's Declare a Pandemic Amnesty', The Atlantic (31 October, 2022).

Owen, Joseph. 'States of Emergency, Metaphors of Virus, and COVID-19', Verso (31 March, 2020).

Oxfam International, '"Terrifying prospect" of over a quarter of a billion more people crashing into extreme levels of poverty and suffering this year' (12 April, 2022).

Oxford, Professor John. 'A View from the HVIVO', Novus Communications (31 March, 2020).

Patel, Priti. 'Tougher fines ahead of Bank Holiday to crack down on illegal gatherings' (24 August, 2020).

Patrick, Philip. 'Japan's COVID success is a mystery', The Spectator (27 May, 2020).

Pegg, David, and Carole Cadwalladr. 'US data firm admits employee approached Cambridge Analytica', The Guardian (28 March, 2018).

Perolini, Marco. 'France's Permanent State of Emergency', Amnesty International (26 September, 2017).

Pettinger, Tejvan. 'Washington consensus — definition and criticism', *Economics Help* (25 April, 2017).

Plimmer, Gill. 'Mitie criticised for 'insanitary' immigration centre', *Financial Times* (29 February, 2016).

Porta, Miquel. *A Dictionary of Epidemiology*, 6th edition (Oxford University Press, 2014).

Potocnik, Janez, and Julia Okatz. 'How Europe can reshape its cities to boost vibrancy, resilience and climate action', *World Economic Forum* (16 December, 2022).

Prime Minister's Office. 'UK will match record Ukraine support in 2023' (20 September, 2022).

_____. 'UK announces major new package of climate support at COP27' (7 November 2022).

_____. 'US and UK announce new energy partnership' (7 December, 2022).

Public Health England. 'Sources of UK flu data: influenza surveillance data in the UK' (7 January, 2014).

_____. 'Surveillance of influenza and other respiratory viruses in the United Kingdom: Winter 2014 to 2015', *The National Archives* (May 2015).

_____. 'Surveillance of influenza and other respiratory viruses in the UK: Winter 2016 to 2017', *The National Archives* (May 2017).

_____. 'Surveillance of influenza and other respiratory viruses in the UK: Winter 2017 to 2018', *The National Archives* (May 2018).

_____. 'National COVID Surveillance Reports' (23 April, 2020).

_____. 'Daily death reporting now includes all positive COVID-19 deaths' (29 April, 2020).

_____. Public Health England, 'Coronavirus data: Deaths in England'.

Public Health England, Joint Biosecurity Centre, NHS Test and Trace. 'Weekly Coronavirus Disease 2019 (COVID-19) Surveillance Report: Week 32, 2020' (12 August, 2021).

Quality Care Commission. 'Care Quality Commission publishes data showing death notifications involving COVID-19 received from individual care homes' (21 July, 2021).

Quinn, Ben. 'What has happened to England's seven Nightingale hospitals?', *The Guardian* (8 October, 2020).

Raab, Dominic. 'Foreign Secretary's statement on coronavirus (COVID-19): 16 April 2020' (published on 16 April, 2020).

_____. 'United Kingdom Coronavirus Briefing Transcript April 16' (16 April, 2020).

_____. 'Foreign Secretary's statement on coronavirus (COVID-19): 5 May 2020' (published 5 May, 2020).

Rahman, Abdul. 'Opposition political parties banned in Ukraine and 'unified information policy' imposed', *Peoples Dispatch* (21 March, 2022).

Ramakrishnan, Dr. Venki. 'President of the Royal Society urges everyone to wear a face covering', *The Royal Society* (7 July, 2020).

Rashid, Dr. Waqar. 'Is the R number a flawed measure?', *The Spectator* (14 May, 2020).

Rawlinson, Kevin. 'Private firms "are using detained immigrants as cheap labour"', *The Guardian* (22 August, 2014).

Renton, David. 'Thousands of renters could be evicted in June. Will the government protect them?', *The Guardian* (8 May, 2020).

Richards, David, and Konstantin Boudnik. 'Neil Ferguson's Imperial model could be the most devastating software mistake of all time', *The Telegraph* (16 May, 2020).

Robert Koch Institute. 'Bericht zur Epidemiologie der Influenza in Deutschland Saison 2018/19' (2019).

Roeder, Fred. 'What the NHS can learn from Germany's Hospital System', *Comment Central* (8 April, 2020).

Rosano, Aldo, Antonino Bella, Francesco Gesualdo, Anna Acampora, Patrizio Pezzottia, Stefano Marchetti, Walter Ricciardi, Caterina Rizzoa. 'Investigating the impact of influenza on excess mortality in all ages in Italy during recent seasons (2013/14–2016/17 seasons)', *International Journal of Infectious Diseases* (8 August, 2019).

Russ, Katheryn N., Phillip Baker, Manho Kang and David McCoy, 'Corporate Lobbying on U.S. Positions Toward the World Health Organization: Evidence of Intensification and Cross-Industry Coordination', *Global Health Governance*, Vol XVII, No. 1 (Spring 2022).

Scientific Advisory Group for Emergencies. 'Addendum to eighteenth SAGE meeting on Covid-19, 23rd March 2020 Held in 10 Victoria St, London, SW1H 0NN' (23 March, 2020).

Scientific Pandemic Influenza Group on Behavioural Science. 'Options for increasing adherence to social distancing measures' (22 March 2020).

_____. 'Key behavioural issues relevant to test, trace, track and isolate' (6 May, 2020).

_____. 'Public Disorder and Public Health: Contemporary Threats and Risks' (2 July, 2020).

_____. 'Consensus Statement on Local Interventions' (27 July, 2020).

Scottish Parliament. 'The Gender Recognition Reform (Scotland) Bill' (22 December, 2022).

Seddon, Paul, and Rachel Schraer. 'Andrew Bridgen suspended as Tory MP over Covid vaccine comments', *BBC News* (11 January, 2023).

Security Service MI5. 'Threat Levels'.

Shaban, Abdur Rahman Alfa. 'Africa COVID-19 stats: 874,036 cases; 18,498 deaths; 524,557 recoveries', *Africa News* (29 July, 2020).

Shaw, David. 'Vaccination status and intensive care unit triage: Is it fair to give unvaccinated Covid-19 patients equal priority?', *Bioethics* (7 August, 2022).

Sherling, Adrian. 'Muslim and BAME communities not taking coronavirus pandemic seriously, Tory MP says', *LBC Radio* (31 July, 2020).

Sherwood, Harriet. 'Religion: why faith is becoming more and more popular', *The Guardian* (27 August, 2018).

Sidley Austin LLP. 'COVID-19 Control Measures — UK Police Powers' (31 March, 2020).

Smith, Beckie. 'Counter-terrorism director general to lead coronavirus risk response unit', *Civil Service World* (12 May, 2020).

Smyth, Chris. 'Chris Whitty warns of high death rates due to Covid delays', *The Times* (1 December, 2022).

Stanley, Alessandro. 'Russian Banking Scandal Poses Threat to Future of Privatization', *New York Times* (28 January, 1996).

Statista. 'How many mobile phones in total do you and members of your household use?'
_____. 'How often do you attend church or synagogue — at least once a week, almost every week, about once a month, seldom, or never?' (December 2021).

Statistics Sweden. 'GDP largely unchanged in the first quarter of 2020' (29 May, 2020).

Steerpike. 'Six questions that Neil Ferguson should be asked', *The Spectator* (16 April, 2020).

Stevens, Sir Simon and Amanda Pritchard. 'To Chief executives of all NHS trusts and foundation trusts, CCG Accountable Officers, GP practices and Primary Care Networks Providers of community health services' (17 March, 2020).

Sui, Cindy. 'In Taiwan, the coronavirus pandemic is playing out very differently. What does life without a lockdown look like?', *NBC News* (23 April, 2020).

Sullum, Jacob. 'The CDC's New "Best Estimate" Implies a COVID-19 Infection Fatality Rate Below 0.3%', *Reason* (24 May, 2020).

Sumption, Jonathan. 'Former Supreme Court Justice: "This is what a police state is like"', *The Spectator* (30 March, 2020).

Sunak, Rishi. 'PM speech on building a better future' (4 January 2023).

Sweney, Mark. 'Watchdog approves use of UK phone data to help fight coronavirus', *The Guardian* (27 March, 2020).

Synovitz, Ron. 'Russia Has Highest Level Of Wealth Inequality', *Radio Free Europe Radio Liberty* (10 October, 2013).

Taylor, Paul. 'Susceptible, Infectious, Recovered', *London Review of Books* (7 May, 2020).

Thames Valley Police. 'Tell us about a possible breach of coronavirus (Covid-19) measures'.

Thomas, Alex. 'Joint Biosecurity Centre', *Institute for Government* (12 May, 2020);

Tomkins, Professor Adam. 'Legislating against Terror: the Anti-terrorism, Crime and Security Act 2001', *Public Law* (Summer 2002), pp. 205-220.

Thompson, Henry. 'Latest Updates on UK Government COVID-19 Contracts and Spending', *Tussell* (29 March, 2022).

Torres, Anthony. 'Macron to deploy French army against "yellow vest" protests', *World Socialist Website* (21 March, 2019).

Townsend, Mark. 'Detainees at Yarl's Wood immigration centre "facing sexual abuse"', *The Guardian* (14 September, 2013).

Trading Economics. 'United Kingdom Food Inflation' (December 2022).

Transparency International. 'At Your Service: Investigating how UK businesses and institutions help corrupt individuals and regimes launder their money and reputations' (October 2019).

Travis, Alan. 'G4S police control room staff suspended over claims of bogus 999 calls', *The Guardian* (23 May, 2016).

Trebesch, Professor Christophe, Katelyn Bushnell, Lukas Franz, Andre Frank, Bharath Kumar and Ivan Kharitonov. 'Ukraine Support Tracker', *Kiel Institute for the World Economy* (7 December, 2022).

Triggle, Nick. 'Coronavirus: Care homes deaths up as hospital cases fall', *BBC* (28 April, 2020).

UK Cabinet Office. 'Implementing the Sustainable Development Goals' (15 July, 2022).

UK Government. 'Scientific Advisory Group for Emergencies'.

_____. 'Coronavirus (COVID-19) in the UK'.

_____. 'Coronavirus (COVID-19) in the UK (Testing in England)'.

UK Government Chief Scientific Advisor. 'The Internet of Things: Making the most of the Second Digital Revolution' (December 2014).

UK Health Security Agency. 'Notifiable diseases and causative organisms: how to report' (1 May, 2010).

_____. 'Guidance on social distancing for everyone in the UK' (withdrawn on 1 May, 2020).

_____. UK Health Security Agency, 'The R value and growth rate' (15 May, 2020).

_____. 'NHS Test and Trace: what to do if you are contacted' (27 May, 2020).

_____. 'Maintaining records of staff, customers and visitors to support NHS Test and Trace' (2 July, 2020).

_____. 'Stay at home: Guidance for households with possible or confirmed coronavirus (COVID-19) infection' (withdrawn on 24 February, 2022).

UK Parliament. 'Emergency Powers Act 1920', *Hansard* (12 June, 1979).

_____. 'Memorandum to the Joint Committee on the Coronavirus Bill' (20 March, 2020).

_____. 'Update from UK Parliament on coronavirus' (15 April, 2020).

_____. 'Government request call of Parliament' (28 May, 2020).

_____. 'Health Protection (Coronavirus, Restrictions) (England) (Amendment) (No. 2) Regulations 2020. Volume 803: debated on Monday 15 June 2020', *Hansard* (15 June, 2020).

_____. Public Order', (House of Commons, *Hansard* (15 June, 2020).

_____. 'Health Protection (Coronavirus, Restrictions) (England) (Amendment) (No. 3) Regulations 2020', House of Lords, *Hansard* (25 June, 2020).

UK Public General Acts. 'Defence of the Realm Act 1914' (August, 1914).

_____. 'Emergency Powers Act 1920' (29 October, 1920).

_____. 'Public Health (Control of Disease) Act 1984' (26 June, 1984).

_____. 'Police and Criminal Evidence Act 1984' (31 October, 1984).

_____. 'Prosecution of Offences Act 1985' (23 May, 1985).

_____. 'Housing Act 1988 (15 November, 1988)

_____. 'Criminal Justice and Public Order Act 1994' (3 November, 1994).

_____. 'Human Rights Act 1998' (9 November, 1998)

_____. 'Terrorism Act 2000' (20 July, 2000).

_____. 'Regulation of Investigatory Powers Act 2000' (28 July, 2000).

_____. 'Anti-Terrorism, Crime and Security Act 2001' (14 December, 2001).

_____. 'Civil Contingencies Act 2004' (18 November, 2004).

_____. 'Counter-Terrorism Act 2008' (26 November, 2008).

_____. 'Health and Social Care Act 2008' (21 July, 2008).

_____. The Health Protection (Notification) Regulations 2010 (6 April, 2010).

_____. 'Equality Act, 2010' (8 April, 2010).

_____. 'Terrorism Prevention and Investigation Measures Act 2011' (14 December, 2011).

_____. 'Protection of Freedoms Act 2012' (1 May, 2012).

_____. 'Justice and Security Act 2013' (25 April, 2013).

_____. 'Antisocial Behaviour, Police and Crime Act 2014' (13 March, 2014).

_____. 'Data Retention and Investigatory Powers Act 2014' (17 July, 2014).

_____. 'Counter-Terrorism and Security Act 2015' (12 February, 2015).

_____. 'Recall of MPs Act 2015' (26 March, 2015).

_____. 'Investigatory Powers Act 2016' (29 November, 2016).

_____. 'Data Protection Act 2018' (23 May, 2018).

_____. 'Coronavirus Act 2020' (25 March, 2020).

_____. 'Police, Crime, Sentencing and Courts Act 2022' (28 April, 2022).

UK Statutory Instruments. 'The Data Retention and Acquisition Regulations 2018' (31 October, 2018).

_____. 'The Health Protection (Coronavirus) Regulations 2020' (10 February, 2020).

_____. 'The Health Protection (Notification) (Amendment) Regulations 2020' (6 March, 2020).

_____. 'The Health Protection (Coronavirus, Business Closure) (England) Regulations 2020' (23 March, 2020).

_____. 'The Health Protection (Coronavirus, Restrictions) (England) Regulations 2020' (26 March, 2020).

_____. 'The Investigatory Powers (Temporary Judicial Commissioners and Modification of Time Limits) Regulations 2020' (27 March, 2020).

_____.'The Coronavirus (Retention of Fingerprints and DNA Profiles in the Interests of National Security) Regulations 2020' (2 April, 2020).

_____. 'The Investigatory Powers (Communications Data) (Relevant Public Authorities and Designated Senior Officers) Regulations 2020' (21 April, 2020).

_____. 'The Health Protection (Coronavirus, Restrictions) (England) (Amendment) Regulations 2020' (22 April, 2020).

_____. 'Investigatory Powers (Communications Data) (Relevant Public Authorities and Designated Senior Officers) Regulations 2020' (24 April, 2020).

_____. 'Health Protection (Coronavirus, Restrictions) (England) (Amendment) (No. 2) Regulations 2020' (13 May, 2020).

_____. 'The Health Protection (Coronavirus, Restrictions) (England) (Amendment) (No. 3) Regulations 2020' (31 May, 2020).

_____. 'The Health Protection (Coronavirus, Restrictions) (England) (Amendment) (No. 3) Regulations 2020' (1 June, 2020).

_____. 'The Health Protection (Coronavirus, Restrictions) (No. 2) (England) Regulations 2020' (3 July, 2020).

_____. 'The Health Protection (Coronavirus, International Travel) (England) Regulations 2020' (3 June, 2020).

_____.'The Health Protection (Coronavirus, Wearing of Face Coverings on Public Transport) (England) Regulations 2020' (15 June, 2020).

_____. The Health Protection (Coronavirus, Restrictions) (No. 2) (England) Regulations 2020, (3 July, 2020)

_____. 'The Health Protection (Coronavirus, Restrictions) (England) (No. 3) Regulations 2020' (18 July, 2020).

_____. 'The Health Protection (Coronavirus, Wearing of Face Coverings in a Relevant Place) (England) Regulations 2020' (23 July, 2020).

_____. 'The Health Protection (Coronavirus, Restrictions) (Blackburn with Darwen and Bradford) Regulations 2020' (31 July, 2020).

_____. 'Health Protection (Coronavirus, Restrictions on Gatherings) (North of England) Regulations 2020' (4 August, 2020).

_____. 'The Health Protection (Coronavirus, Wearing of Face Coverings in a Relevant Place) (England) (Amendment) Regulations 2020' (6 August, 2020).

_____. 'The Health Protection (Coronavirus, Wearing of Face Coverings in a Relevant Place) (England) (Amendment) Regulations 2020' (8 August, 2020).

_____. 'The Health Protection (Coronavirus, Restrictions on Gatherings) (North of England) (Amendment) Regulations 2020' (8 August, 2020).

_____. 'The Health Protection (Coronavirus) (Restrictions on Holding of Gatherings and Amendment) (England) Regulations 2020' (28 August, 2020).

_____. 'The Health Protection (Wearing of Face Coverings in a Relevant Place and on Public Transport) (England) (Amendment) Regulations 2020' (27 August, 2020).

_____. 'The Health Protection (Coronavirus, Restrictions) (No. 2) (England) (Amendment) (No. 4) Regulations 2020' (14 September, 2020).

_____. The Health Protection (Coronavirus, Restrictions) (No. 2) (England) (Amendment) (No. 4) Regulations 2020 (13 September).

United Nations. 'Convention on the Prevention and Punishment of the Crime of Genocide' (9 December, 1948).

_____. 'Kyoto Protocol to the United Nations Framework Convention on Climate Change' (1998).

_____. 'Transforming our world: the 2030 Agenda for Sustainable Development', Department of Economic and Social Affairs (Resolution adopted by the General Assembly on 25 September, 2015).

University of Oxford, Blavatnik School of Government. 'COVID-19 Government Response Tracker' (March 2020-December 2022).

VST Enterprises. 'COVI-PASS™ Digital Health Passport', *YouTube* (26 May, 2020).

Wachman, Richard. 'AstraZeneca agrees to pay £505m to settle UK tax dispute', *The Guardian* (23 February, 2010).

Waldron, Ben. 'Holland and Barrett worker in Burton tests positive for coronavirus', *Derby Telegraph* (29 May, 2020).

Walker, Amy. 'NHS gives Amazon free use of health data under Alexa advice deal', *The Guardian* (8 December, 2019).

Wang, Chen, Peter W. Horby, Frederick G. Hayden and George F. Gao. 'A novel coronavirus outbreak of global health concern', *The Lancet* (15 February, 2020).

Warner, Jeremy. 'Only now are the crippling costs of lockdown becoming fully apparent', *The Telegraph* (20 August, 2022).

Warrell, Helen, and Sarah Neville. 'Senior spy appointed to lead the UK's joint biosecurity centre', *Financial Times* (5 June, 2020).

Wedel, Janine R. 'The Harvard Boys Do Russia', *The Nation* (14 May, 1998).

West, Dave. 'NHS hospitals have four times more empty beds than usual', *HSJ* (13 April, 2020).

Williams, Martin. 'UK billionaires see personal wealth grow by £25bn during pandemic lockdown', *The Herald Scotland* (14 June, 2020).

Williams, Oscar. 'Secret data and the future of public health: why the NHS has turned to Palantir', *The New Statesman* (21 May, 2020).

Wilson, Rhoda. 'Council claims it is a "Victim of Abuse" following new Policy to enforce Climate Lockdowns without consent of the Public', *The Exposé* (9 December, 2022).

_____. 'Covid Vaccine News: How much longer can Covidians keep up appearances?', *The Exposé* (4 January, 2023).

Wood, David. 'Coronavirus: UK could be "worst affected country in Europe', *ITV News* (12 April, 2020).

Woodcock, Andrew. 'Scathing report blasts "unimaginable" £37bn cost of coronavirus test and trace system', *Independent* (10 March, 2021).

Woodrow, Pippa, and Kirsty Brimelow, QC. 'Guide to Coronavirus Offences: Help for the public, police and lawyers', Doughty Street Chambers (7 May, 2020).

World Council for Health. 'Press Conference: Dr. Aseem Malhotra's New Peer-Reviewed Paper Calls for Immediate and "Complete Suspension" of Covid-19 Vaccine' (27 September, 2022).

World Economic Forum. '1500 organizations working together in the COVID Action Platform' (6 May, 2020).

_____. 'Our Partners' (2023).

_____. 'Measuring Stakeholder Capitalism: Towards Common Metrics and Consistent Reporting of Sustainable Value Creation' (2023).

World Health Organization. 'International Guidelines for Certification and Classification (Coding) of COVID-19 as Cause of Death' (20 April, 2020).

_____. 'WHO launches first ever global report on infection prevention and control' (6 May, 2022).

Worldometer. 'COVID-19 Coronavirus Pandemic'.

World Population Review. 'GDP per Capita by Country 2023'.

Wright, Nicholas. 'Coronavirus and the Future of Surveillance: Democracies Must Offer an Alternative to Authoritarian Solutions', *Foreign Affairs* (6 April, 2020).

Xie, Weizhen, Stephen Campbell and Weiwei Zhang. 'Working memory capacity predicts individual differences in social-distancing compliance during the COVID-19 pandemic in the United States', *PNAS* (10 July, 2020).

Yau, Cannix. 'Hong Kong government temporarily suspends two consultancy firms from making bids for projects', *South China Morning Post* (27 March, 2017).

Younger, Rachel. 'Coronavirus: Shops can call police if customers fail to wear face covering, Hancock says', *ITV News* (14 July, 2020).

Zbytniewska, Karolina. 'Coronavirus: Which European countries introduced the state of emergency?', *Euractiv* (6 May, 2020).

Žižek, Zlavoj. 'Monitor and Punish? Yes, Please!', *The Philosophical Salon* (16 March, 2020).

Zylberman, Patrick. *Tempêtes microbiennes. Essai sur la politique de sécurité sanitaire dans le monde transatlantique* (Paris, Gallimard, 2013).

L - #0459 - 200323 - C0 - 229/152/19 - PB - DID3524507